RADIOIMMUNOLOGY 1979

RADIOIMMUNOLOGY 1979

Proceedings of the IVth International Symposium on Radioimmunology held in Lyon (France) 19-21 April 1979.

Sponsored by Institut National de la Recherche Médicale et Délégation Générale à la Recherche Scientifique et Technique.

Edited by:

Ch.A. BIZOLLON

Scientific Committee:

R.S. YALOW	P.E. HALL
G.E. ABRAHAM	G. HEYNEN
P. FRANCHIMONT	R. MORNEX
	J.C. SCHWARTZ

Organizing Committee:

Ch.A. BIZOLLON	J. CORNIAU
H. BORNET	C. GHARIB
B. CLAUSTRAT	J. SASSARD
R. COHEN	M. VINCENT

1979

ELSEVIER/NORTH-HOLLAND BIOMEDICAL PRESS
AMSTERDAM · NEW YORK · OXFORD

ISBN: 0-444-80154-5

Published by:
Elsevier/North-Holland Biomedical Press
335 Jan van Galenstraat, P.O. Box 211
Amsterdam, The Netherlands

Sole distributors for the USA and Canada:
Elsevier North-Holland Inc.
52 Vanderbilt Avenue
New York, N.Y. 10017

Library of Congress Cataloging in Publication Data

International Symposium on Radioimmunology, 4th, Lyons, 1979.
Radioimmunology, 1979.

Includes bibliographies and indexes.
1. Radioimmunoassay--Congresses. 2. Hormones--Analysis--Congresses. 3. Endorphins--Analysis--Congresses. I. Bizollon, Charles A. II. Institut national de la santé et de la recherche médicale. III. France. Délégation générale à la recherche scientifique et technique. IV. Title.
QP519.9.R3I58 1979 616.07'56 79-18266
ISBN 0-444-80154-5

Printed in The Netherlands

PREFACE

This volume serves as the proceedings for the IVth International Symposium on Radioimmunology of Lyon (France). These Symposia, which started in 1972 soon after the wide development of radioimmunoassays in France, were firstly devoted to the technical problems of the methodology. In the following years it appeared to us useful to join together the methodological and pathophysiological aspects of the research made available by radioimmunology.

The comparison of the papers of the present meeting with those of the previous one, held two years ago, shows that substantial progress has been made in many areas. Of the major interests of the Symposium was not only the possibility of direct and friendly contacts, but above all the possibility of comparison between the procedures used and the data obtained in different laboratories.

The conclusion of the Session devoted to the quality control could be that the adolescent (i.e. radioimmunoassay) suffering from gigantism described a few years ago by G.E. Abraham has now the size and the experiences of an adult. The reading of the session on thyroid hormones, hormones regulating calcium and phosphate homeostasis and reproduction are very attractive in this point of view. But there are still several problems to be clarified and important questions to be answered : this was the case of the session on endorphins. This was also the aim of the opening lecture of Dr. R.S. Yalow on *"Radioimmunoassay of some peptides in the brain"* which gave the state of the art in studies which would not have been possible without radioimmunology.

It is a great pleasure for the Organizing Committee to acknowledge its great debt to Dr. R.S. Yalow who is now Doctor Honoris Causa of the Claude Bernard University (Lyon) and to Dr. G.E. Abraham, P. Franchimont, P.E. Hall, G. Heynen, R. Mornex and J.C. Schwartz for chairing with attention and skill the five sessions of the Symposium.

Our thanks goes to those whose moral and financial support allowed the broad international representation gathered in this meeting, especially the Hospices Civils de Lyon.

The Organizing Committee

ACKNOWLEDGEMENTS

This Symposium was aided by contributions from :

ABBOTT
ALLARD
AMERSHAM
BECKMAN INSTRUMENTS
BERTHOLD FRANCE
BIOLYON
BIOMERIEUX
BIOSYSTEMES-UNION CARBIDE
BRISTOL
CEA
CLINICAL ASSAYS
COMPTOIR LYONNAIS DE VERRERIE
CORNING-SOVIREL
DELAGRANGE
EUROBIO
FLAMMARION
GILSON
GUERBET TESTS
HEWLETT-PACKARD
HOECHST-BEHRING
ICI-PHARMA
INFORMATEK
INSTITUT PASTEUR PRODUCTION
KONTRON
LABAZ
LEDERLE
LEPETIT
LIPHA
L.K.B. INSTRUMENTS
MERCK-SHARP-DOHME-CHIBRET
MERRELL-TORAUDE
PACKARD INSTRUMENTS
PHARMACIA
PRECIBIO
RADIOIMMUNOASSAY LIMITED
RHÔNE-ALPES CHIMIE
ROHM-HAAS-MICROMEDIC
SANDOZ
SPECIA
TECHNICON
TEKTRONIX
TRAVENOL-HYLAND
WINTROP

CONTENTS

Radioimmunology 1979, Ch. A. Bizollon, editor.

RADIOIMMUNOASSAY OF SOME PEPTIDES IN THE BRAIN.

R.S. YALOW, E. STRAUS
Veterans Administration Medical Center, Bronx, New York 10468
The Mount Sinai School of Medicine, City University of New York, New York, New York 10029.

Radioimmunoassay has for many years had a central role in endocrinology. It has made possible the acquisition of virtually all the information now known about the regulation of hormonal secretion and the interrelationship among the hormones. Recently it has been applied to studies of the localization, concentration and chemical forms of peptides arising in or having effects on the central nervous system (CNS). This report summarizes the contributions from our laboratory to this very active field.

There have been a number of reports[1-4] suggesting that peptide hormones such as β-lipotropin, ACTH, and peptides structurally related to them are widely distributed in the brain of the rat in extra-hypothalamic regions. We considered that this distribution might be a consequence of the small dimensions of the rodent brain. We therefore undertook to investigate whether the distribution of pituitary peptides in the much larger brains of man, monkey and dog resembled the distribution in the brains of rodents such as rat and rabbit. We observed that the dimensions within which ACTH is found is about the same for all these species but that the particular anatomical regions which contain ACTH depend on the brain size[5] (fig. 1). We subsequently observed[6] that the distribution of TSH closely paralleled that of ACTH. Both these peptides are widely distributed in the brain of the rat but are found only in the hypothalamic regions of the primate brain. Since there is no reason to assume that the synthetic mechanisms are different in small-brained animals than in primates, we believe that these studies are consistent with our hypothesis that the pituitary is the sole site of synthesis of these pituitary peptides and that they are found in other cranial sites due to mechanisms other than synthesis. We are not familiar with any reports of the distribution of peptides such as lipotropin or the endorphins in the primate brain.

The persistence of pituitary peptides in the brains of commercially prepared hypophysectomized rats has been taken as evidence for de novo synthesis of such peptides in the brain. In general it is more difficult to evaluate the turnover of brain peptides than of circulating peptides. The turnover times in the brain might be measured in days not minutes as in the periphery. Although

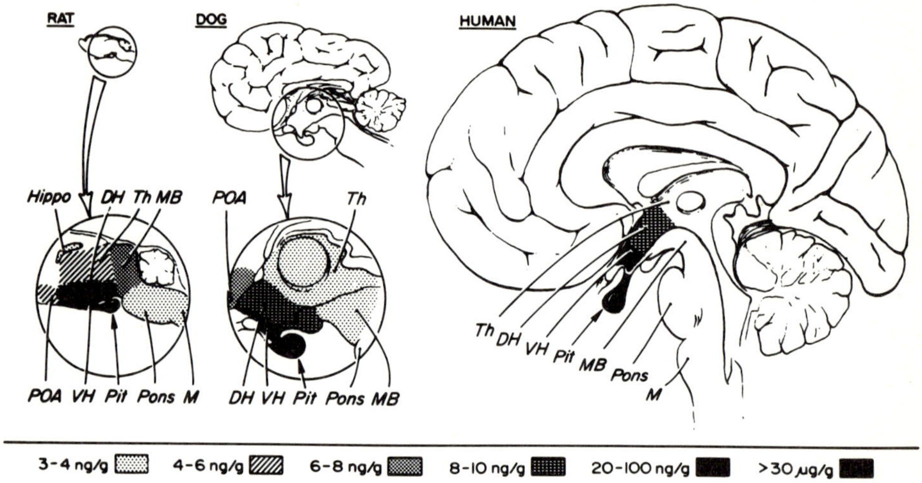

Fig. 1 - Distribution of immunoreactive ACTH in the pituitary and brain of several animal species. The rat, dog and human brains are drawn to scale. The regions shown in circles have been enlarged to show in better detail the concentrations of ACTH in the brain of the rat and dog. ACTH was not detectable in regions shown in white. Abbreviations : Pit, pituitary gland; VH, ventral hypothalamus; DH, dorsal hypothalamus; POA, preoptic area; MB, midbrain; M, medulla; TH, thalamus; Hippo, hippocampus. (reproduced from ref. 5)

we also have noted that residual pituitary tissue is rarely detected upon visual inspection of the sella, scrapings of the sella contain ACTH amounting to as much as 5% that of the intact pituitary[5]. This represents a considerable residual source of ACTH since the hypothalamic content of this peptide is only about 0.1% that of the pituitary. Furthermore, although there is an immediate decrease in stress-stimulated ACTH release in hypophysectomized rats, after 2 months the plasma ACTH can be stress-stimulated to about 80% of the level found in intact rats[5] (fig. 2). Thus even in these "*hypophysectomized*" rats we believe that residual pituitary fragments are the source of the brain ACTH.

What are the possible routes for transport of pituitary peptides to the brain ? Mezey et al[7] have demonstrated a significant flow of labeled peptides from the pituitary to the brain, particularly to the hypothalamus and suggested that this transfer is partly vascular via the stalk. They believe that

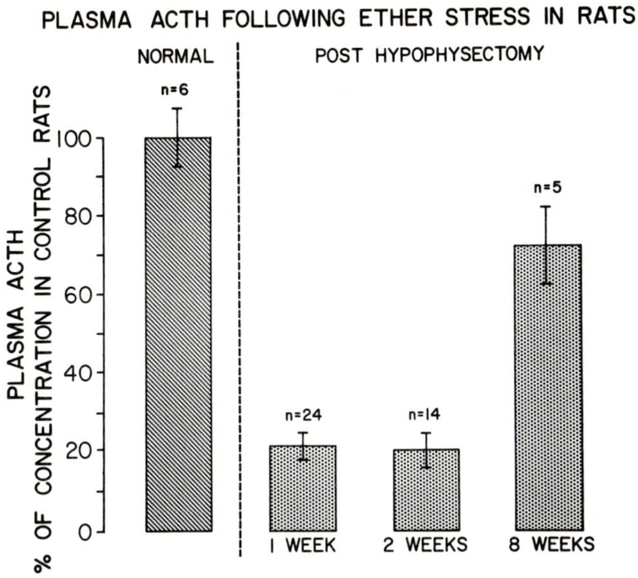

Fig. 2 - Plasma ACTH following ether stress in control and hypophysectomized rats. (reproduced from ref. 5)

transport to other areas may occur via the cerebrospinal fluid but do not rule out the possibility of a neural route. Bergland and Page[8] have asked the question "*Can the pituitary secrete directly to the brain ?*" and provided anatomical evidence which answered this question in the affirmative. These data taken together suggest a lesser role for pituitary peptides in the regulation of CNS function than was considered in the earlier reports[1-4].

Recently Havrankova et al[9] have reported that insulin concentration in acid-ethanol extracts of whole rat brain were on the average 25 times higher than plasma insulin levels and have suggested that insulin might be synthetized by cells in the nervous system. However the concentrations of insulin in extracts of the brains of larger animals such as the rabbit and dog is lower than plasma insulin[10] (table 1). However the insulin contents of extracts of heart, liver and kidney are 2 to 6 fold higher than plasma levels[10]. It is quite likely that insulin is not synethetized in any of these tissues but is derived simply by extraction from receptor sites[10].

Synthesis in one anatomical region and transport to or concentration in another cannot account for the observations that several peptides are common to the brain and gastrointestinal tract. Our interest in this field was derived from the initial finding by Vanderhaegen et al[11] of a peptide in the central nervous system which reacts with a gastrin antiserum and the subsequent report of Dockray[12] who suggested on the basis of immunologic evidence that the brain peptide resembled cholecystokinin (CCK)-like peptides more closely that it did gastrin-like peptides.

For our work in this field we employed two different radioimmunoassay systems. The homologous system employed an antiserum prepared in a goat by immunization with intact porcine cholecystokinin (pCCK33) and ^{125}I-pCCK33 as tracer. In this system no crossreaction is observed with CCK octapeptide (CCK8) or the gastrins (big, G34 or little, G17) in spite of their sharing a common COOH-terminal pentapeptide or with any other of the gut hormones. Thus this antiserum appears to be directed towards the NH_2 portion of intact pCCK. The other radioimmunoassay system employs an antiserum from a rabbit (rabbit B) immunized with gastrin tetrapeptide amide coupled through carbodiimide to bovine serum albumin and ^{125}I-G17 as tracer. In this system the crossreactivities of pCCK33 and CCK8 are identical on a molar basis; G17 is slightly more immunoreactive and CCK variant (CCK39) is slightly less immunoreactive.

Using the rabbit B antiserum, we have observed that in all animal species studied the immunoreactive content as measured in the CCK-8 assay averaged about five-fold greater in gut extracts than in brain extracts (table 2). However the concentrations in the gut and brain extracts were comparable among the different species and did not change significantly on tryptic digestion[13,14] (table 2).

In the same monkey and dog extracts in which CCK-like material was present in about the same concentration as in the pig extracts we failed to detect immunoreactivity with the anti-pCCK serum (table 2). The immunoreactive CCK in extracts of the gut and brain of the pig were comparable when measured with either antiserum[13, 14] (table 2). The failure to detect immunoreactive CCK in dog and monkey brain and gut extracts, which were proven to have this hormone when measured in the CCK8 assay, forms the basis for our prediction based on RIA that there are major differences between pig and the other animal cholecystokinins in the NH_2 portions of the molecule. Since this portion of the molecule is not directly involved in its biologic action, it is not surprising that the amino acid sequences in this region of the molecule have diverged during the course of evolution.

Table 1 - Insulin recoverable from the circulation and tissue extracts.

	RABBITS (Av. of 2)	DOG (1)
	ng/ml	
Plasma	1.0	1.8
Blood	1.0	1.2
	ng/g	
Cortex	.6	.2
Hypothalamus	.8	.2
Cerebellum	.5	.2
Brain Stem	.5	.5

Table 2 - Immunoreactive content of brain and gut extracts.

		Goat 1 ASSAY μg pCCK equivalent/ml		Rabbit B ASSAY μg CCK8 equivalent/ml	
SPECIES	ORGAN	BEFORE TRYPSIN	AFTER TRYPSIN	BEFORE TRYPSIN	AFTER TRYPSIN
Pig (2) *	Brain	0.80±0.05†	ND	0.20±0.01	0.15±0.01
	Gut	1.80±0.1	ND	0.60±0.05	0.50±0.03
Monkey (1)	Brain	ND	ND	0.05±0.01	0.05±0.02
	Gut	ND	ND	0.40±0.05	0.35±0.05
Dog (2)	Brain	ND	ND	0.10±0.01	0.10±0.01
	Gut	ND	ND	0.70±0.02	0.70±0.05

( )* no of animals
ND = not detected
†mean ± standard error of the mean of multiple assays.

Our observations that extracts of the pig brain and gut react in the homologous pCCK33 assay system, although CCK8 does not, demonstrate that intact CCK33 is present in both anatomical regions[13]. Furthermore Sephadex gel fractionation and assay in the COOH-terminal assay reveal that in brain and gut extracts of all species studied CCK33 is present in amounts quite comparable to those of the COOH-terminal fragments[14] (fig. 3). These results differ from those of Dockray[12] who reported no immunoreactivity in the region of CCK33 and Rehfeld[15] who reported that the molecular form behaving like CCK33 accounted for only 2% to 5% of the total immunoreactivities in porcine and human brains.

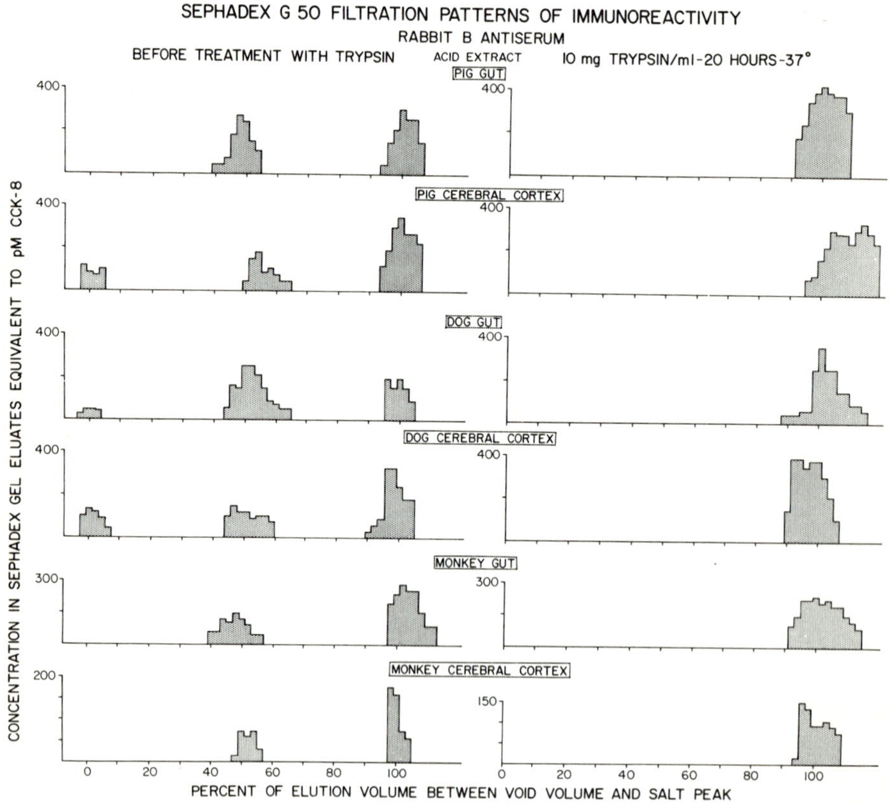

Fig. 3 - Immunoreactivity in eluates following Sephadex G50 gel filtration was determined using an antiserum which reacts identically on a molar basis with intact porcine cholecystokinin (pCCK) and its COOH-terminal octapeptide (CCK8). Purified pCCK has an elution volume midway between the void volume and the salt peak and CCK8 coelutes with the salt peak in this system. Shown are the patterns for pig, dog and monkey brain and gut extracts before (left) and after (right) prolonged tryptic digestion. Note the complete conversion to a CCK8-like peptide with no loss in immunoreactivity.
(Reproduced from Yalow : Radioimmunoassay : A probe for fine structure of biologic system. In *Les Prix Nobel. En 1977*. The Nobel Foundation, Stockholm, Sweden, 1978, pp 243-264).

We believe that CCK33 is a prominent component of brain CCK-like immunoreactivity and consider that the failure of the other groups to confirm our observations is due to the existence in the brain of a very active converting enzyme 16. If this enzyme is not inactivated during the extraction process a higher fraction of CCK8 than is present in vivo would be generated. We have partially purified a specific converting enzyme from canine and porcine cerebral cortical extracts[16]. It is not a non-specific protease nor is it trypsin. This enzyme converts CCK33 to smaller, immunoreactive forms, but fails to convert G34 to G17 (fig. 4). Thus the enzyme is readily distinguishable from trypsin in substrate specificity and differs from it in several physicochemical properties as well. It is not inhibited in the presence of lima bean trypsin inhibitor at a concentration sufficient to inhibit 1 mg trypsin/ml incubation mixture. It is inactivated when incubated with substrate at 45°C for one hour whereas trypsin remains fully active when incubated under the same conditions at 55°C. On sucrose gradient ultracentrifugation the proteolytic activity associated with trypsin is, as expected, recovered above albumin; the activity associated with the solubilized brain enzyme is recovered below γ-globulin. Thus the solubilized enzyme appears to be larger in molecular weight even than γ-globulin. The enzyme does not appear to be species specific since conversion of pCCK33 to the smaller hormonal forms is observed whether the enzyme is derived from the canine or porcine cerebral cortex. Further investigation is required to determine whether the enzyme in the gut that converts CCK33 to the C-terminal fragments resembles or is different from that found in the brain.

Where in the brain is CCK found ? Its concentration is highest in the cerebral cortex[13, 15]. Our immunohistochemical studies which were performed using the rabbit B antiserum suggest that CCK8, at least, appears to be concentrated in cortical neurons[17] (fig. 5). More recently subcellular fractionation of the rat cerebral cortex demonstrated the presence of immunoreactive cholecystokinin in the pellet identified by electron microscopy to contain a high proportion of synaptic vesicles[18]. The recovery in this pellet of 40% of the total immunoreactivity in the initial cortical extract (fig. 6) is quite comparable to that of other peptides such as VIP[19, 20] and somatostatin[21] which have also been reported to localize in the synaptosomes. The concentration of CCK-like peptides in the synaptosomal pellet from the rat cerebral cortex is consistent with our immunohistochemical demonstration of its localization in rabbit cerebral cortex[17].

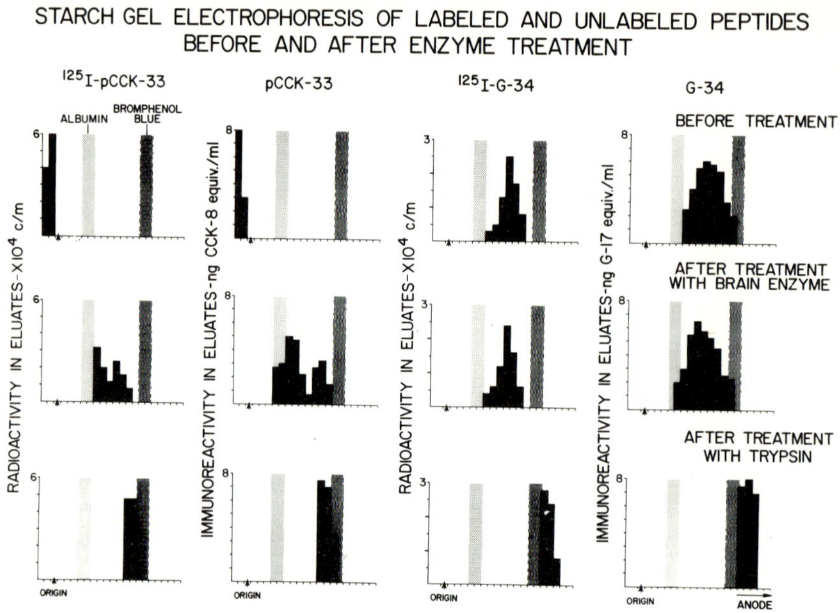

Fig. 4 - Starch gel electrophoresis of ^{125}I-labeled and unlabeled CCK and of ^{125}I-labeled and unlabeled gastrin-34 before (top) and after treatment with brain converting enzime (middle) or with trypsin (bottom). Trypsin converts labeled and unlabeled CCK to fragments with starch gel electrophoretic mobility resembling CCK8 and labeled and unlabeled gastrin-34 to fragments resembling gastrin-17. The brain converting enzyme does not alter gastrin-34 but converts CCK to fragments with starch gel electrophoretic mobility resembling CCK12 and CCK8. 0, origin (reproduced from ref. 16).

Although roles as neuroregulators or neurotransmitters have been postulated for several neuropeptides there has been no direct evidence for their involvement in physiologic or pathophysiologic processes. However we now have direct evidence of abnormalities in brain CCK-like immunoreactivity in obese mice who are markedly hyperphagic[22, 23].

It has long been known that there are several inbred strains of rodents which manifest hyperphagia, hyperglycemia and obesity and that damage in and around the ventromedial hypothalamus is followed by a similar clinical syndrome. Furthermore there are some reports suggesting that intracranial administration of CCK or related peptides was more effective than systemic administration of the same peptides in limiting appetite[24, 25]. It therefore seemed of interest to determine whether hyperphagic rodents have abnormalities in brain CCK. The Obese (ob) and Diabetes (db) strains are known to be single-gene mutants with different loci whose mode of inheritance is autosomal recessive. Extracts of the brains of ob/ob mice contain about 1/3 the immunoreactive CCK of their non-obese littermates[22]; CCK in extracts of the brains of db/db mice does not differ significantly from that of their non-obese litterlates[23] (fig. 7). We therefore hypothesize that the hyperphagia of ob/ob mice is due to a deficient signal to the hypothalamic satiety center because of diminished brain content of CCK. The hyperphagic db/db mice do not have diminished immunoreactive brain CCK, but this does not rule out the possibility of other abnormalities in the cerebral cortex-hypothalamic axis. These data demonstrate that the shared phenotype of hyperphagic, obese mice does not express a common genetic defect. Gold thioglucose lesioned mice with obesity have significantly more brain CCK than do their control non-lesioned littermates, suggesting the possible involvement of an interrupted feed-back loop involving the cerebral cortex-hypothalamic axis[23] (fig. 7).

These findings taken together are evidence of the direct role of CCK in the coarse regulation of appetite. Whether it has any role in what may be called the fine-tuning of the system, i.e., the diurnal regulation of appetite, is not determined by these studies.

It is of interest to speculate whether some cases of marked obesity in humans (body weights greater than twice normal) may be associated with abnormalities in brain CCK. Since there is not a common genetic defect in all strains of genetically obese mice and since humans are of diverse genetic backgrounds it is unlikely that all human obesity would be related to the same abnormality. It is obviously not practical to test the human system using methods similar to those we employed for the animal model but other approaches are possible.

CCK was long considered to be a gut hormone. Yet the major portion of CCK is now known to reside in the brain. Is this peptide involved only in the regulation of appetite or does it have other functions ? Unfortunately the classic methodology of endocrinology, extirpation of an organ and demonstration of a deficiency disease, is not readily applicable in neuroendocrinology. Nonetheless with perspicacious experimentation the complete picture will eventually by revealed.

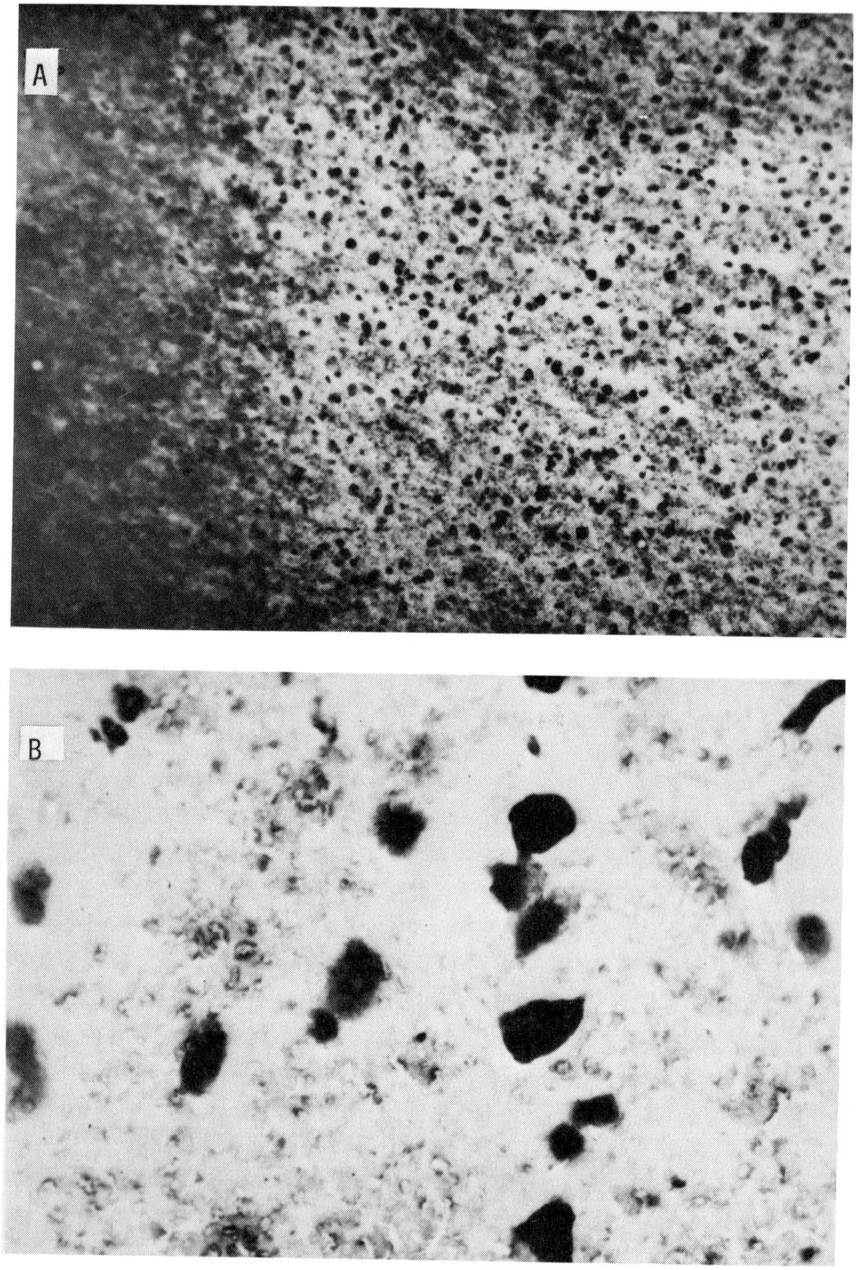
A
B

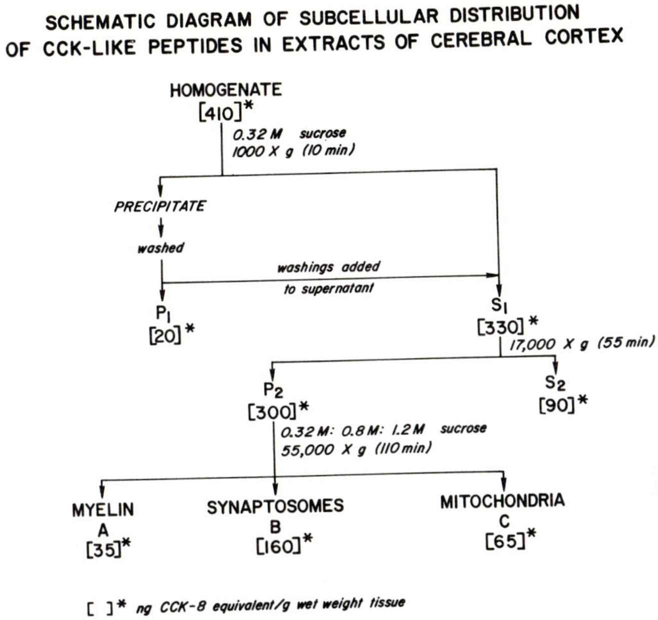

Fig. 6 - Flow diagram and recovery of CCK-like immunoreactivity for subcellular fractionation of a rat cerebral cortical extract.
* Numbers in brackets are ng of CCK8 equivalent per g wet weight of tissue. (reproduced from ref. 18)

Fig. 5 - A : Low power photomicrograph of rabbit cerebral cortex (frontal lobe). The tissue was stained by the immunoperoxidase technique using rabbit B antiserum in a 1:10 dilution. Staining of individual cell bodies can be seen in all layers of cortical grey matter and diffuse staining can be seen at the bottom in subcortical white matter (X33).

B : Higher-power photomicrograph showing staining of cell bodies in cortical grey matter (X208).
(Reproduced from Yalow : Radioimmunoassay : A probe for fine structure of biologic systems. In *Les Prix Nobel En 1977*. The Nobel Foundation, Stockholm, Sweden, 1978, pp 243-264

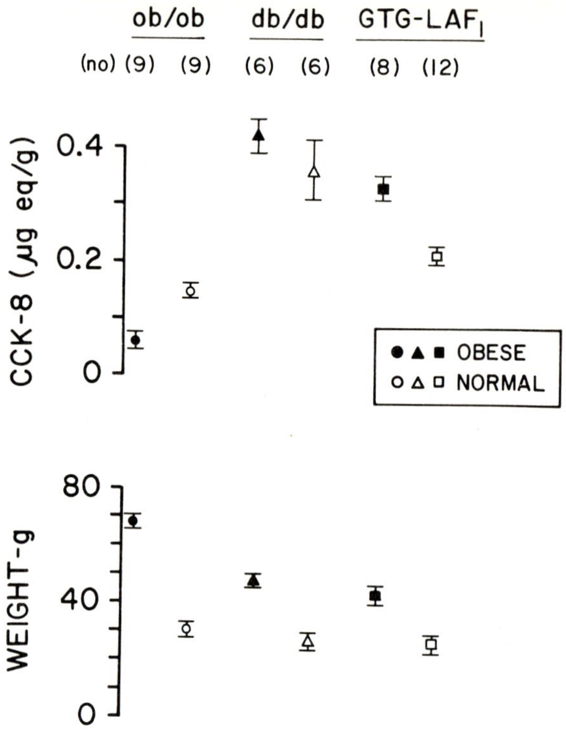

Fig. 7 - Weight and brain immunoreactive CCK content in obese, hyperphagic mice and their control littermates. The Obese (ob/ob) and Diabetes (db/db) strains are single-gene mutants with different loci whose mode of inheritance is autosomal recessive. The LAF_1 mice developed obesity and hyperphagia subsequent to gold thioglucose (GTG) lesioning of the ventromedial hypothalamus.

Supported by the Medical Research Program of the Veterans Administration.

REFERENCES -

1 - Simantov, R., Kuhar, M.J., Uhl, G.R. and Snyder, S.H. (1977) - Proc. Natl. Acad. Sci. USA, 74, 2167

2 - Cheung, A.L. and Goldstein, A. (1976) - Life Sci., 19, 1005

3 - Krieger, D.T., Liotta, A. and Brownstein, M.J. (1977) - Proc. Natl. Acad. Sci. USA, 74, 648

4 - Krieger, D.T., Liotta, A. and Brownstein, M.J. (1977) - Brain Res. 128, 575

5 - Moldow, R. and Yalow, R.S. (1978) - Proc. Natl. Acad. Sci. USA, 75, 994

6 - Moldow, R. and Yalow, R.S. (1978) - Life Sci., 22, 1859

7 - Mezey, E., Palkovits, M., de Kloet, E.R., Verhoef, J. and De Wied, D. (1978) Life Sci., 22, 831

8 - Bergland, R.M. and Page, R.B. (1978) - Endocrinology, 102; 1325

9 - Havrankova, J., Schmechel, D., Roth, J. and Brownstein, M. (1978) - Proc. Natl. Acad. Sci. USA, 75, 5737

10 - Eng, J. and Yalow, R.S. (1979) Endocrinology (supplement) Abstract *To be published*

11 - Vanderhaeghen, J.J., Signeau, J.C. and Gepts, W. (1975) - Nature (London) 257, 604

12 - Dockray, G.J. (1976) - Nature (London), 264, 568

13 - Muller, J.E., Straus, E. and Yalow, R.S. (1977) - Proc. Natl. Acad. Sci. USA, 74, 3035

14 - Straus, E. and Yalow, R.S. (1978) - Proc. Natl. Acad. Sci. USA, 75, 486

15 - Rehfeld, J.F. (1978) - J. Biol. Chem., 253, 4022

16 - Straus, E., Malesci, A. and Yalow, R.S. (1978) - Proc. Natl. Acad. Sci. USA 75, 5711

17 - Straus, E., Muller, J.E., Choi, H-S, Paronetto, F. and Yalow, R.S. (1977) - Proc. Natl. Acad. Sci. USA, 74, 3033

18 - Pinget, M., Straus, E. and Yalow, R.S. (1979) - Proc. Natl. Acad. Sci. USA, 75, 6324

19 - Giachetti, A., Said, S.I., Reynolds, R.S. and Koniges, F.C. (1977) - Proc. Natl. Acad. Sci. USA, 74, 3424

20 - Besson, J., Rotszteun, W., Laburthe, M., Epelbaum, J., Beaudet, A., Kordon, C. and Rosselin, G. (1979) - Brain Res. *To be published*

21 - Epelbaum, J., Brazeau, P., Tsang, D., Brawer, J. and Martin, J.B. (1977) - Brain Res., 126, 309

22 - Straus, E. and Yalow, R.S. (1979) - Science, 203, 68

23 - Straus, E. and Yalow, R.S. (1979) - Endocrinology (Supplement) Abstract, *To be published*

24 - Stern, J.J., Cudillo, C.A. and Kruper, J. (1976) - J. Comp. Physiol. Psychol., 90, 484

25 - Maddison, S. (1977) - Psychol. Behav., 19, 819

ENDORPHINS

© 1979 Elsevier/North-Holland Biomedical Press
Radioimmunology 1979, Ch. A. Bizollon, editor.

OPIOID PEPTIDES AS INTERCELLULAR MESSENGERS

JEAN-CHARLES SCHWARTZ
Unité 109 de Neurobiologie, Centre Paul Broca de l'I.N.S.E.R.M., 2ter rue d'Alésia 75014 Paris, France.

INTRODUCTION

In retrospect it could be stated that the existence of opioid peptides i.e. of endogenous substances mimicking the various actions of morphine-like agents could have been hypothesized several years before 1975 : exogenous molecules modify the activity of biological systems generally by interfering with endogenous messengers like neurotransmitters or hormones. In fact the decisive finding was in 1973 that synthetic or semi-synthetic opiates interact with receptors located at the surface of the responding cells as shown by ^{3}H-ligand binding studies in the laboratories of E. Simon, S.H. Snyder and L. Terenius. The presence of endogenous ligands for these receptors in various tissues and CSF was almost simultaneously reported in 1975 in the laboratories of A. Kosterlitz, S.H. Snyder, A. Goldstein and L. Terenius.

Due to the fact that these endogenous opioid peptides are relatively abundant in nervous and pituitary tissues, their isolation (followed during the procedure by biological tests) was not an extremely difficult analytical task, at least as compared to the isolation of peptide hormones like CRF which still remains to be performed.

The first identified "endomorphins" were the enkephalins i.e. the two pentapeptides Methionine-Enkephalin and Leucine-Enkephalin. Hughes et al. remarked that the sequence of Met-Enkephalin was present in β-lipotropin, a 31 amino-acid peptide hormone discovered several years ago in the pituitary by Li (1964). From this time, a large body of experimental data has confirmed that the substances shared most of the known actions of synthetic morphine-like agents on a variety of test-systems. The structural analogy between a prefered conformation of enkephalins and potent opiates easily accounted for the recognition of both classes of compounds by the same receptors.

In 1975, i.e. during the same year as the identification of enkephalins by Hughes and his colleagues, A. Goldstein and his colleagues detected in pituitary extract the presence of peptides with morphine-like activity. In the following year Li and Cheung, Bradbury et al. and Guillemin et al. identified several fragments of the β-lipotropin molecule sharing morphine-like activity. These fragments termed α-, β- and γ-endorphin were also demonstrated to share the actions of opiates regarding receptor binding or elicitation of biological responses. However recent data suggest that, whereas the 31 aminoacid peptide, β-endorphin, has to be regarded as a true messenger substance, the two shorter endorphins are probably isolation artifacts.

Hence three well-established opioid peptides remain as messenger candidates : the two enkephalins and β-endorphin.

What is their functional role ? To answer this question requires that should be identified i) the kind of cells storing and releasing the putative messenger ii) the physiological conditions under which release is elicited iii) the nature of responding cells and biologic responses. Whereas the latters are relatively well-known from a large body of experiments with synthetic opiates, the formers are being currently unraveled because the identification of opioid peptides has provided experimental tools to localize and assay these substances. Many excellent reviews (see Reading List) have been recently devoted to this subject and only an overview of the more significant conclusions will be attempted here.

Thus it appears that enkephalins are to be considered as neurotransmitters i.e. messengers involved in neuro-neuronal communication, whereas β-endorphin is both a neurotransmitter and a hormone. This statement might be an oversimplification but, at the present stage, has perhaps the merit of clarification of concepts for a non-directly concerned reader facing an overflow of scientific literature. More precise data and subtle considerations are to be found in the Reading List.

ENKEPHALINS AS NEUROTRANSMITTERS

The idea that enkephalins should be considered as neurotransmitters in mammalian brain is suggested by a variety of experimental data that will be summarized under the following headings.

Cellular localization

Both enkephalins are widely distributed in the brain and spinal cord and are found in a variety of peripheral tissues like the gastrointestinal tract and the adrenals. Met-Enkephalin is generally more abundant than Leu-Enkephalin but since the ratio of the two pentapeptides is somewhat variable between one cerebral region to the other, this suggests that they might be held in distinct cellular stores.

That enkephalins are contained in neurons in the Central Nervous System was suggested by the early findings that, upon subcellular fractionation of brain tissues, these substances were mainly recovered in fractions enriched in nerve-endings. The intraneuronal localization of enkephalins is also suggested by their decreased levels in brain areas in which kainic acid, a substance ablating selectively neurons, is injected.

These assumptions were soon confirmed when antibodies to enkephalins were raised which allowed their immunofluorescent localization within discrete sets of neurons in the CNS as well as in peripheral organs. Because of the limited specificity of antisera against each of the two enkephalins, their respective localizations have not yet been clearly differentiated. As is the case with other brain peptides, the enkephalins can be easily visualized in axons and nerve-terminals but pretreatment of the animals with colchicine, an agent blocking the axoplasmic transport, is required to evidence them within perikarya.

It is already difficult to summarize the findings provided by the application of these methods but it appears that i) enkephalin-containing neurons are widespread within the brain and not restricted to areas thought to be involved in the control of pain mechanisms, ii) high differences exist in the density of enkephalin-containing neurons in brain, which seems to parallel the distribution of opiate receptors, iii) in a large number of cases enkephalin neurons seem to be short interneurons, iv) lesion experiments have, in a few cases, suggested the presence of enkephalin pathways (in the stria terminalis and in the pallidum).

Biosynthesis and Turnover

A number of peptide hormones appear to be stored in the form of large inactive precursors, from which they are released by proteolytic cleavage. It is clear that the origin of cerebral enkephalins is not circulating β-lipotropin or β-endorphin originating from the pituitary because long-term hypophysectomy does not alter the levels of the pentapeptides in brain.

In the case of Met-Enkephalin the precursor might be β-lipotropin because this molecule has been immunohistochemically evidenced in brain but there are clear differences in the distribution of the two immunoreactive substances. In the same way it is unlikely that β-endorphin is a metabolic precursor of Met-Enkephalin because the antibodies to β-endorphin reveal neurons with a distribution distinct from that containing the pentapeptide.

Following intracerebral injection of ^{3}H-tyrosine or ^{3}H-glycine or incubation of brain slices or isolated organs with these ^{3}H-precursors, a small incorporation into the Met-Enkephalin molecule has been demonstrated. However in all cases, it occured after a lag period of about 1h, suggesting that the pentapeptides derive from a larger precursor. The latter might be a protein synthesized in ribosomes since the incorporation is blocked in the presence of cycloheximide or puromycin. Preliminar in vivo experiments have indicated a rather slow decline in the brain level of ^{3}H-enkephalins labeled after administration of ^{3}H-tyrosine, suggesting a rather slow turnover. In contrast, acute administration of cycloheximide, used as a potential synthesis inhibitor, results, in about 1h, in a significant decrease in endogenous enkephalin level in mouse striatum : this could reflect the rate of utilisation of the pentapeptide and would be compatible with an half-life of the cerebral pentapeptides in the same range as that of "classical" neurotransmitters like the monoamines, i.e. only a few hours. However, it is clear that the methodology for such studies has to be improved before definite conclusions can be made in this respect.

Release

One of the criteria a putative neurotransmitter has to fulfill is that of release from the alleged pathway.

Indirect evidence was already provided, before the discovery of enkephalins, when it was observed that the opiate receptor antagonist, naloxone, elicited some physiological effects opposite to those of opiates : for instance this antagonist diminishes the nociceptive threshold in mice or enhances the release of acetylcholine from the guinea-pig myenteric plexus during nerve-stimulation.

More direct evidence for the neuronal release of enkephalin has been provided by the observations, made in several laboratories, that endogenous Met- and Leu-Enkephalin are released in the incubation medium from depolarized brain slices or synaptosomes by a calcium-dependent process.

Interestingly enough this release was demonstrable only when the incubation medium contained a high concentration of dipeptides acting as competitive inhibitors of peptidases : this suggests that released enkephalins are immediately recognized by inactivating enzymes localized in the vicinity of enkephalinergic terminals.

Inactivation

Neurotransmitter messages are rapidly turned off : for instance released acetylcholine is immediately hydrolyzed by acetylcholinesterase whereas monoamines are submitted to an active reuptake. Whereas the latter process is unlikely to be involved in peptide inactivation, this is not the case for the proteolytic cleavage which has been shown to occur (and has been a disturbing factor) in early research on enkephalins. When the pentapeptides are exposed to proteolytic activity in serum or brain homogenates, the first step in the progressive cleavage of the molecule consists in the release of tyrosine, the N-terminal aminoacid of the molecule, as shown in various laboratories.

Recently we have evidenced the presence in the CNS of a peptidase which is likely to be involved in the control of enkephalinergic transmission. This "enkephalinase" is a dipeptidyl-carboxypeptidase (it releases ^{3}H-Tyr-Gly-Gly from ^{3}H-enkephalins) which presents a high affinity for the two enkephalins (Km around 0.1μM) contrasting with the much lower affinity of other enkephalin-degrading enzymes, i.e. aminopeptidases. In contrast with the latters, it is selectively associated with membrane-enriched fraction from brain tissues. Structure-activity studies indicate that this metallo-enzyme (probably a zinc-containing protein) has a clear chemical specificity towards the entire enkephalin molecule. Furthermore, its regional distribution, parallel to that of opiate receptors, as well as the similar percent decreases in the number of these receptors and in the activity of the enzyme following selective lesions suggest that both membrane components are held on the same neurons, possibly in vicinity. Finally enkephalin-dipeptidylcarboxypeptidase activity is selectively and markedly increased in animals chronically treated with morphine. Such change might reflect an adaptation of the enkephalin-sensitive cells to an excessive stimulation mediated by opiate receptors.

If our hypothesis that enkephalin-dipeptidyl-carboxypeptidase is the "acetylcholinesterase of enkephalins" is confirmed, this would imply that inhibitors of this enzyme might constitute a new class of antinociceptive agents.

Enkephalin Receptors

It is likely that opiate receptors i.e. binding sites in the CNS recognized by morphine-like agents and opioid peptides in fact represent at least in part post-synaptic receptors for putative enkephalinergic neurons. Indeed, as already stated, the respective distribution of the pentapeptides and the receptors, the latters revealed either biochemically or autoradiographically, are generally in rather good agreement.

From lesion studies, it appears that on a variety of neuronal systems opiate receptors are located presynaptically : for instance this appears to be the case for substance P neurons projecting in the dorsal horn of the spinal cord (and carrying nociceptive messages at this level) as well as for catecholaminergic (noradrenergic and dopaminergic) neurons in the brain. This presynaptic localization probably reflects one of the major mode of action of enkephalins (and opiates), i.e. the "presynaptic inhibition" of transmitter release. Such presynaptic inhibition, a well-established function of short interneurons, might well account for the analgesic actions of opioids (at least at the level of the spinal cord) as well as for their mood-modifying properties (possibly mediated by presynaptic inhibition of catecholamine release).

Classical pharmacological tests as binding studies suggest that opiate receptors in various tissues (and possibly various parts of the CNS) are constituted by an heterogenous population of binding sites. It is not yet clear whether this heterogeneity reflects that of their endogenous ligands or the existence of sub-populations of sites recognizing the same endogenous ligand (like in the case of α- and β-adrenergic receptors). In any case this obviously interesting concept demands to be clarified that more selective antagonists should be developed and their physiological actions assessed.

β-ENDORPHIN AS HORMONE AND NEUROTRANSMITTER

A difficulty in establishing the cellular stores of β-endorphin has been, and largely remains the lack of specificity of antibodies raised towards this molecule. The main identified cross-reacting substances are the parent molecule β-lipotropin as well as the myelin basic protein, both to be found in significant amounts in neuroendocrine tissues.

β-Endorphin in the pituitary

The pituitary peptide, β-lipotropin, isolated by Li in 1964, has lipolytic activity and contains the sequence of β-melanocyte stimulating hormone (β-MSH) which is devoid of opiate-like activity. On the other hand, β-endorphin, which corresponds to the 61-91 sequence, can interact with opiate receptors by its N-terminal moiety and appears on some systems to be much more potent than enkephalins, a feature probably related in great part to its higher resistance to tissue peptidases.

Both RIA and immunocytochemical data indicate that β-endorphin is absent from the neurohypophysis but located in the adenohypophysis and intermediate lobe of several animal species.

In the adenohypophysis, the peptide is stored in corticotrophs, probably in the form of a large molecular weight precursor. The latter, termed pro-opiocortin has a molecular weight of 31.000 and contains the ACTH molecule in its sequence. Recently in a very elegant work Nakanishi et al. (1979) succeeded in purifying the mRNA for pro-opiocortin and by recombinant DNA techniques described its full sequence. The corresponding aminoacid sequence of pro-opiocortin reveals that the molecule is composed of four repetitive structures, each having a MSH sequence or its analogue ; each unit is flanked on both sides by a pair of basic aminoacid residues at the level of which proteolytic processing probably takes place. ACTH and β-lipotropin exist as contiguous peptides also separated by the Lys-Arg sequence. From the work of Rossier, Bloom, Guillemin and their colleagues it appears that β-endorphin is released in blood, together with ACTH during stressful situations and that the levels of the two circulating hormones are parallel. Splitting from pro-opiocortin could occur during the release process because a peptidase activity releasing β-endorphin has been detected in the pituitary.

Whereas the function of released ACTH is well established, this is not the case for β-endorphin. It is not yet clear whether the maximal concentrations of β-endorphin evaluated in blood are sufficient to activate opiate receptors in brain or even in peripheral tissues.

β-Endorphin in Brain

As shown by RIA, brain contains significant amounts of β-endorphin and these levels are unchanged after hypophysectomy. The regional distribution shows no parallelism with that of enkephalins and many areas rich in the pentapeptides are devoid of detectable β-endorphin.

Furthermore careful immunocytochemical studies have revealed β-endorphin-containing neuronal perikarya and fiber tracts throughout the diencephalon. Perikarya are mainly localized in the tuberal hypothalamus and seem to project to midline areas throughout the diencephalon as well as to the pons, especially at the level of periaqueducal gray. The distribution of these fibers recall that of LHRH-containing neurons but with some differences. It is likely that this neuronal system also stores β-endorphin in the form of pro-opiocortin. The function of β-endorphin in this system might be that of a neurotransmitter but, at the present time, this is largely an assumption.

READING LIST

. Costa, E. and Trabucchi, M.D. (1978) The Endorphins vol. 18, Raven Press, New York, pp. 1-379.

. Goldstein, A. (1976) Science, 193, 1081-1086.

. Iversen, L.L. and Dingledine, R. (1976) Nature, 262, 738-739.

. Klee, W.A. (1977) Endogenous opiate peptides. In Peptides in Neurobiology (H. Gainer ed.), Plenum Press, New York, pp. 375-396.

. Marx, J.L. (1976) Science, 193, 1227-1229.

. Snyder, S.H. and Simantov, R. (1977) J. Neurochem. 28, 13-20.

. Van Ree, J.M. and Terenius, L. (1978) Characteristics and Function of Opioids, Elsevier/North Holland, Amsterdam, pp. 1-509.

. Uhl, G., Childers, S.R. and Snyder, S.H. (1978) Opioid Peptides and the Opiate Receptor, Frontiers in Neuroendocrinology (W.F. Ganong and L. Martini eds), pp. 289-329.

. Usdin, E., Bunney, W.E. and Kline, N.S. (1979) Endorphins in Mental Health Research, Mc Millan, London, pp. 1-618.

Radioimmunology 1979, Ch. A. Bizollon, editor.

RADIOCOMPETITIVE ASSAY OF ENDOMORPHINS

CLAUDE GROS
FRA n° 8 INSERM, Unite de Radioimmunologie Analytique, Institut Pasteur
28 Rue du Docteur Roux, 75724 Paris Cedex 15.

INTRODUCTION

The study of endomorphins and of their levels after various pharmacological treatments has rapidly required the development of an analytical system more sensitive and more specific than the biological tests which had originally allowed the demonstration of these substances[1]. The introduction of methods using competition between a labelled and an unlabelled ligand for specific binding sites has allowed development of the microassays required for such investigation, in particular for the assay of cerebral neuropeptides.

Two types of radiocompetitive assay have been developed for these substances, the radioreceptor assay and the radioimmunoassay.

RADIORECEPTOR ASSAY

The presence in the central nervous system of specific opiate receptors which are also specific for endogenous endomorphins provides the binding reagent of choice for radiocompetitive assay of these substances. It was using the competition of (^{3}H) opiates for these recognition sites that Terenius and Wahlstrom[2] and Pasternak et al.[3] first characterized endogenous ligands in brain extracts.

Using a particular fraction of rat striatum and (^{3}H) leu-ENK as a ligand, Audigier et al.[4] have shown, alongside a low-affinity non-specific binding, the presence of a saturatable binding corresponding to two types of binding site with different Kd values: a high affinity (Kd = 5nM) for which the binding of (^{3}H) leu-ENK is inhibited by morphine or by naloxone, which is in fact the specific opiate receptor, and another low affinity receptor (40nM) insensitive to morphine and its antagonists. Using a concentration of (^{3}H) leu-ENK such that only the specific site is involved (5nM), it has been possible to assay total endomorphin levels in biological extracts for comparison with the standard curve obtained by displacement of the binding of the tritiated ligand by increasing known doses of leu-ENK (figure 1)[5].

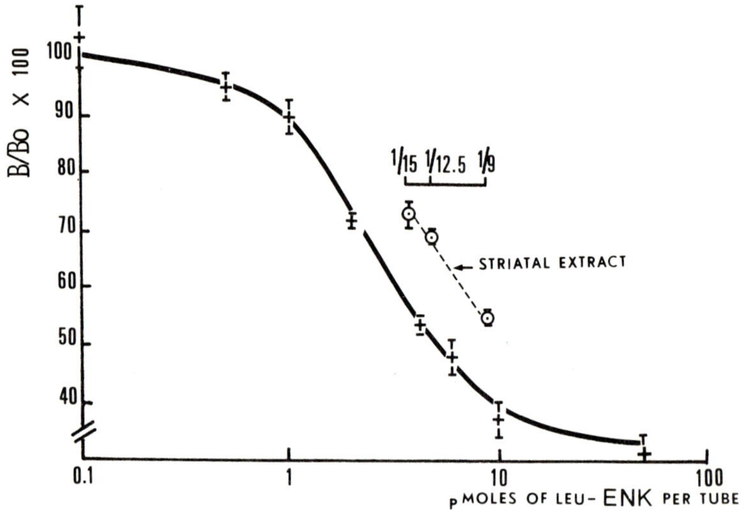

Fig. 1. Radioreceptor assay of endomorphins. Inhibition of (^{3}H) leu-ENK binding to rat striatal membranes by leu-ENK (+——+) and tissue extract (⊙----⊙)

Other authors have carried out this assay using radioactive ligands such as (^{3}H) morphine[6], (^{3}H) etorphine[7], (^{3}H) met-ENK, (^{3}H) naloxone and (^{3}H) hydromorphine[8,9], (^{125}I) DAla$_2$D leu$_2$-ENK[10] or (^{3}H) dihydromorphine and (^{3}H) naltrexone[11], with sensitivity of the same order as that shown in table 1.

RADIOIMMUNOASSAY

The endomorphins have amino acid sequences identical to those found in the hypophysial hormone β-lipotropine (β-LPH) whose role is as yet poorly understood (fig. 2)

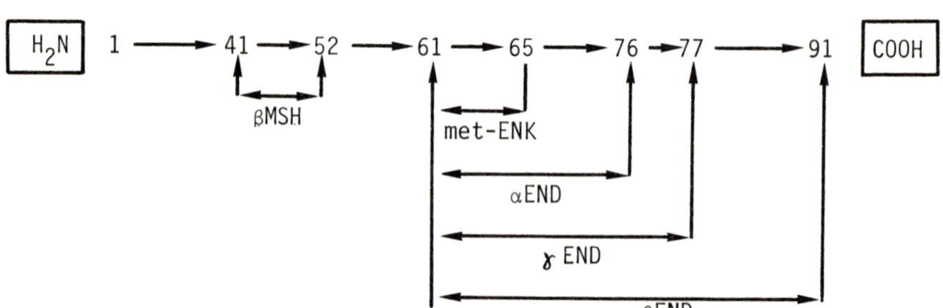

Fig. 2. Relationships between βLPH and endomorphins sequences.

TABLE 1

PERFORMANCE OF RADIORECEPTOR ASSAYS USING DIFFERENT LABELLED LIGANDS

LABELLED LIGANDS	IC 50 (nM)			REFERENCES
	Met-ENK	Leu-ENK	βEND	
(^{3}H) Morphine * 4nM	36 - 111		120 - 370	Doneen et al. (1977) [6]
(^{3}H) Dihydromorphine*	17			Terenius (1977) [11]
(^{3}H) Naltrexone*	460			
(^{3}H) leu-ENK* 5nM	22.5	15	12	Gros et al. (1978) [5]
(^{3}H) Met-ENK* 2nM	3	5	2	Simantov et al. (1978) [8]
(^{3}H) Naloxone* 1.5nM	8	20	3	
(^{3}H) Dihydromorphine*	12.5	12.5	3	
(^{125}I) $Dala_2$ $Dleu_2$ ENK** 2. 10^5 cpm		1		Miller et al. (1978) [10]

* binding to rat brain membranes

** binding to N_4TG_1 (neuroblastoma) cells

While this sequence homology poses problems of specificity discussed later, the interest of the radioimmunoassay is that it allows selective measurement of each of these peptides using specific antibodies. In addition, the use of (^{125}I) iodinated tracers allows sensitivities much greater than that obtained with the radioreceptor assay.

ENKEPHALINS

These are two pentapeptides varying only by their C-terminal amino acid (leu or met), having in common an iodinable tyrosyl residue in the N-terminal position.

Preparation of radioactive tracers. The tritiated derivatives of enkephalin are commercially available, with a specific radioactivity ranging between 30 and 40 Ci/mmole. In a radiocompetitive immunoassay, the more tracer added, the more unmarked antigen will be required to displace it from the antibody. Thus, the use of the (^{125}I) iodinated derivative with a specific activity generally 50 times higher than that of the tritiated derivative allows considerably better sensitivity, provided that the iodination does not change the recognition of the antigen by the antibody.

The iodinated enkephalin derivatives are prepared by the classic chloramine T method and purified, either by gel filtration chromatography[12,13], or by thin-layer chromatography allowing the elimination of degradation and non-iodinated products[5]. The specific radioactivity of the tracers thus obtained ranges between 1,000 and 2,000 Ci/mmole.

Preparation of anti-enkephalin antibodies. So as to render the enkephalins immunogenic in the rabbit, they must be coupled to a protein carrier. The coupling position on the enkephalin molecule is a determining factor for the specificity of the assay; it is essential that the C-terminal portion of the molecule be preserved so as to allow differentiation between the enkephalins. Figure 3 shows the various coupling possibilities used for met-ENK.

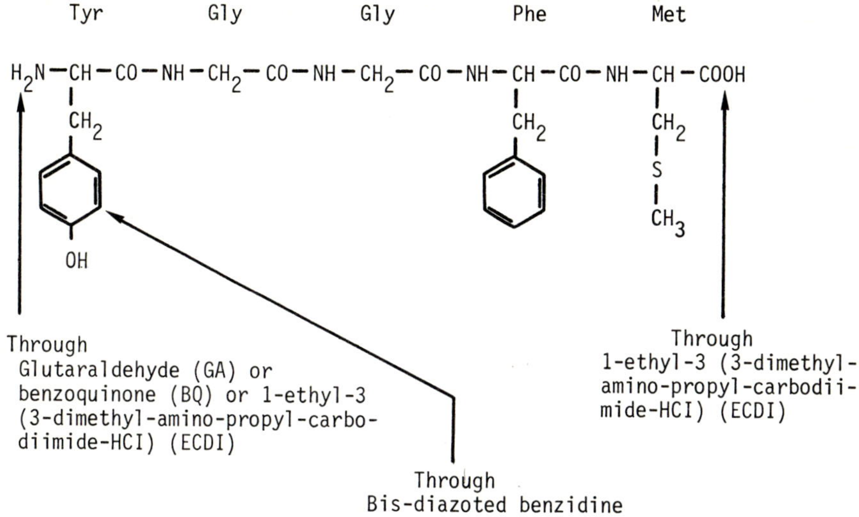

Fig. 3. Various coupling points for immunogen preparation (met-ENK).

In our laboratory, we have obtained antibodies by the immunisation of rabbits with enkephalins carbodiimide-coupled to ovalbumine. The N-terminal end of the enkephalin is preferentially coupled, as shown by the low cross-reaction with the corresponding analogues[5].We have shown that neither enkephalin fragments nor the various endorphins or morphine have any cross-reaction,and this up to micromolar concentrations

The standard curve which we have obtained with the anti met-ENK antiserum, shown in figure 4, shows the increase in sensitivity obtained by using an iodinated tracer as contrast with that obtained with a tritiated tracer. This allows assay of enkephalin obtained in milligram quantities of rat striatum. The parallel values of the standard curve and the various dilutions of striatal is a good index for the specific recognition of enkephalins in the extract. This point will be discussed below.

Table 2 shows the results obtained by various authors using different immunogens.

TABLE 2

PERFORMANCE OF RADIOIMMUNOASSAYS FOR ENKEPHALINS USING DIFFERENT LABELLED TRACERS, AND IMMUNOGENS.

LABELLED LIGANDS	IMMUNOGEN	IC 50 (nM)	Lower detection limit(pg)	CROSS REACTIONS*		REFERENCES
				Met-ENK	Leu-ENK	
(^{3}H) leu-ENK 4nM	BSA + ECDI	1	50	20	100	Weissman et al.(1976)[14]
(^{3}H) Met-ENK	Suc.hemocyanin + ECDI		2500	100	10	Yang et al.(1977)[15]
(^{3}H) leu-ENK	Suc.hemocyanin + ECDI		500	10	100	
(^{3}H) Met-ENK 2nM	Thyroglobulin + ECDI		100	100	0.3	Wesche et al.(1977)[16]
(^{3}H) leu-ENK 1nM	Thyroglobulin + ECDI		30	0.1	100	
(^{3}H) Met-ENK 4.6nM	Hemocyanine + ECDI	50	5700	100	1	Simantov et al.(1977)[17]
(^{3}H) leu-ENK 4.6nM	Hemocyanine + ECDI	20	2000	< 1	100	
(^{125}I) leu-ENK	BSA + BDB	0.05	2	3.3	100	Rossier et al.(1977)[12]
(^{125}I) Met-ENK	BSA + GA	0.5	20	100	< 0.1	Miller et al.(1978)[10]
(^{125}I) leu-ENK	BSA + GA	0.4	10	< 0.1	100	
(^{125}I) Met-ENK	Ovalbumine + ECDI	0.57	10	100	7	Gros et al.(1978)[5]
(^{125}I) leu-ENK	Ovalbumine + ECDI	0.55	10	5	100	

* Calculated from the molar ratios of IC50 x 100.

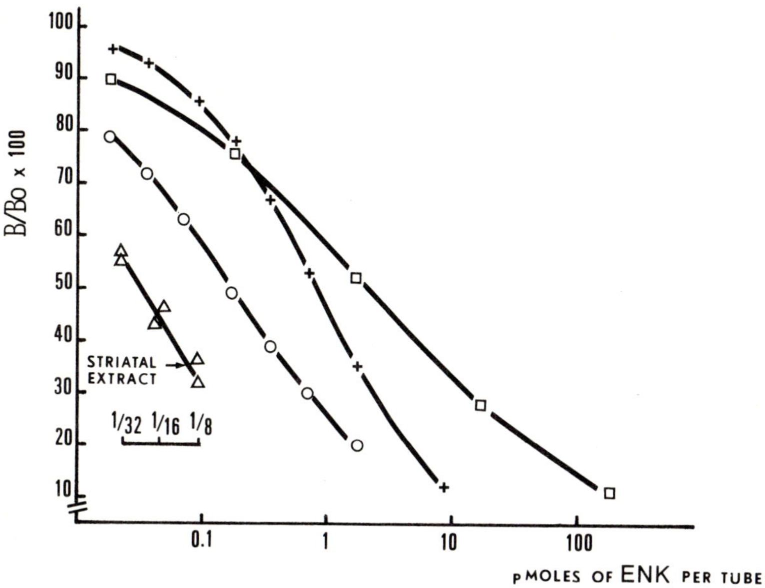

Fig. 4. Radioimmunoassay of met-ENK. Inhibition of (^{125}I) met-ENK binding to anti met-ENK serum by unlabelled met-ENK (○—○), leu-ENK (□—□) and rat striatal extract (△—△). Inhibition of (^{3}H) met-ENK binding by met-ENK (+—+).

β-ENDORPHIN

For radioimmunoassay of β-endorphin, (^{125}I) iodinated tracers (chloramine T method and gel filtration purification) and immunogen preparation using the same coupling methods as for enkephalins are used.

The performance of assays by various group of researchers are shown in table 3. The fact that β-END is identical to the C-terminal fraction of β-LPH induces a major cross-reaction with this hormone in all cases. On the other hand, the cross-reaction between the enkephalins and the other endorphins (α and γ) are in general almost negligible.

Using an immunogen obtained by coupling β-END to BSA with benzoquinone, linking the amine groups of the carrier with those of the antigen by formation of a bridge, we have produced antibodies allowing a sensitivity of 20 pg (figure 5).

TABLE 3

PERFORMANCE OF RADIOIMMUNOASSAYS FOR βENDORPHINS (βEND)* USING DIFFERENTS IMMUNOGENS

ANTIGEN	IMMUNOGEN	IC50 (nM)	Lower detection limit(ng)	CROSS REACTIONS**				REFERENCES
				h-βEND	p,c-βEND	h-βLPH	p,o-βLPH	
h-βEND	h γglobulin + ECDI	0.28	0.1	100	100	10		Li et al.(1977)[18]
p-βEND	b thyroglobulin + BDB	0.33	0.05		100		100	Guillemin et al.(1977)[19]
p-βEND	crude porcine ACTH preparation (Organon)	0.01	0.005	100			5.5	Yoshimi et al.(1978)[20]
p-βEND	Aminobenzyloxymethyl cellulose	1.1			100		8	Ross et al.(1978)[21]
c-βEND	αEND+bovine thyroglobulin + ECDI	0.18		78	100	22	33	Ross et al.(1978)[21]
h-βEND	Bovine thyroglobulin + ECDI	0.2	0.025	100		50		Höllt et al.(1978)[22]
c-βEND	Ovalbumine + BQ	0.13	0.02	100	100	+	45	Gros et al.(1979)[23]
h-βEND	Ovalbumine + BQ	0.20	0.04	100	0	+	0	Gros et al.(1979)[23]

* h : human; p : porcine; c : camel; o : ovine.

** Calculated from the molar ratios of IC50 x 100.

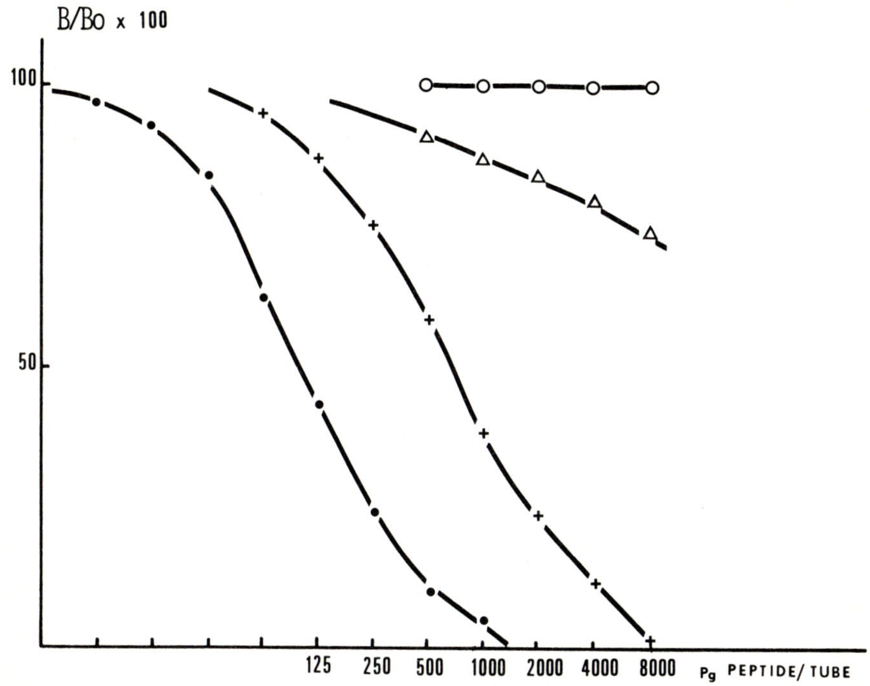

Fig. 5. Radioimmunoassay of β-END. Inhibition of (^{125}I) h-βEND binding to anti c-βEND serum by unlabelled h- or c-βEND (•——•), p-βLPH (+——+), γEND (Δ——Δ) and met-ENK (O——O).

DISCUSSION

Two essential points must be taken into consideration to validate results of radiocompetitive assays: the conditions for preparation of biological extracts and the interpretation of the results of radioimmunoassay.

1) Preparation of biological extracts. It should be carried out so as to maintain the integrity of the endogenous products, and their extraction should be complete.

After sacrifice of the animals, the tissue should be homogenised in an acid medium (0.1N HCl) so as to avoid degradation by cerebral peptidases. After heat-treatment at 95° for 15 minutes, neutralization in Tris pH 7.4 buffer, and centrifugation, the endomorphins may be assayed in the supernatants, and we have shown that under these conditions, their degradation is negligible[5].

2) Interpretation of the results obtained with radioimmunoassay. We have shown that the parallelism of the standard curve and the curve of the various dilutions assayed is due to their recognition with equal affinity by the antibody. We cannot however affirm with certainty that the standard and assayed substance are identical, and this data must be supplemented with other tests for identity, for example chromatography (gel filtration, partition chromatography or HPLC). As we have stated above, for β-END assay, the major cross-reaction with β-LPH will provide erroneous results if extracts are assayed directly, without previous purification. In various structures including the bovine caudate nucleus[24], the sympathetic ganglia of the rat, the quinea pig, or the rabbit[25], the pig hypothalamus[26], and the chiken embryo retina[27] enkephalin-like substances have been shown. These substances are recognised by anti-enkephalin antibodies, but they correspond not to the native enkephalins but to a higher-weight molecular species. We may consider that while these substances may be enkephalin precursors, a specific neurotransmettor role has not yet been shown.

Using radioreceptor and radioimmunoassay numerous authors have studied the distribution of endomorphins in the brain and in the pituitary of the rat and have shown major regional variations in enkephalin levels, independent of endorphin levels[5,12,15,16,28,29,30]. The amounts of enkephalins and endorphins assayed by radioimmunoassay represents only a fraction of endomorphin levels measured by radioreceptor assay, regardless of the region. This would appear to indicate the existence of other morphinomimetic substances, the importance of which remains to be determined.

REFERENCES

1. Hughes, J. (1975) Brain Res. 88, 295-308.
2. Terenius, L. and WAHLSTROM, A. (1974) Acta Pharmacol. Tox. 35, 1, 55-60.
3. Pasternak, G.W. et al. (1975) Life Sci. 16, 1765-1769.
4. Audigier, Y. et al. (1977) Eur. J. Pharmacol. 41, 247-248.
5. Gros et al. (1978) J. Neurochem. 31, 29-39.
6. Doneen, B.A. et al. (1977) Biochem. Biophys. Res. Com. 74, 656-662.
7. Cheung, A.L. et al. (1977) Life Sci. 20, 1285-1290.
8. Simantov, R. et al. (1978) Eur. J. Pharmacol. 47, 319-331.
9. Akil, H. et al. (1976) Opiates and endogenous opioid peptides. Elsevier/ North Holland Biochemical press Amsterdam, pp. 63-70.

10. Miller, R.J. et al. (1978) Life Sci. 22, 379-388.
11. Terenius, L. (1977) Psychoneuroendocrinology, 2, 53-58.
12. Rossier, J. et al. (1977) Proc. Natl. Acad. Sci. USA, 74, 5162-5165.
13. Miller, R.J. et al. (1978) J. Biol. Chem., 253, 531-538.
14. Weissman, B.A. et al. (1976) FEBS letters, 70, 245-248.
15. Yang, H.Y. et al. (1977) Neuropharmacology, 16, 303-307.
16. Wesche, D. et al. (1977) Naunyn-Schmiedeberg's Arch. Pathol., 30, 79-82.
17. Simantov, R. et al. (1977) Brain Research, 134, 358-367.
18. Li, C.H. et al. (1977) Biochem. Biophys. Res. Com., 75, 576-579.
19. Guillemin, R. et al. (1977) Biochem. Biophys. Res. Com., 77, 361-366.
20. Yoshimi, H. et al. (1977) Life Sci., 22, 2189-2196.
21. Ross, M. et al. (1977) Life Sci., 22, 1123-1130.
22. Höllt, V. et al. (1978) Naunym-Schmiedeberg's Arch. Pharmacol., 303, 171-174.
23. Gros, C. et al. (1979) in preparation.
24. Yang, H.-Y.T. et al. (1978) Neuropharmacology, 17, 433-438.
25. Di Giulio, A.M. et al. (1978) Neuropharmacology, 17, 989-992.
26. Kangawa, K. and Matsuo, H. (1979) Biochem. Biophys. Res. Com., 86, 153-160.
27. Humbert, J. et al. (1979) Neuroscience letters, accepted for publication.
28. Simantov, R. and Snyder, S.H. (1976) Opiates and endogenous opioid peptides North-Holland Biomedical Press, Amsterdam, pp. 41-48.
29. Hong, J.S. et al. (1977) Brain Research, 134, 383-386.
30. Duka, T. et al. (1978) Biochem. Biophys. Res. Com., 85, 1119-1127.

Radioimmunology 1979, Ch. A. Bizollon, editor.

ENDORPHINS IN HUMAN CEREBROSPINAL FLUID (CSF) AS INDICATORS OF CENTRAL ENDORPHIN ACTIVITY

LARS TERENIUS and A. WAHLSTRÖM
Department of Pharmacology, University of Uppsala, Sweden

The term endorphin is used to characterize endogenously occurring substances with morphino-mimetic properties. These substances are peptides. Since their discovery in 1975 (1,2), it has become clear that there are in fact several endorphin systems. At the present stage of knowledge three different systems have been described (Table 1).

TABLE 1
ENDORPHIN SYSTEMS

Peptide	No. of amino acid residues	Occurrence
Leucine- and methionine-enkephalin	5	CNS, gastrointestinal tract, peripheral nerves and ganglia, adrenal medulla
β-Endorphin	31	Brain, pituitary
Kyotorphin	2	Brain

We have to-day no information about the potential importance of Kyotorphin (3), while the enkephalin and β-endorphin systems are better characterized. Specific antibodies have been raised against these latter peptides and used to map their distribution with immunohistochemical techniques. The enkephalins show a wide distribution in the CNS and occur at all levels. Furthermore they can be found in peripheral nerve tissue and also in non-neuronal tissue such as the adrenal medulla and gastrointestinal gland cells. β-Endorphin occurs in the brain in much less abundance and mainly in a diffuse projection from hypothalamic to thalamic areas. In the pituitary it occurs in several cell types with preponderance for corticotrophs.

The differences between β-endorphin and the enkephalins in chemistry and distribution is coupled with differences in activity profiles. While the enkephalins are fairly easily degraded, β-endorphin is a rather stabile compound with a half-life in plasma of 10-15 minutes and with long-lasting effects if introduced directly into the brain. It may therefore be appropriate to consider the enkephalins as shortacting and local messengers, in the nervous system perhaps of a neurotransmitter type, while β-endorphin may give more general and sustained effects suggesting a role as a hormone or neuromodulator. The more general aspects of the endorphin field have been covered recently in several reviews (4-6).

Measurements of endorphin activity in man

The wide-spread distribution of endorphins suggest that their functional role may be extensive. Also a consideration of the wide range of effects of morphine (7) would draw attention to studies on their functional role in physiologic and pathophysiologic situations. For instance, the regulation of pain and mood may be influenced by endorphins as may pituitary function. It is therefore easy to see clinical entities which would be of interest to study. Essentially two different methods are available (8), a) the use of the narcotic antagonist naloxone to block endorphin activity or b) the measurement of endorphin levels. Each approach has its limitations. Naloxone will affect every endorphin system and is therefore unable to discriminate between different systems. Chemical measurements have a limited applicability in humans, because one is restricted to body fluids. While levels in body fluids may accurately reflect the activity in hormonal systems, they may not do so in locally acting systems as those with enkephalins. Moreover, we have to face the problem of various sites of production. For instance, measurements of CNS endorphin activity should preferably be concentrated to the analysis of cerebrospinal fluid (CSF) to avoid blurring by peripheral sources. Interest has so far been focused on CNS endorphins and most studies have consequently been directed to CSF analysis. Table 2 illustrates the endorphin concentrations measured by radioimmunoassay (enkephalin and β-endorphin, respectively) and by radioreceptorassay.

TABLE 2

NORMAL LEVELS OF ENDORPHINS IN HUMAN CSF

Method Measured activity	pmol/ml range	Number of patients	Author
RIA Met-enkephalin	0.3-11.6	10	Akil et al.[9]
RIA β-endorphin	0.05-0.15	17	Jeffcoate et al.[10]
RRA Fraction I	0.4-1.6[x]	19	Lindström et al.[11]

[x] Expressed as methionine-enkephalin equivalents

It should be remembered that the RIA-methods give immunoactive material while the RRA gives receptoractive material. The exact chemical nature of the immunoreactive material has not been characterized. In the β-endorphin assay, which crossreacts extensively with β-lipotropin, corrections are done by the use of several antibodies directed against different fragments of β-lipotropin (10). The measurements of endorphin activity by RRA has been the favoured approach in this laboratory (11,12). An active fraction, termed Fraction I, has been characterized and measured in a large series of patients (Table 3).

TABLE 3

SUMMARY OF PROPERTIES OF FRACTION I

Chemistry:	Not identical to hitherto described endorphins Probably peptide of molecular weight ∿ 1000
Receptor interaction:	More like β-endorphin than enkephalin
Site of production:	Brain? and spinal cord

Although some of our experimental evidence would suggest a relationship to the β-endorphin system, the spinal site of production strongly suggests that Fraction I is related to the enkephalin system since β-endorphin has not been found in the spinal cord (4). We are presently trying to establish the structure of the active material.

Functional studies and CSF levels of endorphins

Probably the best evidence for a functional relevance of β-endorphin in a clinical context comes from studies on pain relief induced by intracerebral electrical stimulation. This technique utilizes electrodes implanted into paraventricular brain areas. The induced pain relief is long-lasting. Frequently, a naloxone injection will cause the recurrence of pain. Concomittantly, there seems to be an increase in CSF β-endorphin levels, suggesting a causal relationship (Table 4).

TABLE 4

EFFECT OF INTRACEREBRAL STIMULATION ON CSF β-ENDORPHIN LEVELS

Before stimulation fmol/ml	15 min after stimulation fmol/ml	Number of patients	Author
<25	250-500	5	Akil et al.[13]
49-60	77-206	3	Hosobuchi et al.[14]

β-Endorphin in CSF seems to be of brain origin, since patients with hyper- or hypo- pituitarism have normal levels (10). On the other hand, serum levels of β-endorphin reflect pituitary function. However, these studies are outside the scope of this paper.

The mesurement of endorphin activity with a radioreceptorassay, started at a time when the chemical structures of endorphins were unknown (12). In retrospect, this approach should be a valid one, in view of the chemical complexity of endorphins and the potentially large number of endorphin fragments. Empirically it was found that the levels of a chromatographic fraction, called Fraction I, related to certain clinical variables. A very significant observation in this regard was the finding of an elevation of Fraction I levels in lumbar CSF after low-frequency, high-intensity transcutaneous nerve stimulation (lo-TNS) in patients with chronic pain (15). The effect seemed to be a specific phenomenon segmentally related to the stimulation area. The effects of this procedure for clinical pain relief, have been found to be naloxone-reversible (16,17), thus linking the two phenomena. Further strengthening the connection between lo-TNS, induced pain relief and endorphins is the observation that TNS using high frequency (hi-TNS) gives adequate pain relief without affecting Fraction I levels or to be naloxone-reversible (17,18). The results are summarized in Table 5.

TABLE 5
ENDORPHINS AND TNS MECHANISMS

Stimulation mode	Effect of naloxone	Effect on Fraction I
hi-TNS	None	None
lo-TNS (electro-acupuncture)	Reversal	Increase

hi-TNS = high-frequency, low-intensity transcutaneous nerve stimulation
lo-TNS = low-frequency, high-intensity transcutaneous nerve stimulation

It was observed during these studies that patients with chronic pain tended to have comparatively low levels of Fraction I endorphin. More detailed studies revealed, that low levels were characteristic of patients with neurogenic pain while in patients where the pain syndrome could not be ascribed to peripheral nerve lesions, the levels were in the normal range (Table 6).

TABLE 6
FRACTION I ENDORPHIN AND CHRONIC PAIN (11,19)

Subjects	Fraction I (pmol/ml) ≤ 0.6	>0.6
Neurogenic pain	28	5
Psychogenic pain	1	16
Healthy volunteers	2	17

These data suggest, that chronic neurogenic pain is frequently associated with low endorphin levels. This indicates a peripheral defect in mechanisms activating endorphin systems. Patients with low endorphin levels are frequently good responders to TNS, indicating that the endorphin systems are intrinsically active but the peripheral triggering systems inadequate. So far, no information is available as to the nature of these systems. However, there may be a connection between serotonin metabolites in the CSF and Fraction I (20).

The levels of Fraction I also seem to reflect responsiveness to experimental pain. Both experimental pain thresholds and tolerance limits tend to be high in a population of patients with chronic pain with high Fraction I levels (21). Another psychophysical variable is visual average evoked potentials. Patients with high endorphin levels (and high pain measures) are less sensitive to increases in visual stimuli than those with low (22). Finally, there was a significant correlation between depressive symptomatology and Fraction I (19). Thus, both measures of sensory reactivity and mood levels seem to be related to a single biochemical variable, the levels of Fraction I. This purely empirical finding lends itself to speculations regarding the regulation of mood and behaviour in more general terms. The identification of the chemical structure of Fraction I is a much needed prerequisite for further progress in our understanding of these phenomena.

The observations reviewed here, and several experimental observations regarding opiates and their effects on mood and behaviour, prompted us to extand the measurements of Fraction I to patients with psychiatric disorders. The best evidence for a link between endorphins and these disorders comes from work on schizophrenia. Several arguments were put forward to predict such a link (Table 7).

TABLE 7
THE ENDORPHIN HYPOTHESIS OF SCHIZOPHRENIA (11,23,24)

1. CSF endorphins (Fraction I) frequently high
2. CSF endorphins tend to decline on neuroleptic medication
3. Antagonist-analgesics produce psychoto-mimetic effects
4. Intraventricular injection of β-endorphin produces catatonia

The hypothesis led to the testing of naloxone in schizophrenia with some positive results (23,25). Recent therapeutic studies with an endorphin analogue, des-tyrosine-γ-endorphin, also support the hypothesis that endorphins are linked to schizophrenia (26). Further studies will be needed to clarify the causal relationships.

CONCLUSIONS

The endorphins constitute a class of compounds which are widely distributed in the body. It is likely that they are directly involved or influenced indirectly in several clinically important conditions. This paper has focused on the evaluation of endorphins in central nervous function. It has been found emperically that various CNS mechanisms can be followed by measurement of CSF endorphin levels. Correlations exist between such levels and various psychophysical variables. Endorphin measurements in CSF may serve a role in the subdiagnosis of various clinical syndromes affecting mood and behaviour.

ACKNOWLEDGEMENTS

This work is supported by the Swedish Medical Research Council.

REFERENCES

1. HUGHES, J. (1975) Brain Res., 88, 295-308.
2. TERENIUS, L. and WAHLSTRÖM, A. (1975) Acta Physiol, Scand., 94, 74-81.
3. TAKAGI, H., SKIONI, H., UEDA, H. and AMANO, H. (1979) Eur. J. Pharmacol., 55, 109-111.
4. TERENIUS, L. (1978) Ann. Rev. Pharmacol. Toxicol., 18, 189-204.
5. Van REE, J. and TERENIUS, L. (1978) Characteristics and Function of Opioids, Elsevier/North-Holland, Biomedical Press.
6. HUGHES, J. and KOSTERLITZ, H.W. (1977) Br. Med. Bull., 33, 157-161.
7. JAFFE, J.H. and MARTIN, W. (Goodman, A. and Gilman, A., ed.) (1975) The Pharmacological Basis of Therapeutics, Mac Millan, New York, p. 245-283.
8. TERENIUS, L. and WAHLSTRÖM, A. (1978) in Centrally Acting Peptides (Hughes, J., ed.), McMillan, London, pp. 161-178.
9. AKIL, H., WATSON, S.J., SULLIVAN, S. and BARCHAS, J.D. (1978) Life Sci., 23, 121-126.
10. JEFFCOATE, W.J., REES, L.H., LOWRY, P.J., Mc LOUGHLIN, L., RATTER, S.J., HOPE, J. and BESSER, G.M. (1978) Lancet, July 15, 119-121.
11. LINDSTRÖM, L.H., WIDERLÖV, E., GUNNE, L.-M., WAHLSTRÖM, A. and TERENIUS, L. (1978) Acta Psychiat. Scand. 57, 153-164.
12. TERENIUS, L. and WAHLSTRÖM, A. (1975) Life Sci., 16, 1759-1764.
13. AKIL, H., RICHARDSON, D.E., BARCHAS, J.D. and LI, C.H. (1978) Proc. Natl. Acad. Sci., 75, 5170-5172.
14. HOSOBUCHI, Y., ROSSIER, J. BLOOM, F. and GUILLEMIN, R. (1978) Soc. Neuroscience Abstr., 4, 410-413.
15. SJÖLUND, B., TERENIUS, L. and ERIKSSON, M. (1977) Acta Physiol. Scand., 100, 382-384.

16.SJÖLUND, B. and ERIKSSON, M. (1976) Lancet i.i., 1085.

17.SJÖLUND, B. and ERIKSSON, M. (1979) Brain Res., in press.

18.Unpublished observations.

19.ALMAY, B.G.L., JOHANSSON, F., von KNORRING, L., TERENIUS, L. and WAHLSTRÖM, A. (1978) Pain, 5, 153-162.

20.Unpublished observations.

21.von KNORRING, L., ALMAY, B.G.L., JOHANSSON, F. and TERENIUS, L. (1978) Pain, 5, 359-365.

22.von KNORRING, L., ALMAY, B.G.L. and TERENIUS, L. (1978) Neuropsychobiology, in press.

23.GUNNE, L.-M., LINDSTRÖM, L. and TERENIUS, L. (1977) J. Neural. Transm., 40, 13-19.

24.BLOOM, R. SEGAL, D., LING, N. and GUILLEMIN, R. (1976) Science, 194, 630-632.

25.TERENIUS, L. (1978) in Characteristics and Function of Opioids (van Ree, J. and Terenius, L., eds.). Elsevier/north-Holland Biomedical Press, Amsterdam pp. 143-158.

26.VERHOEVEN, W.M.A., van PRAAG, H.M., BOTTER, P.A., SUNIER,A., van REE, J.M. and de WIED, D. (1978) Lancet, i., 1046-1047.

© 1979 Elsevier/North-Holland Biomedical Press
Radioimmunology 1979, Ch. A. Bizollon, editor.

EFFECT OF ADRENALECTOMY AND GLUCOCORTICOID TREATMENT UPON ACTH, α-MSH, β-MSH, β-LPH, β-ENDORPHIN AND γ-ENDORPHIN-LIKE IMMUNOREACTIVITIES IN THE ANTERIOR LOBE OF THE PITUITARY.

SYLVIE JEGOU[x], JEROME LEPINE[¶], JEAN COTE[¶], ANDRE DUPONT[¶], MARIE-CHRISTINE TONON[x]
GEORGES PELLETIER[¶], HUBERT VAUDRY[x] AND FERNAND LABRIE[¶]
[x]Laboratoire d'Endocrinologie, Département de Biochimie et de Physiologie Cellulaire, Faculté des Sciences 76130 Mont-Saint-Aignan (France)
[¶]Groupe de Recherche en Endocrinologie Moléculaire, Le Centre Hospitalier de l'Université Laval, Quebec G I V 1 G 2 (Canada).

INTRODUCTION

The demonstration of parallel release of adrenocorticotropin (ACTH), β-melanotropin (β-MSH), β-lipotropin (β-LPH) and β-endorphin immunoreactivities in human[1-7] and other mammalian species [8] led to the discovery of a common precursor molecule (31 K precursor) which contains the entire amino-acid-sequences of β-LPH and ACTH[9-13]. These findings are in total agreement with immunohistochemical data which provide evidence that ACTH and β-LPH are contained within the same pituitary cells[14-17], and are even present within the same secretory granules [17-18]. They were recently confirmed by the most elegant work of Nakanishi *et al*[19], who have determined the sequence of the RNA messenger coding for the ACTH-LPH precursor molecule.

The presence of an endopeptidase in the adenohypophysis which selectively splits the Leu^{77}-Phe^{78} peptide bond of β-LPH has been demonstrated[20]. Purification and identification of other cleavage products of β-LPH indicate that pituitary peptidases may split other bonds of the hormone[21], such as Lys^{46}-Met^{47}, Arg^{60}-Tyr^{61},Lys^{79}-Asn^{80}. Tonin, a proteolytic enzyme purified from rat submaxillary gland[22] has been found to cleave specifically β-LPH and to generate an opiate-like peptide (β-LPH^{61-78})[23]. γ-endorphin (β-LPH^{61-77}), α-endorphin (β-LPH^{61-76}) and Met-enkephalin (β-LPH^{61-65}) are the principal fragments issued from β-LPH degradation by brain proteases[24].

It has been recently demonstrated that parallel release of ACTH, β-LPH, β-MSH and β-endorphin immunoreactivities occurred from rat anterior pituitary cells in primary culture : similar stimulation was observed with various CRF preparations, with dibutyryl cyclic AMP and with theophylline, whereas preincubation of the cells with 10 nM dexamethasone reduced about 50% the secretion of all peptides[25-27]. The enzymatic cleavage of the 31 k precursor molecule leads to the maturation of different hormonal peptides in the intermediate lobe and in the distal lobe of the pituitary gland[28-31]. Therefore, it is important to determine if the inhibitory feedback of dexamethasone is exerted only on the biosynthesis of the precursor molecule or whether glucocorticoids may also control the biosynthesis or the activity of the proteolytic enzymes involved in the processing of the 31 K.

The aim of the present study was the development of five specific and sensitive radioimmunoassay (RIA) methods which make possible simultaneous measurement of various peptides related to β-LPH and ACTH in the distal lobe of normal rats, adrenalectomized (ADX) rats, or ADX rats under chronic dexamethasone treatment.

MATERIALS AND METHODS

Animals. Forty adult male Sprague-Dawley rats, weighing 190 to 230 g, were used for this study. A fisrt group was composed of 20 normal control rats. A second group was composed of 10 ADX rats which received sub-cutaneous injections of saline twice a day for 15 days. A third group was composed of 10 ADX rats which received sub-cutaneous injections of dexamethasone (80 μg dexamethasone per injection and per rat in saline) twice a day, for 15 days.

The brains were rapidly removed after decapitation, the *pars distalis* was carefully separated from the *nervosa intermedia* and the distal lobes were collected on dry-ice. The pituitaries were weighed while frozen and immediately homogenized in 5 ml of 2 N acetic-acid (4°C ; 30 sec). The homogenates were transferred into 20 ml boiling acetic-acid and kept at 90°C for 5 min. After centrifugation at 5,000 g for 15 min, the supernatants were lyophilized.

Sephadex G-75 chromatography. Each lyophilised extract was dissolved in 200 μl of distilled water, and submitted to gel filtration, at 4°C, on a Sephadex G-75 (1.5 x 90 cm) column using 0.05M, pH 7.6 phosphate buffer as an eluent. One hundred fractions (1.8 ml/fraction) were set apart and stored at - 20°C until measurement of peptide contents. Synthetic α- and β-*h*MSH, *p*ACTH, β-*h* and γ-endorphins and purified β-*o*LPH were used as markers.

Peptide radioimmunoassays.

α-MSH RIA. The antiserum used for α-MSH RIA was developped in rabbits using synthetic α-MSH conjugated to bovine serum albumin[32]. The iodination and RIA procedures were the same as recently described, except that separation of bound and free α-MSH was performed with polyethylene-glycol 6000

(PEG)[33].

ACTH RIA. The antiserum used for ACTH RIA was developped in sheep according to Orth[34]. The RIA procedures were the same as previously described[35] except that the duration of the incubation was reduced to 24 hours and precipitation of free ACTH was performed with charcoal.

β-MSH RIA. Antiserum against β-MSH was developped in guinea-pig[36] and was a generous gift from Dr M. Donnadieu (Hopital Saint-Vincent de Paul, Paris).

β-Endorphin RIA. Antiserum against porcine β-endorphin was raised in rabbits. Synthetic β-*p*endorphin was conjugated to bovine serum albumin with bis-diazotized benzidine. PEG was used to separate bound from free hormone.

γ-Endorphin RIA.The radioimmunoassay method for γ-endorphin measurement has been recently described in details[37]. Antibodies have been raised in rabbits using synthetic γ-endorphin conjugated to bovine serum albumin by the ethyl-carbodiimide method.

Calculations. Radioimmunoassay data were calculated and analyzed with a Hewlett-Packard calculator, model 9830, using a program based on model II of Rodbard and Lewal[38].

RESULTS

Characterization of antibodies. Evaluation of antibody specificity has been achieved by use of 41 synthetic or purified peptides related to ACTH or to β-LPH. The results are summarized in table I. The sequence recognized by α-MSH ; ACTH ; β-MSH ; β-endorphin ; and γ-endorphin antibodies were respectively : ACTH $^{10-11}$; ACTH$^{18-24}$; β-LPH$^{51-58}$; β-LPH$^{70-91}$ and β-LPH $^{68-77}$. On a weight basis, cross-reactions of α-MSH antibodies with synthetic porcine and human ACTH were 0.1%. Cross-reaction of ACTH antibodies with synthetic α-MSH ; β-*h*MSH ; and ACTH$^{17-39}$ were 0.0017% ; <0.0001%, and <0.0001%, respectively. Cross-reactivity between β-MSH antibodies and γ-*p*LPH was 14%. Cross reactivity between β-*p*endorphin antibodies and β-*o*LPH was 15% ; conversely very weak cross-reaction occurred between β-*p*endorphin antibodies and synthetic γ-endorphin (<0.06%) or α-endorphin (0.06%). Cross-reaction of γ-endorphin antibodies with purified β-*o*LPH, synthetic α-endorphin, and synthetic β-*p*endorphin were 1.39%, 0.4%, and 9.4%, respectively.

Sephadex G-75 gel chromatography of pituitary extracts from normal rats. Two major peaks of β-endorphin and β-MSH immunoreactive material which co-migrated exactly with purified β-*o*LPH and β-*h*MSH were detected, as previously described[29]. A small peak of immunoreactive ACTH eluted before

TABLE 1

EVALUATION OF ANTIBODIES ACTH, α-MSH, β-MSH, β-ENDORPHIN AND γ-ENDORPHIN : TITER, SENSITIVITY AND SPECIFICITY.

	antiserum	ACTH AS	α-MSH AS	β-MSH AS	β-pendo AS	γ-pendo AS
	working titer	1/350,000	1/40,000	1/40,000	1/4,700	1/35,000
	sensitivity threshold (pg)	20	3	7	50	10
CROSS-REACTIVITIES BETWEEN ANTIBODIES AND VARIOUS ACTH AND βLPH RELATED PEPTIDES (mass /mass).	*h*ACTH synthetique	1	10^{-3}			
	*p*ACTH synthétique		5 x10^{-4}			
	*p*ACTH naturelle	0.37	1.2 x10^{-2}			
	*r*ACTH naturelle	0.13				
	α-MSH	1.7 x 10^{-5}	1			
	$^{1-10}$ACTH	< 10^{-6}	2 x10^{-6}			
	$^{1-16}$ACTH amide	2.4 x 10^{-4}	2 x10^{-3}			
	$^{1-19}$ACTH amide		2 x10^{-4}			
	$^{1-24}$ACTH	1	10^{-3}			
	$^{4-10}$ACTH	< 10^{-6}				
	$^{11-19}$ACTH amide	0.38	1.5 x10^{-6}			
	$^{11-24}$ACTH	6.5 x 10^{-3}				
	$^{17-39}$ACTH amide	< 10^{-6}	8 x10^{-6}			
	β-*h*LPH			2.6 x 10^{-3}		
	β-*o*LPH		5 x10^{-6}	4.5 x 10^{-3}	0.15	1.3 x 10^{-2}
	γ-*p*LPH			0.14		
	γ-*o*LPH			8.7 x 10^{-5}		
	β-*h*MSH	< 10^{-6}	3 x10^{-6}	1		
	β-*b*MSH	10^{-5}				
	β-*p*endorphine (61-91)				1	9.4 x 10^{-2}
	γ-*p*endorphine (61-77)				< 0.6 x 10^{-3}	1
	α-*p*endorphine (61-76)				< 0.6 x 10^{-3}	4 x 10^{-3}
	$^{61-62}$ β-*p*LPH				< 0.6 x 10^{-3}	< 10^{-5}
	$^{61-63}$ β-*p*LPH				< 0.6 x 10^{-3}	< 10^{-5}
	$^{61-68}$ β-*p*LPH				< 0.6 x 10^{-3}	1.2 x 10^{-3}
	$^{61-69}$ β-*p*LPH				< 0.6 x 10^{-3}	< 10^{-5}
	$^{61-79}$ β-*p*LPH				< 0.6 x 10^{-3}	1.5 x 10^{-1}
	$^{61-87}$ β-*p*LPH				0.27	6 x 10^{-2}
	$^{62-91}$ β-*p*LPH				0.27	0.070
	$^{66-76}$ β-*p*LPH				< 0.6 x 10^{-3}	2 x 10^{-3}
	$^{66-91}$ β-*p*LPH				1	9 x 10^{-2}
	$^{68-76}$ β-*p*LPH				< 0.6 x 10^{-3}	2 x 10^{-3}
	$^{68-91}$ β-*p*LPH				1	3.4 x 10^{-2}
	$^{70-76}$ β-*p*LPH				< 0.6 x 10^{-3}	4.5 x 10^{-5}
	$^{70-91}$ β-*p*LPH				1	1.2 x 10^{-4}
	$^{72-76}$ β-*p*LPH				< 0.6 x 10^{-3}	< 10^{-5}
	$^{72-91}$ β-*p*LPH				0.57	< 10^{-5}
	$^{74-91}$ β-*p*LPH				1.8 x 10^{-3}	< 10^{-5}
	$^{75-77}$ β-*p*LPH				0.6 x 10^{-3}	< 10^{-5}
	$^{76-91}$ β-*p*LPH				0.6 x 10^{-3}	< 10^{-5}
	$^{78-91}$ β-*p*LPH				0.6 x 10^{-3}	2.2 x 10^{-5}

the β-oLPH marker while two other major components with apparent molecular weights of ≃ 12K and ≃ 4K were observed. Owing to the extrem specificity of the α-MSH RIA system, all the α-MSH immunoreactive material co-migrated with synthetic α-MSH. A small amount of γ-endorphin like immunoreactivity, eluted in the same position as authentic γ-endorphin was also detected.

Sephadex G-75 gel chromatography of pituitary extracts from adrenalectomized rats. Fifteen days after adrenalectomy, a 4 to 10 fold increase in all peptide contents was recorded : the two major peaks of ACTH increased 4 fold, the peak of α-MSH increased 5 fold, the peak of γ-endorphin increased 10 fold.

It was also observed that, in the intermediate lobe, α-MSH content was not modified by glucocorticoid level.

Sephadex G-75 gel chromatography of pituitary extracts from ADX rats treated with glucocorticoids. When adrenalectomized rats received long term dexamethasone treatment (160 µg dexamethasone per animal and per day for 15 days), the pituitary content in all peptides returned to normal value : as compared with adrenalectomized rats β-LPH and β-endorphin-like materials were reduced 3 times ; α-MSH was reduced 4 times.

The present data show that combination of gel filtration and specific radioimmunoassay methods will prove useful for the determination of the cellular and molecular mechanisms controlling biosynthesis and/or release of ACTH and β-LPH related hormones.

Our results clearly demonstrate that long term alteration of glucocorticoid levels are accompanied by parallel changes of cell content of ACTH, β-LPH, β-endorphin, γ-endorphin and α-MSH. Parallel changes of the above-mentioned peptides indicate that the inhibitory feedback action of glucocorticoids in the anterior pituitary gland is exerted mainly, if not exclusively, on the formation of the 31 K precursor rather than on the biosynthesis or activity of the proteolytic enzymes involved in its processing.

ACKNOWLEDGEMENTS

This work was supported by grants from INSERM (contrat 58-78-90) and from the Medical Research Council of Canada.

We are indebted to Dr D. Coy (Veterans Administration Hospital, New-Orleans) Dr N. Ling (Salk Institute, San Diego) Drs P.A. Desaulles and W. Rittel (Ciba-Geigy, Basel) for their most generous gift of synthetic ACTH and β-endorphin and other short chain analogues.

The authors thank C. Delarue, F. Leboulenger, J. Lecourt and P. Leroux for skillful technical assistance.

S. Jegou and M.C. Tonon were recipient of DGRST Graduate Fellowship.

REFERENCES

1. Abe, K., Nicholson, W.E., Liddle, G.W., Orth, D.N. and Island, D.P. (1969) J. Clin. Invest., 48, 1580-1585.
2. Sawin, C.T., Abe, K. and Orth, D.N. (1970) Arch. Intern. Med., 125, 708.
3. Kastin, A.J., Beach, G.D., Hawley, W.D., Kendall, J.W., Edwards, M.S. and Schally, A.V. (1973) J. Clin. Endocrinol. Metab., 36, 770.
4. Donald, R.A. and Toth, A. (1973) J. Clin. Endocrinol. Metab., 36, 925-930.
5. Kastin, A.J., Hawley, W.D., Miller, M.C. and Schally, A.V. (1974) Endocrinol. Exp., 8, 97.
6. Hirata, Y., Matsukura, S., Imura, H., Nakamura, M. and Tanaka, A. (1976) J. Clin. Endocrinol. Metab., 42, 33-40.
7. Tanaka, K., Nicholson, W.E. and Orth, D.N. (1978) J. Clin. Endocrinol. Metab., 46, 883-890.
8. Guillemin, R., Vargo, T., Rossier, J., Minick, S., Ling, N., Rivier, C., Vale, W. and Bloom, F. (1977) Science, 197, 1367-1369.
9. Roberts, J.L. and Herbert, E. (1977) Proc. Natl. Acad. Sci.USA, 74, 5300-5304.
10. Roberts, J.L. and Herbert, E. (1977) Proc. Natl. Acad. Sci. USA, 74, 4826-4830.
11. Mains, R.E., Eipper, B.A. and Ling, N. (1977) Proc. Natl. Acad. Sci. USA, 74, 3014-3018.
12. Rubinstein, M. Stein, S. and Udenfriend, S. (1978) Proc. Natl. Acad. Sci. USA, 75, 669-671.
13. Eipper, B.A. and Mains, R.E. (1978) J. Biol. Chem., 253, 5732-5744.
14. Dubois, P., Varques-Regairas, H. and Dubois, M. (1973) Z. Zellforsh. 145, 131-143.
15. Moriarty, G. (1973) J. Histochem. Cytochem, 21, 855-894.
16. Phifer, R.F., Orth, D.N. and Spicer, S. (1974) J. Clin. Endocrinol. Metab, 39, 684-692.
17. Pelletier, G., Leclerc, R., Labrie, F., Cote, J., Chretien, M. and Lis, M. (1977) Endocrinology, 100, 770-776.
18. Tramu, G. and Beauvillain, J.C. (1978) "Biochemical endocrinology : Synthesis and release of adenohypophyseal hormones, cellular and molecular mechanisms "Plenum New-York Mc Kerns & M. Jutisz eds, in press.

19. Nakanishi, S., Inouc, A., Kita, T., Nakamura, M., Chang, A.C.Y., Cohen, S.N. and Numa, S. (1979) Nature, 278,423-427.
20. Gráf, L. and Kenessey, A. (1976) Febs Letters, 69, 255-260.
21. Gráf, L., Kenessey, Ā. , Berzétei, I. and Rónai, A.Z. (1977) Biochem. Biophys. Res. Commun, 78, 1114-1123.
22. Boucher, R., Demassieux, S., Garcia, P. and Genest, J. (1977) Circ. Res., 41, 26-29.
23. Seidah, N.G., Chan, J.S.D., Martini, G., Benjannet, S., Chretien, M., Boucher, R. and Genest, J. (1979) Biochem. Biophys. Res. Commun, 86, 1002-1013.
24. Austen, B.M., Smyth, D.G. and Snell, C.R. (1977) Nature, 269, 619-621.
25. Allen, R., Herbert, E., Hinman, M., Shibuya, H. and Pert, C.B. (1978) Proc. Natl. Acad. Sci. USA, 75, 4972-4976.
26. Vale, W., Rivier, C., Yang, L., Minick, S. and Guillemin, R. (1978) Endocrinology, 103, 1910-1915.
27. Raymond, V., Lépine, J., Lissitsky, J.C., Côte, J. and Labrie, F. (1979) Mol. Cell. Endocrinol., in press.
28. Crine, P., Gianoulakis, C., Seidah, N.G., Gossard, F., Pezalla, P.D., Lis, M. and Chretien, M. (1978) Proc. Natl. Acad. Sci. USA, 75, 4719-4723.
29.Eipper, B. and Mains, R.E. (1978) Journal of Supramolecular Structure, 8, 247-262.
30.Lissitsky, J.C., Morin, O., Dupont, A., Labrie, F., Seidah, N.G., Chretien, M., Lis, M. and Coy, D.H. (1978) Life Sci., 22, 1715-1722.
31.Lissitsky, J.C., Lépine, J., Raymond, V., Dupont, A., Côte, J. and Labrie, F. (1978) Endocrinology, in press.
32. Vaudry, H., Tonon, M.C., Delarue, C., Vaillant, R. and Kraicer, J. (1978) Neuroendocrinology, 27, 9-24.
33. Dubé, D., Lissitsky, J.C., Leclerc, R., Pelletier, G. (1978) Endocrinology, 102, 1283-1291.
34. Orth, D.N. (1974) Jaffe and Behrman "Methods of Hormone Radioimmunoassay" Academic Press, New-York.
35. Vaudry, H., Vague, P., Dupont, W., Leboulenger, F. and Vaillant, R. (1975) Gen. Comp. Endocr., 25, 313-322.
36. Donnadieu, M. and Servaux, D. (1973) Biomedicine, 19, 272-274.
37. Jegou, S., Tonon, M.C., Leboulenger, F., Delarue, C. and Vaudry, H. (1978) Biochem. Biophys. Res. Commun, 83, 201-208.
38. Rodbard, D. and Lewald, J.E. (1970) 2nd Karolinska Symposium on Research Methods in Reproductive Endocrinology, Geneva, Diczfaluzy, E. ed, 79-103.

Radioimmunology 1979, Ch. A. Bizollon, editor.

METHIONINE ENKEPHALIN AND RELATED SUBSTANCES WITHIN CHICKEN EMBRYO RETINA.

Jeanne HUMBERT, Philippe PRADELLES and Fernand DRAY
INSERM FRA n° 8, Unite de Radioimmunologie Analytique, Institut Pasteur,
28 Rue du Dr. Roux, 75724 PARIS Cedex 15.

INTRODUCTION

The last several years have seen an increase in the evidence for a functional role of opioid peptides such as methionine-enkephalin (met-ENK) in neural processes [1]. The vertebrate retina is a typical example of a system rich in interconnections which analyses and integrates physiological stimuli; however, our knowledge of its neurotransmitters and neuromodulators remains fragmentary[2].

We have previously reported a major decrease in met-ENK and substance P-like material in the amygdaloid and striatal structures of rats subsequent to visual deprivation either by enucleation or darkness[3]. Although stereospecific binding of etorphin has been demonstrated in rat retina[4], the probable existence of enkephalins, generally associated with the opiate receptors[5], has not been investigated. We have thus undertaken an immunologic study of retinal neuropeptides and we here report results showing the presence of met-ENK and related molecules in the chicken embryo retina.

MATERIALS AND METHODS

Sampling and extraction procedures. Eyes of chicken embryos (13 days old) were quickly excised and transferred into ice-cold saline (NaCl 0.15 M) to limit enkephalin degradation during the dissection of neural retina. Tissues were then disrupted with an ultrasonic probe in the presence of 0.1 N HCl, and aliquots were taken for protein determination as described by Löwry et al.[6], using bovine serum albumin as standard. Acid homogenates were heated to 95°C for 15 min.,buffered and centrifugated. Enkephalins were recovered in the clear supernatant.

Radioimmunoassay. A highly sensitive radioimmunoassay (RIA) for met-ENK has been previously described[7]. Briefly : radioiodination of met-ENK at the tyrosyl residue was performed according to the method of Hunter et al.[8] using chloramine T. ^{125}I-monoiodo-met-ENK (2000 Ci/mmole) was first purified by thin-layer chromatography on Silica gel (nBuOH, HOAc, H_2O / 4:1:1; Rf = 0.38) and was then extracted with a methanol-water solution (v/v).

For rabbit immunisations, met-ENK was conjugated to ovalbumin using carbodiimide. The antiserum showing the best binding parameters (40% binding at the 1:6000 final dilution) and the hightest sensitivity (IC_{50} = 0.6 nM, lowest detection limit = 10 pg per tube) was selected. Although this antiserum showed significant cross-reactivity with leu-ENK (7%), cross-reactivity with either the C- or N-terminal fragments of enkephalins as well as with α- or β-endorphin was negligible (less than 0.1%) suggesting that C-terminal residues are involved in the binding by the antibodies. Ovalbumin did not crossreact.

Chromatography. High performance liquid chromatography (HPLC) was performed on a μBondapak C_{18} column (0.7 x 30 cm, Waters Instruments) using a MeOH, H_2O, NaAc (55:40:5, pH 4) mobile phase. The retinal extracts were also fractionated on a Sephadex G 50 column (1.76 x 73 cm) equilibrated in NH_4CO_3 0.5 M, pH 8.5. Radioimmunoassay for met-ENK was carried out for each of the eluted fractions.

RESULTS

The retina extracts inhibit binding of ^{125}I met-ENK to the specific antibodies. Response curves obtained with increasing dilutions (up to 1/32) closely parallel that of the standard (figure 1 A). Substracting for leu-ENK cross-reactivity (leu-ENK has been previously shown in the chicken embryo retina[9]) 600 ± 100 pg of met-ENK equivalent were found per mg protein (6 experiments, n=84 retina). This level was dramatically altered after cyanogen bromide treatment, without modification in the leu-ENK content, or by incubation of the homogenized retina at 37°C before acidification (half-life of approximatively one minute).

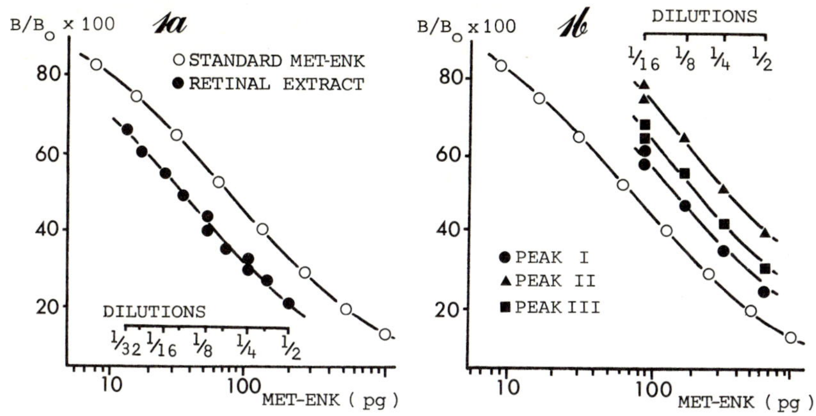

FIGURE 1 Binding of ^{125}Imet-ENK to specific antibodies in the presence of unlabelled met-ENK (open symbols) or biological extracts (closed symbols) *a*: Crude extract assay *b*: Assays of G 50 peaks (as defined by fig. 2A)

The performance of the C_{18} column with our experimental conditions (pressure = 1000 psi, flowrate = 0.5 ml/min.) was defined by the retention time for various peptides : TRH = 5.5 to 6 min., leu-ENK = 9 to 9.5 min., and met-ENK = 7.5 to 8 min. For injection, the retinal extracts were lyophilized before being dissolved in the mobile phase. RIAs showed a single sharp peak eluting in 7.5 to 8 min., to be the true met-ENK. A major loss of total antigenic retinal material was seen.

Crude extracts were chromatographed on a Sephadex G_{50} column. At least three eluted peaks were able to displace ^{125}I met-ENK binding to specific antibodies. The apparent molecular weight were : for peak I (eluted with the void volume) up to 30,000, for peak II, 5,000 to 3,000, and for peak III, 500 to 300 (fig. 2A). Dose-response curves for each of these peak remained closely parallel to the standard curve (fig. 1B).

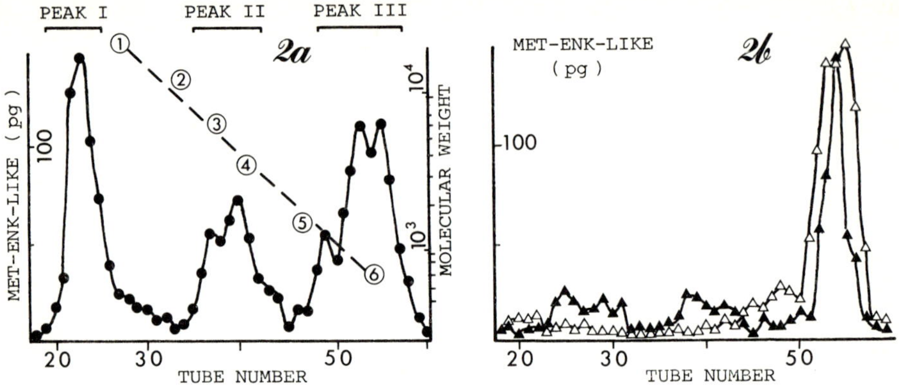

FIGURE 2 G 50 CHROMATOGRAPHY. Calibration (– –) : ① Human Growth Hormon ② Cytochrom C ③ Aprotinin ④ ^{125}I-β-Endorphin ⑤ Actinomycin ⑥ ^{125}I-monoiodo-met-ENK. Met-ENK immunoreactivity (—) : *a* Retinal extract elution *b* Monkey retina (▲) and Chicken brain (△) extracts elutions.

DISCUSSION AND CONCLUSION

Our data strongly suggest that one fraction of the retinal extracts posesses some characteristics of authentic met-ENK :

i) similar dose-response parameters in the RIAs,

ii) identical retention time in HPLC, and

iii) same molecular weight as shown by gel filtration (peak III).

The high sensitivity to cyanogen bromide treatment and the short half-life of the antigenic molecules, as preliminary observed, are in good agreement with the specificity of our antiserum and with other reports[10,11]. Although unambiguous identification, by isolation and structural analysis, has not been performed, we may assume that the retina contains true met-ENK, this being consistent with the presence of opiate receptors within the retina[4].

Sephadex G50 chromatography reveals high molecular weight substances able to inhibit the binding of labelled tracer to anti met-ENK antibodies, with the same affinity as the standard. The extraction and chromatographic procedures could produce some unrelated substances which interfere with the RIA, or induce the molecular aggregation of peak III into larger molecules. However, gel filtration of met-ENK rich extracts of either embryonic chicken brain or monkey retina did not show such a complex elution pattern, but rather a single peak III (fig. 2B). Retinal peaks II and I could have the met-ENK antigenic determinants on a longer sequence, suggesting the existence of a met-ENK embryonic retinal precursor.

In conclusion, we have attempted to show that RIA requires validation by further analysis. We are currently using these techniques for the study of the substance P, which is often associated with enkephalins in the central nervous system[12]. Some positive preliminary results encourage us in the belief that the retina will be a fruitful tool in the study of the functional interaction of neuropeptides.

REFERENCES

1. Barker, J.L., Neale, J.H., Smith, T.G. and Mac Donald, R.L. (1978) Science, 199, 1451-1453.
2. Rodieck, R.W. (1973) The vertebrate retina, Freeman W.H. Ed. pp.514-525.
3. Pradelles, P., Gros, C., Humbert, J., Le Gal La Salle, G. and Ben-Ari, Y. (1979) Brain Res. 166, 192-194.
4. Medzihradsky, F. (1976) Brain Res., 108, 212-219.
5. Snyder, S.H. and Simantov, R. (1977) J. Neurochem., 28, 13-20.
6. Löwry, O.H., Rosenbrough, N.H., Farr, A.L. and Randall, R.J. (1951) J. Biol. Chem., 193, 265-275.
7. Gros, C., Pradelles, P., Rougeot, C., Bepoldin, O., Dray, F., Fournie-Zaluski, M.C., Roques, B.P., Pollard, H., Llorens-cortes, C. and Schwartz, J.C. (1978) J. Neurochem., 31, 29-39.
8. Hunter, W. and Greenwood, F. (1964) J. Biochem., 91, 43-55.
9. Humbert, J., Pradelles, P., Gros, C. and Dray, F. Neuroscience letters to be publish ed.
10. Simantov, R., Childers, R.S. and Snyder, H.S. (1977) Brain Res., 135, 358-367.
11. Hughes, J. (1975) Brain Res., 88, 295-308.
12. Hökfelt, T., Ljungdahl, A., Terenius, L., Elde, R. and Nilsson, G. (1977) Proc. Nat. Acad. Sci., 74, 3081-3985.

THYROID HORMONES

Radioimmunology 1979, Ch. A. Bizollon, editor.

MEASUREMENT OF SERUM THYROID HORMONES AND THYROGLOBULIN BY RADIOIMMUNOASSAY TECHNIQUES

INDER J. CHOPRA, M.D.
Department of Medicine UCLA Center for the Health Sciences, Los Angeles, California, U.S.A.

INTRODUCTION

Application of radioimmunoassay (RIA) techniques to study of endocrine pathophysiology began in 1960 when Berson and Yalow developed a RIA for study of insulin concentration in biological fluids[1] . Odell et al were among the first to apply a RIA for thyroid related studies in 1964-65 when they employed TSH RIA in the study of the pituitary-thyroid axis[2] . However, it was not until 1970-71 that RIAs were used for study of thyroid hormone physiology[3-8] . This delay appears related to two factors : i) the classical belief that iodothyronines, which are characterized by their small molecular weight, are non-antigenic[9] ; and ii) reasonably convenient and sensitive competitive protein binding assay (CPBA) had become available for study of at least one of the two thyroid hormones, i.e., T_4[10] and attempts were underway to use CPBA for study of the role of T_3 in thyroid hormone economy as well[11]. Several groups were, however, not quite satisfied by the then available competitive binding methods for study of T_3 concentration in plasma. Requirement of large volumes of sample, and methodological artifacts were some matters of concern[12, 13]. Additionally, the procedure was so time consuming that it could take almost 6 full days to get data on T_3 concentration in 6 sera[14] . Studies in 1970 by Brown, Ekins and their coworkers and by Gharib et al[3, 4] revealed that it is feasible to produce T_3 binding antisera by immunization of rabbits with conjugates of T_3 with bovine or human serum albumin. We approached the situation by depending more on nature's ability rather than our own to produce conjugates of T_3 with a larger protein. We immunized rabbits with crude human or bovine thyroglobulin which holds T_3 and T_4 in a natural covalent linkage . It was interesting that serum of rabbits so immunized contained antibodies which could bind quite specifically T_3 , T_4 as well as thyroglobulin[5] . These studies indicated quite clearly that at least 3 different populations of antibodies can be produced when rabbits are immunized with thyroglobulin : one that binds T_3 specifically, another that binds T_4 specifically and yet another that binds thyroglobulin specifically. It seemed possible then to develop three different RIAs using the serum of a rabbit immunized with thyroglobulin. This possibility has actually been verified in subsequent studies[5-8, 15, 16].

Even though specific antibodies had become available, RIAs of thyroid hormones in 1970-71 [3,5,6] were still relatively cumbersome because of the need for extraction of the iodothyronines from serum prior to quantitation. This had to be done because of an unusual difficulty in RIA of thyroid hormones which was not experienced in then well-known RIAs of polypeptide hormones. It related to a very avid binding of thyroid hormones to a transport protein in serum, i.e., thyronine binding globulin (TBG). TBG interferes in RIA of thyroid hormones in two ways[15] : i) it competes with the antibody for the radioactive ligand and ii) it does not release T_4 and T_3 in serum for reaction with the antibody. These problems have now been essentially solved by recognition and use of several compounds, e.g., 8-anilino-1-naphtalene sulfonic acid (ANS), sodium salicylate, dilantin[7,8, 17-19].

T_4 RADIOIMMUNOASSAY

The basic principle of T_4RIA is similar to that of other RIA's in that it compares the ability of standards and unknowns to compete with radioactive T_4 for binding sites on a T_4-binding antiserum. The simple steps required for performance of a T_4RIA[7] are as follows :

The various reagents are added in 10 x 75 mm glass tubes in the following order : i) 0.075 M barbital buffer containing 2 % normal rabbit serum, 150 µg of ANS and about 10,000 counts per min of ^{125}I-T_4 (S.A. - 100 mCi/mg or greater), 385 µl. ii) Standards (0.5 to 40 µg T_4/100 ml of charcoal (or resin) treated, T_4-free, human serum) and unknows, 15 µl. iii) 100 µl of a diluted T_4-binding rabbit antiserum known to bind about 30-40 % of added 125 I-T_4. The tubes are incubated at room temperature for 1 hr and at 4 C for 5 min and goat anti-rabbit gamma globulin (second antibody) is added to separate bound from free radioactivity. The per cent bound radioactivity in the standards is plotted on the ordinate against their concentration (µg/100 ml) to plot a standard curve. The per cent bound radioactivity in the unknowns is then used to read their serum T_4 concentration from the standard curve. The T_4 RIA can usually measure T_4 accurately between concentrations of 1 and 40 µg/100 ml. This sensitivity and assay range allow accurate determination of T_4 in one attempt in most clinical situations of hypo-, eu- or hyperthyroidism[7].

In general there is a reasonable comparability of the results of T_4 RIA and GPBA of T_4. However, there are some drawbacks of CPBA compared to RIA. These include : 1. CPBA requires extraction of T_4 from serum and extraction efficiency of different batches of reagents can vary. 2. CPBA requires evaporation of serum extracts; evaporation is time-consuming. 3. The separation of bound from free radioactive T_4 in the final step of CPBA[10] requires precise timing of contact of reaction mixture with resin. 4. Sera with T_4 concentration < 3 and > 20 μg % require re-assay with CPBA for accurate determinations.

T_4 measurement is the most commonly employed test of thyroid function. Several studies using T_4RIA have shown that RIA allows in general a quite clear separation of hypo-and hyperthyroid patients from euthyroid subjects[7,19,20]. However, alterations in serum concentration of TBG exert an important influence on serum T_4 concentration . Thus, serum T_4 concentration is increased when TBG is increased and vice-versa. Serum concentration of TBG may be increased during estrogen administration, pregnancy or because of an x-linked inherited disorder of TBG synthesis. On the other hand, serum concentration of T_4 is reduced in euthyroid subjects when serum concentration of TBG is subnormal. Serum TBG concentration may be decreased in association with nephrotic syndrome,androgen treatment or an inherited disorder of TBG synthesis. When serum TBG is abnormal, appropriate interpretation of serum total T_4,as measured by RIA (or CPBA),requires either determination of free T_4 using measurements of free fraction of T_4 (e.g., by equilibrium dialysis) or assessment of free T_4 index using T_3^- resin uptake. The latter approach is simpler, less expensive and, therefore, more popular than the former for clinical purposes.

Recently, abnormalities in serum T_4 concentration in non-thyroidal systemic illnesses have attracted considerable attention. Thus, while serum T_4 is within the normal range in the majority of patients with nonthyroidal illness, some cases demonstrate low as well as high values[21,22].Additionally, when agents such as gall bladder dyes have been administered,serum T_4 may be elevated in absence of hyperthyroidism. This increase apparently reflects a decrease in metabolism of T_4 caused by gall bladder dyes[23,24].

Key advantages of the T_4 RIA include its exquisite sensitivity, allowing T_4 measurements in all states of thyroid function using only 10-25 μl of unextracted serum and its remarkable simplicity rendering it suitable for processing of large numbers of samples in a short period of time and for automation.These special advantages of T_4 RIA have been best utilized in programs for screening of newborns for hypothyroidism using only a few μl of blood, transported dry on a filter paper to the laboratory.Based on studies of over 200,000 newborns, Dr. Dussault and co-workers have reported an incidence of neonatal hypothyroidism of 1 in 6000 live births in Quebec[25];studies in other areas of North America have supported this fining[26,27].It turns out that this incidence of neonatal hypothyroidism is nearly 2-2 1/2 time that of phenylketonuria, which like hypothyroidism, is a potential cause for mental deficiency and for which routine screening of the newborns is mandatory in several countries.

RIA of T_4 has also been considered useful in the diagnosis of thyroid functional status in individuals receiving treatment with exogenous T_3[28]. Thus, Duick et al observed that while serum T_4 is suppressed clearly in euthyroid individuals receiving 100 μg/day of T_3 for 28 days, its concentration is usually over 2 μg/100 ml. Interestingly, however, serum T_4 of hypothyroid patients as a group was significantly less than in euthyroid controls. This suggested that with a sensitive T_4-RIA at hand it may not be necessary for patients to go off thyroid replacement for determination of their thyroid function status.

T_3 RADIOIMMUNOASSAY

T_3 is present in serum in quantities much smaller, 1/70 or so that of T_4. However, its significance in overall calorigenic effect of thyroid hormones is heightened by its greater biological potency. Some have proposed that T_3 may be the sole thyroactive material and the biological effect of T_4 may be mostly due to its *in vivo* conversion to T_3.

Until 1971 the popular technique for quantitating serum T_3 was the one devised by Sterling and co-workers[11]. It consisted of three steps: 1) extraction of thyroid hormones from 5 to 10 ml serum by column chromatography using Dowex AG 50 W-X_2 (H^+ form). 2) T_3 was then separated from T_4 by descending paper chromatography. 3) In the final step, T_3 was quantitated by a sensitive CPBA using human serum TBG. The mean serum T_3 by this method was 200 ng/100 ml. However, several investigators observed that despite adequate precautions, paper chromatography may be associated with two problems, one of which is incomplete separation of T_4 from T_3 while the other is an *in vitro* deiodination of T_4 to T_3 during chromatography[12,13]. These difficulties appeared to lead to a falsely high estimate of serum T_3 by CPBA and served to stimulate research on development of RIA methods for measurement of T_3. Several RIA procedures are now available which can measure T_3 quite accurately using only 20 to 400 μl of unextracted serum. The basic principle of many of these RIAs is similar in that they employ an agent which can displace T_3 from TBG, but which does not appreciably interfere with antibody binding of T_3. The various compounds used include T_4, tetrachlorthyronine, dilantin, salicylate and ANS[8, 15,17,18,29]. Some T_3RIA have employed extracts of sera[3,30] while still others have attempted to inactivate TBG e.g. by heat treatment[31]. T_3 binding antisera have been obtained by immunization of rabbits with conjugates of T_3 with human or bovine serum albumine or thyroglobulin. Cross reaction of T_4 with T_3 antibodies used in most published T_3RIAs has been 0,1 % or less

Normal serum T_3 by RIA used in our laboratory[8] ranges between 50 and 200 ng/100 ml. Serum T_3 is elevated in nearly all cases with Graves' hyperthyroidism unless serum TBG is low or another systemic illness complicates hypothyroidism. Overall experience indicates that serum T_3 measurement may be the single most sensitive test for the diagnosis of hyperthyroidism. Sterling and coworkers first described the existence of a syndrome of clinical hyperthyroidism associated with normal T_4 in which hyperthyroidism is attributable to elevated serum T_3. They have termed this syndrome as T_3-thyrotoxicosis[32]. On the basis of studies using T_3RIAs it has been estimated that 5-10 % hyperthyroid patients in iodine-sufficient areas may manifest T_3-thyrotoxicosis at the time of their first presentation.

Serum T_3 measurement has not proved to be a good test for diagnosis of hypothyroidism. About 20 % of clinically hypothyroid patients have serum T_3 concentrations which fall within the normal range[33] . On the basis of the findings indicating that some 1/3 of T_4 produced daily in normal man may be converted to T_3 and that T_3 is 3-4 times as potent as T_4, it has been proposed that T_3 may be the sole biologically active thyroid hormone and that T_4 functions merely as a prohormone for T_3. However, the finding of normal T_3 in several clinically hypothyroid cases questions this thesis. The data actually suggest that the hypothyroid patients with normal total and also free T_3[33] are hypometabolic because they lack in their circulation adequate amounts of the other thyroactive substance i.e. T_4.

Importance of T_4 as a hormone is underscored also by recognition in recent years a number of situations (v.i.) in clinically euthyroid individuals where serum total or free T_3 is markedly decreased but serum T_4 is normal and free T_4 is normal or high [34-37]. These situations have been collectively referred to as low T_3 syndrome. T_3 syndrome may be seen in normal fetus and newborn, a variety of systemic illnesses including liver and kidney failure, febrile illnesses and malignancy , caloric deprivation states including fasting, protein-calorie malnutrition and anorexia nervosa, burns , major surgical operation and during administration of several drugs. Serum TSH is typically normal in patients with low T_3 syndrome but is moderately elevated in some cases[35, 36]. Additionnally, when we studied OKd interval, it was normal or reduced , the latter finding would be consistent with some degree of hyperthyroidism[34]. However the test may be influenced by factors other than circulating thyroid hormone levels. It is evident, however, that the laboratory data do not offer any support to the possibility of hypothyroidism in nonthyroid illnesses. It seems possible that patients with low T_3 syndrome remain euthyroid despite very low total or free T_3 because serum concentration of free T_4 is normal or high and may compensate for the decrease in serum free T_3 concentration.

REVERSE T_3 RADIOIMMUNOASSAY

RIA methods have been important to the understanding of thyroid physiology and pathophysiology pertaining not only to the conventional thyroid hormones, T_4 and T_3, but also to other iodothyronines, such as reverse T_3 (rT_3) and various diiodothyronines, (T_2s)[38, 39]. Reverse T_3 was first considered to be present in rat thyroglobulin and serum by Roche et al in 1956[40]. However, its presence in human serum was considered unlikely. Similarly, Roche et al had described the presence of 3,3'-T_2 in circulation of the rat in 1956 and Flock et al made this observation in the dog in 1960[41]. However, since sensitive methods for precise quantitation were not available and since it did not appear likely that T_2 will be present in human circulation, the interest in this compound was very limited. Recent demonstration by RIAs that rT_3 as well as several T_2's are normal components of human circulation and that important changes occur in their serum concentration in the thyroid and systemic disease and during administration of some drugs has stimulated new interest in the role of these iodothyronines in thyroid hormone physiology[37]. It is clear that rT_3 and T_2 are both very weak, essentially inert, in calorigenesis or suppression of TSH. However, the questions now being raised ask whether these and other iodothyronines are involved in important functions other than calorigenesis or TSH suppression. Research on these and related matters should broaden our perspective on the biological purposes to iodothyronines.

Normal serum rT_3 in our laboratory averages around 40 ng/100 ml with a range of 20-60 ng/100 ml. Reverse T_3 is increased in hyper- and decreased in hypothyroidism. Serum rT_3 is increased moderately when TBG concentration is increased as in normal pregnancy. Reverse T_3 is detected consistently in serum of hypothyroid patients receiving replacement treatment with synthetic T_4. Interestingly, serum rT_3 in these individuals is similar to or sometimes even higher than in normal individuals. This indicates that peripheral metabolism of T_4 must be an important source of rT_3[37, 38].

Perhaps the most interesting information obtained with regard to rT_3 is that its serum concentration is increased in a number of situations (low T_3 syndrome, v.s.) where there is a selective deficiency of T_3 in serum and serum T_4 is normal. This is true in the case of the normal fetus and the newborn, in calorie deprivation states, and in a variety of systemic illnesses and after administration of drugs like dexamethasone, radiocontrast agents used for cholecystography, amiodarone (an antianginal agent), propanolol and propylthiouracil[36, 37]

While there are reasonably clear changes in serum rT_3 in states of thyroid dysfunction, measurement of rT_3 is not proposed as a routine test for diagnosis of thyroid disease. Measurement of serum T_3 and T_4 for diagnosis of hyperthyroidism and of serum T_4 and TSH for diagnosis of hypothyroidism would be more helpful and practical than measurement of rT_3. Measurement of rT_3 may aid the diagnosis of hypothyroidism in the presence of a systemic illness, however. Thus, when serum T_3 is low and serum T_4 low or low normal in a patient with a systemic (nonthyroidal) illness, findings of a high or high normal serum rT_3 and normal TSH would favor the diagnosis of euthyroidism whereas findings of low or low normal serum rT_3 and high TSH would suggest associated hypothyroidism[21].

The finding that serum rT_3 is characteristically elevated in the term fetus prompted a study of rT_3 in amniotic fluid. The data indicated that rT_3 concentration is very high in amniotic fluid as early as 15-20 wk of gestation and decreases gradually thereafter[42]. The mean amniotic fluid rT_3 value at 15-20 wk gestation was approximately 5 fold that in maternal serum while the mean value in term amniotic fluid was approximately one and one half times that in maternal serum. These data have raised a possibility that measurement of amniotic fluid rT_3 may assist in prenatal diagnosis of thyroid dysfunction, especially hypothyroidism.

THYROGLOBULIN (Tg) RADIOIMMUNOASSAY

Beside study of iodothyronines, RIA methods have also been applied to study of another thyroidal product namely, thyroglobulin. Thyroglobulin was once considered to be a secluded thyroidal antigen that does not enter circulation. However, studies from several laboratories have indicated that Tg is indeed a normal component of human serum and that its serum concentration is increased in hyperthyroidism and in subacute thyroiditis. Studies have also documented an increase in serum Tg after TSH administration and a decrease in its levels after administration of replacement doses of thyroid hormones to euthyroid subjects[43, 44].

Among the most interesting aspect of studies with thyroglobulin RIA has been the observation that serum Tg levels are increased in patients with thyroid cancers and that the increase is more marked in patients with metastatic carcinoma than in those with localized disease[45]. Some data have questioned the specificity elevated serum Tg levels in diagnosis of thyroid cancer. However, measurement of serum Tg is undoubtedly quite useful as a marker of tumor load in follow up of patients receiving treatment for thyroid cancer. Serum Tg levels fall precipitously when tumor is removed surgically and increase subsequently when ther is reccurrence of the disease[45]. Additionally, in preliminary studies, Drs. Uller and Van Herle have observed that serum Tg levels might be of assistance in predicting remission in Graves' disease patients receiving treatment with antithyroid drugs. They found persistence of very high levels of serum Tg in patients who relapsed after a course of antithyroid drugs whereas serum Tg level was normal or only modestly elevated in patients who stayed in remission following a course of drug treatment[46]. Further studies are needed to substantiate and strengthen these interesting observations.

ACKNOWLEDGEMENTS

Supported in part by USPHS Grants AM 16155 and AM 17251 from the National Institute of Health, Bethesda, Maryland.

REFERENCES

1. Berson, S.A. and R.S. Yalow (1960) J. Clin. Invest.,39 , 1157.
2. Odell, W.D., Wilbur J.F. and Paul W.E. (1965) J. Clin. Endocrinol. Metab., 25, 1179.
3. Brown, B.L., Ekins R.P. , Ellis S.M. and Reith W.S. (1971) Further Advances in Thyroid Research,2, 1107.
4. Gharib , H., Mayberry W.E. and Ryan R.J. (1970) J. Clin. Endocrinol. Metab., 31, 709.
5. Chopra, I.J., Nelson J.C., Solomon , D.H. and Beall G.N. (1971) J. Clin. Endocrinol. Metab.,32, 299.
6. Chopra, I.J., Solomon, D.H. and Ho R.S. (1971) J. Clin. Endocrinol. Metab., 33, 865.
7. Chopra, I.J. (1972) J. Clin. Endocrinol. Metab.,34, 938.
8. Chopra , I.J., Ho , R.S., Lam R. (1972) J. Lab. Clin. Med.,80, 729.
9. Murphy, B.E.P. (1971) in Principles of Competitive Protein Binding Assays (Odell W.D. and Daughaday W.H., eds), J.B. Lippincott Company, Philadelphia p. 108.
10. Murphy, B.E.P. and Pattee C.J. (1964) J. Clin. Endocrinol. Metab.,24, 187.
11. Sterling , K., Brenner D., Newman E.S. and Brenner M.A. (1969) J. Clin. Invest.,48, 1150.
12. Larsen, P.R. (1971) Metabolism,20, 976.
13. Fisher , D.A., and Dussault J.H. (1971) J. Clin. Endocrinol. Metab.,32,675.
14. Dussault, J.H., Lam , R. and Fisher D.A. (1971) J. Lab. Clin. Med .,77, 1039
15. Chopra, I.J., Solomon, D.H., Beall, G.N. (1971) J. Clin. Invest.,50, 2033.
16. Williams, D.E., Chopra, I.J., Orgiazzi, J. and Solomon, D.H. (1975) J. Clin. Endocrinol. Metab., 41, 354.
17. Larsen, P.R. (1971) J. Clin. Invest., 51, 1939.

18. Lieblich, J.M. and Utiger, R.D. (1972) J. Clin. Invest. 51, 157.

19. Larsen , P.R., Dockalova, J., Sipula, D., and Wu , F.M. (1973) J. Clin. Endocrinol. Metab., 37, 177.

20. Chopra, I. J., and Solomon , D.H. (1976) Pharmac. Therap.C., 1, 367

21. Chopra, I.J., Solomon, D.H., Hepner , G.W. and Morgenstein, A. (in Press) Ann. Intern. Med.

22. Birkhauser, M., Busset, R., Burer, R. and Burger A. (1977) Lancet, 2, 53.

23. Burgi, H. , Wimpfheimer , C., Burger , A., Zaunbauer, W., Rosler , H. and Lemarchand-Beraud, T. (1976) J. Clin. Endocrinol. Metab., 43, 1203.

24. Wu, S.Y., Chopra, I.J., Solomon, D.H. and Bennett , L.R. (1978) J. Clin. Endocrinol. Metab., 46, 691.

25. Dussault, J.H., Coulombe , P. and Laberge, C. (1975) J. Pediatrics,86,670.

26. Foley, T.P., Klein, A.H., Augustin, A.U. and Hopwood , J. (1975) in Perinatal Thyroid Physiology and Disease (D.A. Fisher and G.N. Burrow,eds), p. 255, New York.

27. Walfish, P. (1976) Lancet, 1, 1208.

28. Duick, D.S., Stein , R.B., Warren , D.W. and Nicoloff, J.T. (1975) J. Clin. Endocrinol. Metab., 41, 229.

29. Mitsuma, J., Nihei ,N., Gershengorn, M.C. and Hollander C.S. (1971) J.Clin. Invest., 50, 2679.

30. Patel, Y.C., Burger, H.G., Morley, D. and Havlik, H. (1973) J. Clin. Endocrinol. Metab.,36, 187.

31. Sterling, K. and Milch, P.O. (1974) J. Clin. Endocrinol. Metab.,38, 866.

32. Sterling, K., Refetoff, S. and Selenkow, H.A. (1970), J. Amer. Med. Assoc., 213, 571.

33. Chopra, I.J., Solomon, D.H. and Chua Teco, G.N. (1973) J. Clin. Endocrinol. Metab.,36, 1050.

34. Reichlin, S., Bollinger, B.A., Nejad, I. and Sullivan, P. (1973) Mt Sinai Med. J. , 40, 502.

35. Chopra, I.J., Solomon , D.H., Chopra, U., Young, R.T. and Chua Teco, G.N. (1974) J. Clin. Endocrinol. Metab.,39, 501.

36. Chopra, I.J., Chopra,U., Smith, S.R., Reza, M. and Solomon, D.H. (1975) J. Clin. Endocrinol. Metab.,41, 1043.

37. Chopra, I.J., Solomon, D.H., Chopra, U., Wu, S.Y., Fisher, D.A. and Nakamura, Y. (1978) Recent Progr. Horm. Res.,34, 521.

38. Chopra, I.J. (1974) J. Clin. Invest.,54, 583.

39. Wu, S.Y., Chopra, I.J., Nakamura, Y., Solomon, D.H. and Bennet L.R. (1976) J. Clin. Endocrinol.,43, 682.

40. Roche, J., Michel, R., Etling, N. and Nunez, J. (1956) Biochim. Biophys. Acta , 22, 550.

41. Flock, E.U., Bollman, J.L., Grindlay, J.H. and Stoble,G.H.(1961) Endocrinology 69, 626.

42. Chopra, I.J. and Crandall , B.F. (1975) N.Eng. J. Med. 293, 740.

43. Van Herle, A.J., Uller, R.P., Matthews, N.L. and Brown , J. (1973) J. Clin. Invest. 52, 1320.

44. Uller, R.P., Van Herle, A.J. and Chopra, I.J. (1973) J. Clin. Endocrinol. Metab. 37, 741.

45. Van Herle, A.J. and Uller, R.P. (1975) J. Clin. Invest. 56, 272.

46. Uller, R.P. and Van Herle A.J. (1978) J. Clin. Endocrinol. Metab. 46,747.

Radioimmunology 1979, Ch. A. Bizollon, editor.

NON-RADIOACTIVE METHODS FOR THE ASSAY OF THYRONINES, THYROID BINDING PROTEINS AND THYROGLOBULIN

DAVID BOYER RAMSDEN, DAVID NIGEL CROSSLEY, PAUL WILLETTS, WILLIAM ARTHUR BURR, DAVID BURNETT,* ARTHUR RANDELL BRADWELL* and RAYMOND HOFFENBERG
Department of Medicine, University of Birmingham, Birmingham, United Kingdom.

INTRODUCTION

The advent of radioimmunoassay as a measurement technique for compounds of interest in biological material has been a primary factor in developing our understanding of endocrine function and disease. This is exemplified in the thyroid field, where RIA has become the most widely used method for determining the concentration of the thyroid hormones, thyroxine (T4), and 3,3',5-triiodothyronine (T3); metabolites of these such as 3,3',5' - triiodothyronine (reverse T3) and 3,3' -diiodothyronine (split T2), and the most important serum binding protein, thyroxine binding globulin (TBG). As a technique it possesses considerable advantages. It is highly versatile, being applicable to compounds of any molecular weight provided a suitable antiserum can be raised. It is extremely sensitive by comparison with most other techniques, usually not more than a few picogrammes of sample compound being required per tube. Finally, its technical simplicity allows large numbers of samples to be assayed per day. Yet the method does suffer limitations which have to be allowed for or circumvented by the assay procedure.

1. RIA depends on the interaction of antiserum with one or more specific sites on the antigen, and measures compounds containing these sites regardless of the rest of the structure of the molecule. This recognition of determinant sites can give rise to serious cross-reactivity problems, when a molecule is being assayed in the presence of a second molecule in higher concentration possessing the same or a very similar site. An example of this is the cross-reactivity of T4 in the assay of reverse-T3, where the common structure is the β-ring of the thyronine skeleton. This problem was highlighted in a review of reverse-T3 assays by Premachandra[1]. The normal range from different laboratories using a single commercial source of highly purified reverse-T3 differed by as much as 100% among themselves. Although some of this variation could be accounted for by inter-laboratory differences common to all assays, the cross-reactivity of T4 in the assay may be a major feature.

2. RIA usually requires a constant source of pure antigen for radioactive

labelling. These radioactive antigens are particularly unstable, requiring frequent re-labelling of the compound. One ingenuous commercial approach to partially circumvent this, is that employed by Corning Inc. in their TBG assay. Here radioactive TBG is replaced by radioactive T4, which is much more readily prepared. TBG concentration is assayed by the ability of the sample to compete with a saturating dose of albumin for ^{125}I - T4 binding. However, this approach is itself restricted to a very few instances and only serves to highlight the problem.

THYRONINES

In light of the above, one of our major research objectives over the past few years has been the development of gas chromatographic-mass spectrometric (gcms) assays for thyroid hormones in biological samples. It was felt that this approach would obviate some of the objections which can be raised to competitive protein binding and RIA methods. The application of gcms to thyroid hormone assay is not without its difficulties and posed a variety of chemical and technological problems which we have overcome with varying degrees of success. These include extraction, derivative formation, gas chromatographic and mass spectrometric features which are illustrated in assays for two compounds, 3,3',5 5'-tetraiodothyroacetic acid (T4A)[2,3] and the product of the complete T4 deiodination i.e. thyronine (TO).

Internal Standard and Extraction

Most biological material is far from suitable to use directly in a gcms system, thus requiring the compound of interest to undergo some sort of extraction procedure. The objectives of this should be not only to yield as pure a sample as possible but also to achieve as high a yield as possible. In order to monitor this extraction an internal standard is added at the outset, posing a third requirement, that the sample and internal standard be extracted in an identical fashion. In the T4A assay human serum was the starting material and 3,3', 5,5'-tetraiodothyropropionic acid (T4P) was used as internal standard. The multistage extraction procedure, which was ultimately arrived at is tedious and demanding, and to verify it extraction of the two compounds had to be followed through every step using alternatively radioisotopically labelled materials (131-T4P and 125I-T4A) of high specific activity. The mean extraction efficiency for each step was in excess of 88 % and the difference in extraction of the two compounds in any one step was never greater than 1 %.

In the case of TO the starting material was urine. The ease of catalytic reduction of T4 in a deuterium environment enabled the preparation of a much more suitable internal standard. The deutero-TO thus prepared is chemically identical to the endogenous TO except for the small mass difference. Because urine is a slightly 'cleaner' material than serum, a less rigorous extraction procedure was adopted. The efficiency of this was checked by radio-gas chromatography using tritiated TO produced in a similar fashion to the deutero compound. Overall extraction and derivation efficiency was in excess of 60%.

Choice of Derivative

Neither the thyronines nor their acetic acid analogues possess the necessary volatility to make them suitable for gas chromatography. Therefore they need to be converted to more volatile derivatives. This involves blocking the polar functional groups at the two ends of the molecule. In addition to increased volatility, the derivative should possess suitable fragmentation characteristics in the mass spectrometer and stability to water to allow easy storage. In the case of T4A only a carboxylic acid and a phenolic hydroxyl group need to be blocked. A number of reagents singly or in combination are available for this purpose. At the outset of this work we investigated the use of four types of derivative:-

a) Di-Trimethylsilyl
b) O-Pivalyl methyl ester
c) O-Trimethylsilyl methyl ester
d) Dimethyl

Of these the dimethyl derivative, formed by reaction with diazomethane, appeared the most suitable. For a further discussion of these derivatives see Hoffenberg et al (1974)[4]. The dimethyl compound has the additional advantage that it is formed in a single step.

In the mass spectrum of dimethyl T4A the molecular ion ($^m/_e$ 776) is the base peak (most intense ion). The same is true for the molecular ion of dimethyl T4P ($^m/_e$ 790). This confers a still further advantage, since the majority of ions generated by other materials in the sample and by bleed from the gc column are of much lower mass: charge ratio, and consequently do not interfere with the detection of the specific ions referred to.

For TO there is an additional amino group which must be derivatised before successful gas chromatography can occur. In theory the four types of derivative mentioned for T4A may also be formed by TO. However, since TMS derivatives are inherently unstable[5] they were not seriously considered. Reaction with diazomethane resulted in uncontrolled overmethylation and was discounted. More controlled methylating reagents such as methyl-8 appeared not vigorous enough to effect full methylation. Difficulties were experienced with the reaction between pivalic anhydride and iodoamino acids, therefore, although this reagent may be suitable for TO, it was not investigated further. Two reports have outlined the use of heptafluorobutyricacid derivatives for the assay of free T4 and free T3, however, these derivatives were found to be unsuitable for the final step of the extraction procedure outlined here.[6,7]. Therefore, a series of derivatives based on the reaction between amino acids and dichlorotetrafluoro acetone (DCTFA) were investigated. This reaction converts the amino acid function to a substituted oxazolidinone[8]. Subsequent conversion of the phenolic hydroxyl to either the methyl ether or acetyl ester was carried out. Methylation with diazomethane again led to uncontrollable over reaction, but reaction with acetic anhydride gave as the single major product the O-acetyl ester (referred to as Acetyl DCTFA). Although this compound has a gc cut-off point of around 1ng/injection this proved adequate for assay purposes

The major ion in the mass spectrum of the acetyl DCTFA derivative of TO between m/e 50 and the molecular ion was at m/e 199, the tropyllium ion formed by cleavage between the α and β carbon atoms of the thyronine side chain (see reaction scheme 1). Unfortunately this proved susceptible to interference from other materials in the samples and therefore could not be monitored in the assay. The molecular ion was also unsuitable as it was not intense enough. Therefore the ion formed by loss of the acetyl group (m/e 453) was used. The equivalent ion for the internal standard was 3 mass units higher.

Non-Specific Adsorption

A third factor limiting the sensitivity of many gas chromatographic assays is the phenomenon of non-specific adsorption. This results in an abrupt stoppage in the passage of compound along the gc column below a given amount of sample injected, even though this would not be below the limit of sensitivity of the detection system. Both dimethyl T4A and the O-acetyl DCTFA derivative of TO have a pronounced tendency to be adsorbed. To minimise this, all-glass columns and transfer lines were used and these were heavily siliconised. Careful and extensive column conditioning was also necessary. With these precautions samples containing as little as 10pg T4A/injection may be assayed routinely. A transfer efficiency of 30% at the jet separator means that the mass spectrometer is detecting approximately 3pg T4A. For the TO derivative the gc cut-off point was approximately 1ng/injection. This limit was not amenable to further column conditioning.

Clinical Results

Using these assays preliminary investigations on the concentration of T4A in serum and of TO in urine have been made. In 35 healthy euthyroid individuals the serum T4A concentration was found to range between 60 and 160 pmol/l with a mean $\pm$ standard deviation of 114 $\pm$ 26 pmol/l. This contrasts with previous reports where the euthyroid range was considerably higher.[9,10]. In the earlier reports cross-reactivity of T4 or other serum components could not be ruled out, and probably accounts for the higher levels observed. T4A concentration did not correlate highly with other thyroid hormones or binding protein concentration, the highest correlations being between T4A and either total or free T4 ($r = .44$ and $.37$ respectively). In hyperthyroidism T4A concentration ranged between 85 and 357 pmol/l ($n = 25$) and in hypothyroidism between 0 and 65 pmol/l. When compared over the complete range of thyroidal states, the correlation between T4A and T4 concentrations was much higher ($r > 0.7$).

The 24 h urinary excretion of TO was investigated, as it was thought that this might give a good estimate of total thyroidal output of iodothyronines. Complete deiodination of iodoamino acids by peripheral tissue might be anticipated. In 15 euthyroid individuals 24 h TO excretion ranged between 8 and 25 nmol/24 h, with a mean $\pm$ standard deviation of 16.1 ± 4.5 nmol/24 h. Assuming an average daily T4 secretion rate of approximately 100 nmol/24 h it would seem that only 20% is excreted as TO. A number of possibilities exist to account for this surprisingly low value:-

a) most TO may be excreted in faeces.
b) complete deiodination of the majority of T4 does not occur.
c) additional side-chain modification, or phenolic conjugation or other cleavage may assume greater importance as peripheral deiodination proceeds.

The significance of peripheral catabolism of T4 at stages beyond monodeiodination awaits elucidation but these results indicate that this may be more complex than thought hitherto.

<u>Serum Thyroid Hormone Binding Proteins</u>

Of the three major T4 binding proteins in human serum, only assays for thyroxine binding globulin (TBG) and thyroxine binding prealbumin will be discussed. Sufficient data on the third binding protein, albumin, is available elsewhere to warrant no further discussion here. Of the two specific binding proteins TBPA is present in serum in far higher concentration than TBG. Its isolation is technically simple and has been described by a number of authors.[11,12,13]

The role of TBPA in thyroid hormone transport and action is still obscure and because it transports a smaller proportion of T4 than TBG in the vast majority of instances, it tends to be largely ignored. Whilst a knowledge of its concentration may make little contribution to the diagnosis of thyroid dysfunction, it is of interest to note that very low TBPA levels are associated in general with severe illness and undetectable TBPA with a very poor prognosis. We also are unaware of any reported instance of congenital total TBPA deficiency.

Because of its ease of isolation, monospecific antiserum to TBPA has been widely available on a commerical basis for a number of years. Using antiserum, techniques such as single radial diffusion [14] and one dimensional quantitative immunoelectrophoresis[15] are readily applicable. Recent research has shown that one function of TBPA is to transport retinol binding protein (RBP) together with its retinol (ROH) in the form of a bimolecular biligand complex.[16] Apart from inhibiting RBP and ROH loss by filtration through the kidneys, any other physiological significance of this complex awaits elucidation. We were concerned as to whether the presence or absence of this second protein interfered with the TBPA assay. Therefore, we isolated both proteins from serum and assayed standard preparations of TBPA containing graded amounts of RBP with and without ROH. Mixing of RBP and TBPA was carried out under conditions where complex formation could be demonstrated. Altering the RBP concentration by as much as 100% caused the apparent TBPA to vary by only 3.5%, when measured by one dimensional immunoelectrophoresis[17]. Therefore possible RBP interference may be discounted. ROH was without further effect.

TBG until very recently was a far more difficult protein to assay. Only indirect measures of T4 binding capacity being available. This was because of the difficulty of isolating the pure protein from serum. However, the advent of affinity chromatography has allowed an increasing number of authors to achieve this, even though there is still some discrepancy among the different reports as to its precise physico-chemical characteristics. To circumvent the difficulties associated with its isolation, we described a technique which allowed the production of a monospecific anti TBG without recourse to a rigorous purification schedule[18]. The antiserum thus obtained formed the basis of our one dimensional immunoelectrophoretic assay. Using this we have been able to show that in healthy euthyroid subjects serum T4 concentration is linearly related to serum TBG concentration over a range of TBG concentrations ranging from congenital deficiency to the extremes of congenital elevation[19]. This led us to propose the use of a simple T4:TBG ratio to replace the conventional 'Free Thyroxine Index' (FTI). In all but a few instances i.e. except where TBG is below the lower limit of the normal range, T4:TBG ratio can be shown to be parallel to free T4 concentration. As expected in euthyroid pregnant subjects T4:TBG ratio was still within the normal range, although the mean was slightly lower than the normal mean. This contrasts with one commercially available free T4 kit, where these patients could be misdiagnosed as hypothyroid.[20]

Recently we have been interested in developing a screening programme for neonatal hypothyroidism. This was based on a primary T4 screen using heelprick serum left over from an established PKU screening programme. One important cause of false positives in this system was the very low T4 levels associated with congenital TBG deficiency. In order to eliminate the need for patient recall in these instances, the TBG assay was miniaturised so that duplicate measurements could be made on one microlitre of serum. No loss of precision results from this intra-assay variability being approximately 4%. In the brief period this pilot scheme was in operation one TBG deficiency was identified.

Other techniques than single radial diffusion and immunoelectrophoresis are also applicable to the assay of the binding proteins. Bradwell and Deverell (private communication) have developed absorbiometric assays for TBG. In our own experience a nephelometric assay, based on the rate of increase in scattered light as antigen and antibody aggregate, also correlated well with TBG concentration. The sensitivity of the nephelometric assay corresponded to that of the immunoelectrophoretic assay. These latter methods, although requiring slightly more sample than the immunoelectrophoretic and single radial diffusion assays, have the advantage that they give results in a very short space of time. If a rapid T4 assay could be developed for routine use, such as the fluorometric assay described by Smith[21], there is a possibility that a T4:TBG ratio would be available for the clinician at consultation, provided the patient's sample was taken 20 - 30 min earlier.

THYROGLOBULIN (Tg)

The serum concentration of Tg in normal healthy euthyroid adults (0 - 20 μg/ml)[22] is well below that of TBG. Its assay, therefore, by techniques already referred to here is not possible. Only in pathological conditions such as thyroid cancer, where grossly elevated Tg levels occur, is it detectable by single radial diffusion. Even so this method would not always detect such instances and is, therefore, not satisfactory as a simple screening or monitoring technique. A variation of single radial diffusion, where the serum sample was placed in the agarose layer and the antiserum in the well was attempted. This allowed much larger sample volumes to be employed. Although a precipitin ring with normal serum could be seen, this was so feint and the background so intense, that the method was not suitable for routine use.

Apart from classical haemagglutination inhibition[24,25] and immunoelectrophoretic retardation[26] described in the early 1960s, a final possibility for a successful non-radioactive routine assay for Tg is some variation of enzyme immunoassay. In theory this technique should possess the necessary sensitivity and capacity for a routine use, however, we are not aware of any such assay being described. That serum Tg measurement may be of clinical value has been demonstrated by Osotemehin et al (1978)[23]. These authors investigated the use of Tg assay for the detection of neonatal hypothyroidism. Hypothyroid neonates were found to possess either very high levels of Tg, when some functioning thyroid tissue was present, or detectable Tg when thyroid tissue was completely absent. Another use for Tg assay is in the follow-up of patients undergoing total thyroidectomy for thyroid cancer. Serum Tg levels were found to correspond closely with the results of thyroid scans in these patients (unpublished data Black, Masie and Hoffenberg).

CONCLUSIONS

Assays for small molecules, such as thyroid hormones, may be successfully performed using GCMS techniques. Such methods are usually free from interference by factors which would adversely affect RIA techniques, although they lack the sample handling capacity of the latter.

A variety of non-radioactive methods for the assay of TBG and TBPA are available but most lack the sensitivity for a successful Tg assay.

REACTION SCHEME 1

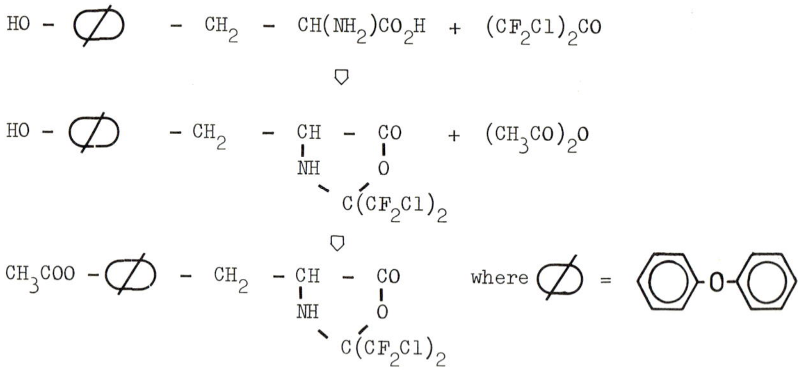

Acknowledgements

We wish to express our gratitude to the Medical Research Council (Grant Nos. G975/315 and G975/885/S) and to the Endowment Fund of the Central Birmingham Health District for their financial support.

References

1. Premachandra, B.N. (1978) Radioimmunoassays of Reverse Triiodothyronine, J. Clin. Endocrinol. Metab., 47, 746 - 50.

2. Crossley, D.N., Ramsden, D.B. and Hoffenberg, R. (1978) Determination of 3,3',5,5' tetraiodothyroacetate (T4A) in human serum by gas chromatography - mass fragmentography (GCMF) Quantitative Mass Spectrometry in Life Sciences II P 219 - 226. Ed. de Leenheer AP. Roncucci RR, van Peteghem C·Elservier.

3. Crossley, D.N. and Ramsden, D.B. Serum tetraiodothyroacetate (T4A) levels in normal healthy euthyroid individuals determined by gas chromatography - mass fragmentography (GCMF). Clin. Chim. Acta (In Press).

4. Hoffenberg, R., Lawson, A.M., Ramsden, D.B. and Raw, P.J. (1974) The application of mass spectrometry to the study of thyroxine and related compounds in biological fluids. In "Mass Spectrometry in Biochemistry and Medicine" pp 303 - 312. Ed. Frigerio A. and Castagnoli N. Raven Press.

5. Lawson, A.M., Ramsden, D.B., Raw, P.J. and Hoffenberg, R. (1975) Mass spectrometric studies of thyroxine and related compounds. Trimethylsilyl derivatives. Biomed Mass Spect 1, 374 - 380.

6. Petersen, B.A. and Vouros, P. (1977) Analysis of thyroid hormones as their heptafluorobutyryl methyl ester derivatives by gas chromatography - mass spectrometry. Anal Chem 49, 1304 - 1311.

7. Petersen, B.A., Hanson, R.N., Giese, R.W. and Karger, B.L. (1976) Picogram analysis of free triiodothyronine and free thyroxine hormones in serum by equilibrium dialysis and electron capture gas chromatography. J. Chromatogr 126, 503 - 516.

8. Husek, P. (1974) Derivatisation of amino acids with 1,3 dichlorotetrafluoroacetone and its use in gas chromatography. J. Chromatogr. 91, 475 - 481.

9. Ramsden, D.B., Raw, P.J. and Hoffenberg, R. (1975) Estimation of tetraiodothyroacetic acid in serum. Proc Roy Soc Med 68, 69 - 70.

10. Burger, A., Nicod, P., Suter, P., Vallotton, M.B., Vagenakis, A. and Braverman, L. (1976) Reduced active thyroid hormone levels in acute illness. Lancet 1, 653 - 655.

11. Tata, J.R. (1961) The purification of thyroxine binding globulin and thyroxine binding prealbumin. Clin Chim Acta 6, 819 - 838.

12. Schultze, H.E., Heimburger, N. and Frank, G. (1962) The aminoacid composition of human prealbumin and human and bovine albumin. Biochem Z 336, 388 - 396.

13. Oppenheimer, J.H., Surks, M.I., Smith, J.C. and Squef, R. (1965) Isolation and characterisation of human thyroxine-binding prealbumin. J. Biol. Chem. 246, 3230 - 3237.

14. Mancini, G., Carbonara, A.O. and Heremans, J.F. (1965) Immunochemical quantitation of antigens by single radial diffusion. Immunochemistry 2, 235 - 254.

15. Laurell, C.B. (1966) Quantilative estimation of protcins by electrophoresis in agarose gel containing antibodies. Annal Biochem 15, 45 - 52.

16. Nilsson, S.F., Rask, L. and Petersen, P.A. (1975) Studies on thyroid hormone binding proteins II. Binding of thyroid hormones, retinol binding protein and fluorescent probes to prealbumin and effect of thyroxine on prealbumin subunit self association. J. Biol. Chem. 250, 8554 - 63.

17. Ramsden, D.B., Prince, H.P., Burr, W.A., Bradwell, A.R., Black, E.G., Evans, A.E. and Hoffenberg, R. (1978) Interrelationship of thyroid hormones, Vitamin A and their binding proteins in acute stress. Clin. Endocrinol (Oxf) 8, 109 - 122.

18. Bradwell, A.R., Burnett, D., Ramsden, D.B., Burr, W.A., Prince, H.P. and Hoffenberg, R. (1976) Preparation of a monospecific antiserum to thyroxine binding globulin for its qunatitation by rocket immunoelectrophoresis. Clin. Chem. Acta 71, 501 - 510.

19. Burr, W.A., Ramsden, D.B., Evans, S.E., Hogan, T. and Hoffenberg, R. (1977) Relationship between Thyroxine binding globulin concentration and T3 uptake: diagnostic value of TBG concentration. Brit. Med. J. 1, 485 - 488.

20. Boss, M., Djahanbakhch, O. and Kingstone, D. (1978) Thyroid disease and pregnancy. Brit. Med. J. (6150) 1496.

21. Smith, D.S. (1977) Enhancement fluoroimmunoassay of thyroxine. FEBS. Letters 77, 25 - 27.

22. Van Herle, H.J., Uller, R.P., Matthews, N.L. and Brown, J. (1973) Radioimmunoassay for measurement of thyroglobulin in human serum. J. Clin. Invest. 52, 1320 - 1327.

23. Osotimehin, B., Black, E.G. and Hoffenberg, R. (1978) Thyroglobulin concentration in neonatal blood: a possible test for neonatal hypothyroidism. Brit. Med. J. (6150) 1467 - 1468.

24. Hjort, T. (1961) Determination of serum thyroglobulin by haemagglutination test. Lancet, 1, 1262.

25. Hjort, T. and Petersen, G.T. (1962) Thyroid antibodies and thyroglobulin in the serum in pregnant and parturient women and in newborn infants. Lancet 2, 259.

26. Assem, E.S.K. (1964) Thyroglobulin in the serum of parturient women and newborn infants. Lancet 1, 139.

* Present address.

Immunodiagnostic Laboratory, Department of Immunology, University of Birmingham, Birmingham, U.K.

Radioimmunology 1979, Ch. A. Bizollon, editor.

IMPLICATIONS FOR THE MEASUREMENT OF THE DIALYSABLE FRACTIONS OF THYROID HORMONES IN THYROID DISEASE.

LINE BALDET et CLAUDE JAFFIOL
- Service de Consultations d'Endocrinologie (Pr. C. Jaffiol)
- Clinique des maladies Métaboliques et Endocriniennes (Pr. J. Mirouze) - Hôpital Saint Eloi - Montpellier 34059 Cedex (France)

Robbins and Rall[1] showed 20 years ago that the thyroid hormones in plasma (T3 & T4) exist in two forms, the one bound to specific plasma proteins (TBG, TBPA and TBA) the other free and directly exchangeable with the tissues. While the bound form is the more important in quantitative terms (50 - 130 ng/ml for T4 ; 0,8 - 2,2 ng/ml for T3) it is the free hormone fraction which is responsible for hormonal action in systemic and pituitary tissues.

Much effort has been spent in trying obtain greatest possible precision for the measurement of free thyroid hormones, and several techniques have been described. The methods currently used fall into two main groups :

1- Indirect measurement of the free fraction by determination of a coefficient of freedom (ultrafiltration, equilibrium dialysis, charcoal adsorption, gel - filtration) which, expressed as a ratio of the total hormone concentration, provides an evaluation of the free hormone level.

2- Direct measurement of the free hormone by radioimmunoassay after separation of free and bound moieties (dialysis, column chromatography).

It is interesting to note that these quite different techniques represent historically the sequence in which free hormone estimation has developed. Thus the indirect measurement of free thyroid hormones came first Sterling et al[2,3] ; Oppenheimer et al[4] ; Ingbar et al[5], followed much more recently by radioimmunoassay Ellis et al[6] ; Weeke et al[7] ; Romelli et al[8].

We have been using equilibrium dialysis to determine free T4 & T3 for several years[9]. The aim of the present study was to establish the influence of certain plasma factors on the dialysable fractions of T4 and T3, and to study the behaviour of these fractions in several thyroid disorders, before and after treatment.

TECHNIQUES

The dialysable fractions of T4 and T3 (DFT4 and DFT3) were measured by a modified Oppenheimer and Surks method.

Labelled thyroid hormones (^{125}I T4 and ^{125}I T3) were obtained from Abbott Laboratories, specific activities 50 - 70 mCi/mg.

Free thyroxine was measured by the addition of ^{125}I T4 at a concentration of less than 1 μg per dl to 1 ml of serum ; ^{125}I T3 at a concentration of less than 2,5 ng per ml was used for the determination of free triiodothyronine. The radioactive tracers were diluted in a 0.125g per dl albumin solution. Tracer-enriched serum was incubed within 30 minutes at room temperature. The labelled serum to be analyzed was diluted to 1/25 in a phosphate buffer (pH7.4-0.025 M) and 5 ml of this mixture was dialysed against 25 ml of the same phosphate buffer. The addition of merthiolate 1/200,000 for T4 and 1/400,000 for T3 was carried out to eliminate bacterial contamination. The duration of the incubation was 16-20 hours at 37°C with constant agitation in a shaker. One ml was collected from the inside of the bag ("in") 3 ml were removed from the outside of the bag ("out") and then transferred to a test tube. A volume of 0.5 ml of a pooled serum was added to each tube. This procedure was followed by one precipitation with trichloracetic acid and then the precipitate was washed twice. The two precipitates were assayed for radioactivity during 5 minutes. The radioactivity of the "out" dialysate precipitate was divided by three to calculate the results for 1ml. The dialysable fraction was thus calculated by using the following formula :

$$DF\ \% = \frac{(V0 + V1) \times {}^{125}\text{I "out"}}{(V0 \times {}^{125}\text{I "out"}) + (V1 \times {}^{125}\text{I "in"})}$$

V0 = volume "out" = 25 ml, V1 = volume "in" = 5 ml

^{125}I "out" :radioactivity of 1 ml of "out"

^{125}I "in" : radioactivity of 1 ml of "in"

Reprodutibility of the method was confirmed from pooled sera introduced into the dialysis series (CV = 8,5 % for DFT4 and 7,5 % for DFT3).

The total plasma concentrations of thyroxine (TT4) and of triiodothyronine (TT3) were determined by specific radioimmunoassay (Abbott Laboratories for TT4 and Lepetit Laboratories for TT3), from which the free hormone concentrations (AFT4 and AFT3) were calculated thus :

$$AFT4\ (pg/ml) = TT4\ (ng/ml) \times DFT4\ \% \times 10^3$$

$$AFT3\ (pg/ml) = TT3\ (ng/ml) \times DFT3\ \% \times 10^3$$

At the same time the free fractions of T4 (FT4) and T3 (FT3) were measured directly by radioimmunoassay after separation on a sephadex column (Lepetit Laboratories).

The maximum binding capacity of TBG (TBG cap.) was measured by a method previously described[10] in which the proteins were separated by reverse-flow electropheresis, in glycine acetate buffer pH 8,6, for concentration of added T4 of 100, 150 and 200 μg/dl. The plasma concentration of TBG was also determined directly by specific radioimmunoassay (Behring Laboratories).

METHODS

Several studies were carried out, both in vivo and in vitro.

1. Influence of T4, T3 and TBG concentration on DFT4 and DFT3

- in vitro study :

Three pools of mixed serum of known TBG cap. were obtained from hyperthyroid (TBG cap. 20,8 μg T4/dl), euthyroid (TBG cap.23,9 μg T4/dl) and hypothyroid subjects (TBG cap. 43,9 μg T4/dl). To each pool were added increasing quantities of cold T4 or T3 (0-60 μg/dl of T4, 0-5 ng/ml of T3). The value of DFT4 and DFT3, and the percentage of ^{125}I T4 bound to TBG were established for the different pools of serum before and after each addition of stable hormone.

- in vivo study :

The concentrations of TBG, TT4, TT3, DFT4, DFT3, AFT4, AFT3, FT4 and FT3 were measured in 49 subjects (10 eu-, 9 hyper-, 10 hypothyroid, 10 women on the contraceptive pill and 10 in their third trimester of pregnancy). From these measurements were derived the correlation between TBG, DFT4 and DFT3 on the one hand, AFT4-FT4 and AFT3-FT3 on the other.

2. Diagnostic value of DFT4, DFT3, AFT4 and AFT3 in divers thyroid disorders.

- Classical hyper- and hypothyroidism

23 thyrotoxic, 20 hypothyroid and 21 euthyroid individuals, classified according to clinical state and either basal TSH or response in the TRH test, were studied. Discriminant analysis[11] was used to rank the diagnostic value of TT4, DFT4 and AFT4, and of TT3, DFT3 and AFT3 in terms of patients known thyroid status.

- Patients with abnormal TRH response.

27 patients, in remission from Graves'disease after radioiodine treatment several months or years previously, were selected on account of an exaggerated response (hyperresponders, 9 cases) or absent response (nonresponders, 18 cases) to TRH. All had normal TT4 and TT3 levels, and none was symptomatic of thyroid

dysfunction. The values for DFT4, DFT3, AFT4 and AFT3 were compared with a normal control population in order to establish whether differences which could emerged to account for the abnormal TRH responses. Wilcoxon's signed ranking test for non-parametric variables[12] was used to look for such differences.

- Hot nodules

18 patients with hot thyroid nodules and negative response to TRH were studied : 9 had typical hyperthyroidism with raised TT3 (groupe I) ; and 9 had normal values of both TT3 and TT4 (groupe II). The values for DFT3 and AFT3 in both groups were compared (by Wilcoxon's test) with those of the control group.

3. Sequential study of DFT4, DFT3, AFT4 and AFT3 during the course of treatment for hyper- and hypothyroidism.

14 thyrotoxicosis patients were studied before and again 3 months after the start of treatment with carbimazole, 30 mg daily.

10 hypothyroid patients (frank myxoedema or total thyroidectomy) were studied before and after treatment for one month first with LT3 (75 μg daily) and then LT4 (200 μg daily). The Wilcoxon test for paired non-parametric data was used for statistical analysis data[12].

RESULTS

1. Influence of T4, T3 and TBG on DFT4 and DFT3

- in vitro study (fig. 1 & 2)

The enrichment of pools of sera from hypo-, hyper- and euthyroid individuals with increasing amounts of LT4 resulted in a fall in the percentage of ^{125}I T4 bound to TBG and a progressive rise in DFT4 and DFT3. This phenomenon occurred at all levels of TBG cap. Thus the rise in DFT4 was related inversely to the initial binding capacity of the serum.

The corresponding results from LT3 enrichment revealed no change in the ^{125}I T4 bound to TBG, nor in the values or DFT4 and DFT3, even in the hyperthyroid patients with low TBG.

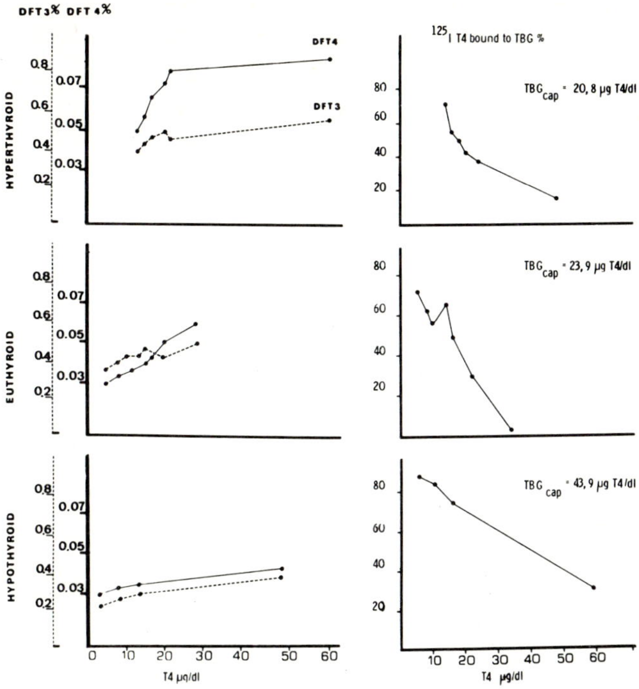

Fig. 1 Variations of DFT4, DFT3 and ^{125}I T4 bound to TBG in relation to the concentration of T4 in serum of hyper-, eu- and hypothyroid patients after addition of T4.

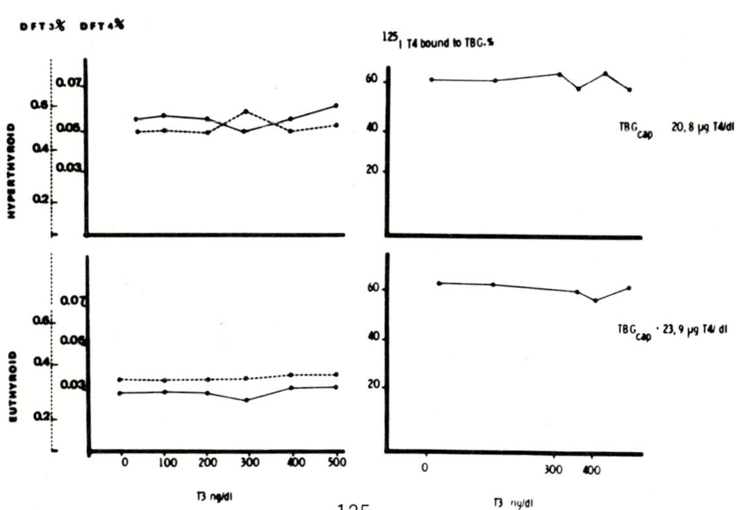

Fig. 2 Variations of DFT4, DFT3 and ^{125}I T4 bound to TBG in relation to the concentration of T3 in serum of hyper- and euthyroid patients after addition of T3.

- *in vivo* study (fig. 3 & 4)

Inverse correlations were found between DFT4 and TBG on the one hand, and between DFT3 and TBG on the other. The scaller of points expressed on arithmetic axes was best described (in the case of both DFT3 and DFT4) by a single exponential according to the equations : DFT4 = 0,035 $e^{-0,02\ TBG}$ (r = -0,71 ; p $<$ 0,001) and DFT3 = 0,38 $e^{-0,02\ TBG}$ (r = -0,85 ; p $<$ 0,001).

Four points (corresponding to the same four patients whether for DFT4 or for DFT3) were clearly independent of the remainder, having greatly elevated levels of DFT4 and DFT3 in respect of their TBG levels. These same four were also found to have particularly high levels of TT4 (170-240 ng/ml) and TT3 (3,5 - 7,25 ng/ml).

In this same group of 49 subjects, the free hormone levels (FT4 & FT3) measured by sephadex filtration showed strong linear correlation with the corresponding concentrations of AFT4/FT4 (r = 0,89 p $<$ 0,001) AFT3/FT3 (r = 0,94 p $<$ 0,001).

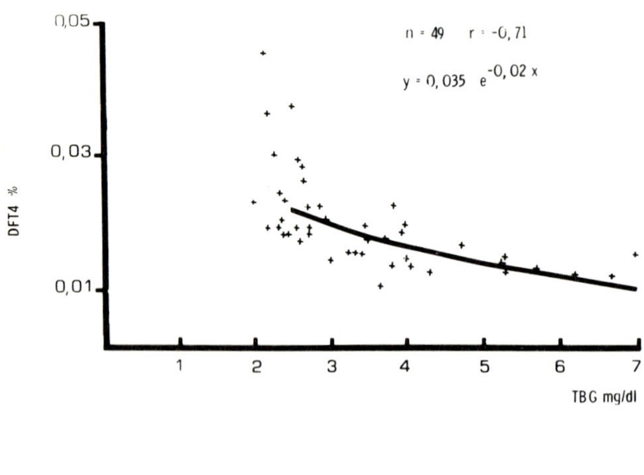

Fig. 3 Correlation between DFT4 and TBG.

TABLE I - THYROXINE BINDING GLOBULIN, TOTAL AND FREE THYROID HORMONES IN FIVE GROUPS OF SUBJECTS.

	TBG mg/dl	TT4 ng/ml	DFT4 %	AFT4 pg/ml	TT3 ng/ml	DFT3 %	AFT3 pg/ml
Controls	n=10	n=21	n=21	n=21	n= 21	n=21	n=21
mean	2.65	83.3	0.020	16.1	1.35	0.21	2.8
SD or range	(2-3.5)	± 13.4	± 0.002	± 3.4	± 0.32	0.02	± 0.7
Thyrotoxic	n=9	n=23	n=23	n=23	n=23	n=23	n=23
	2.46	174 ***	0.034***	60.4***	3.67***	0.30***	11.5***
	(2.2-2.9)	± 29.0	± 0.015	± 29.5	± 1.68	± 0.07	± 7.5
Hypothyroid	n=10	n=20	n=20	n=20	n=20	n=20	n=20
	3.00	23.6***	0.016***	4.2***	0.52***	0.17***	0.9***
	(2.3-4)	± 15.0	± 0.004	± 3.3	± 0.44	± 0.03	± 0.8
Pregnant	n=10	n=10	n=10	n=10	n=10	n=10	n=10
	5.39***	139 ***	0.014***	19	2.10***	0.12***	2.2*
	(3.8-7)	(92-186)	(0.011-0.018)	(15-20)	(1.65-3.25)	(0,09-0.18)	(1.1-3.3)
On contraceptive pill	n=10	n=10	n=10	n=10	n=10	n=10	n=10
	3.62***	115 ***	0.014***	15.5	1.65**	0.17***	2.7
	(2.5-4.3)	(79-147)	(0.010-0.018)	(12-18)	(1.20-2.15)	(0.13-0.23)	(2.3-4.1)

Each group is compared to controls by Wilcoxon's test (*** $p < 0.01$ ** $p < 0.02$ * $p < 0.05$)
n : number of cases ; m = mean ± SD for a number of cases > 20 m (range) for a number of cases < 20

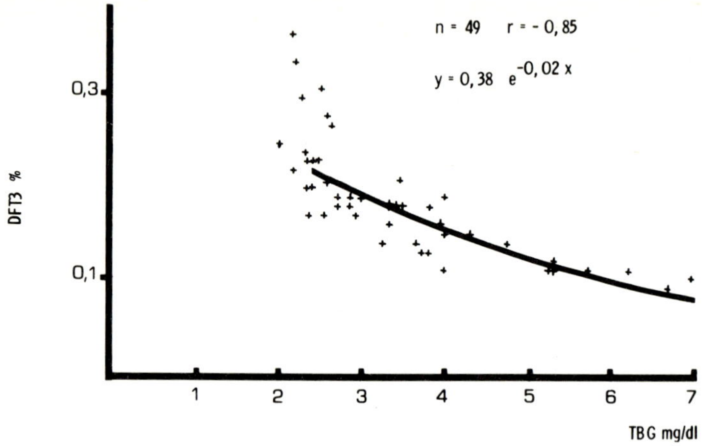

Fig. 4 Correlation between DFT3 and TBG.

2. Diagnostic value of DFT4, DFT3, AFT4 and AFT3 in divers thyroid disorders.
   - Classical hyper - and hypothyroidism.

The results are shown in table I, the statistical significance of differences between patients and controls are indicated. Discriminant analysis suggests the measurement of free thyroid hormones (AFT4 and AFT3) was in no way diagnostically superior to that of total hormones (TT4 and TT3) (Table II).

TABLE II - DISCRIMINANT ANALYSIS OF THE DIAGNOSTIC VALUE OF TOTAL AND FREE THYROID HORMONES IN THYROID DISEASES.

	TT4	DFT4	AFT4	TT3	DFT3	AFT3
Thyrotoxic Controls	97.7 %	84.1 %	86.4 %	88.6 %	88.6 %	79.5 %
Hypothyroid Controls	100 %	65.8 %	95.1 %	85.4 %	78 %	87.8 %

Indicated percentage refers to the correctly classified subjects.

TABLE III - TOTAL AND FREE THYROID HORMONES IN TRH NON-RESPONDERS.

Sujet n°	TT4 ng/ml	DFT4 %	AFT4 pg/ml	TT3 ng/ml	DFT3 %	AFT3 pg/ml	TSH µU/ml	▲TSH µU/ml
1	114	0.012	13.7	1.15	0.17	1.9	1	0
2	116	0.016	18.6	1.40	0.19	2.7	3.4	0
3	119	0.019	22.6	1.77	0.20	3.5	1	1
4	107	0.018	19.3	1.00	0.22	2.2	1	0
5	126	0.015	18.9	1.30	0.22	2.9	2	2
6	92	0.017	15.6	1.20	0.24	2.9	1	0
7	73.5	0.022	16.2	0.70	0.19	1.3	1.9	0.9
8	101	0.020	20.2	1.25	0.22	2.7	1	0
9	100	0.020	20.0	1.30	0.22	2.9	2.5	1
10	93	0.020	18.6	1.10	0.23	2.5	3.8	0.4
11	117	0.020	23.4	1.55	0.20	3.1	1.1	0
12	74	0.020	14.8	1.65	0.20	3.3	1	0.4
13	66	0.021	13.9	1.75	0.22	3.8	4	0.5
14	43	0.021	9.0	2.10	0.24	5	1	0.5
15	84	0.018	15.1	1.10	0.24	2.6	1	0
16	65	0.018	11.7	1.40	0.22	3.1	1.2	0.2
17	83.5	0.018	15.0	1.00	0.21	2.1	1.2	0
18	84	0.021	15.6	1.00	0.17	1.7	1	1.1
Controls n:21	83.3 ± 13.4	0.020 0.002	16.1 3.4	1.35 0.32	0.21 0.02	2.8 0.7	< 5	5 - 20
Significance	NS	NS	NS	NS	NS	NS	NS	p < 0.01

- Patients with abnormal TRH response (Table III, IV)

TABLE IV - TOTAL AND FREE THYROID HORMONES IN TRH-HYPERRESPONDERS.

	TT4 ng/ml	DFT4 %	AFT4 pg/ml	TT3 ng/ml	DFT3 %	AFT3 pg/ml	TSH µU/ml	▲TSH µU/ml
1	65	0.018	11.7	1.5	0.15	2.2	8	78
2	66	0.021	13.8	1.2	1.20	2.4	9	63
3	113	0.025	28.2	2.75	0.22	6	7.5	31.5
4	95	0.020	19	1.5	0.23	3.4	7.5	28
5	67	0.018	12	1.45	0.21	3	23	95
6	65	0.021	13.6	1.65	0.20	3.3	5.75	25
7	82	0.021	17.2	1.15	0.26	3	8	53
8	104	0.017	17.7	1.75	0.21	3.7	18	55
9	83	0.023	19.1	1.45	0.25	3.6	13.5	33
Controls	83.3	0.020	16.1	1.35	0.21	2.8	< 5	5 - 20
n:21	± 13.4	0.002	3.4	0.32	0.02	0.7		
Significance	NS	NS	NS	NS	NS	NS	$p < 0.01$	$p < 0.01$

Statistical analysis revealed no significant differences in DFT4, AFT4, DFT3, AFT3 between patients and controls.

- Hot nodules (Table V)

In Gp. I alone, TT3 and AFT3 were significantly raised ($p < 0.01$) in relation to control values. In gp. II with normal TT3, only the AFT3 was significantly increased ($p < 0.02$).

3. Sequential study of DFT4, DFT3, AFT4 and AFT3 during the course of treatment for hyper- and hypothyroidism.

In the 14 thyrotoxic patients treated with carbimazole, TT4, TT3, DFT4, DFT3, AFT4 and AFT3 fell significantly ($p < 0.01$) by the third month of treatmont (fig.5)

TABLE V - TOTAL AND FREE T3 IN PATIENTS WITH HOT NODULES AND NORMAL OR INCREASED TT3.

		TT3 ng/ml	DFT3 %	AFT3 pg/ml
HOT NODULES AND INCREASED TT3.	1	8.7	0.26	22.6
	2	5.0	0.21	10.5
	3	3.6	0.20	7.2
	4	7.2	0.26	18.7
	5	2.2	0.20	4.4
	6	5.0	0.18	9.0
	7	9.4	0.27	25.4
	8	3.6	0.22	7.9
	9	2.5	0.25	6.3
Significance		$p < 0.01$	NS	$p < 0.01$
HOT NODULES AND NORMAL TT3	10	1.3	0.41	5.3
	11	1.3	0.20	2.6
	12	1.9	0.26	4.9
	13	1.8	0.20	3.6
	14	1.8	0.19	3.4
	15	0.9	0.22	2.0
	16	1.7	0.27	4.6
	17	1.6	0.26	4.2
	18	1.8	0.20	3.6
Significance		NS	NS	$p < 0.02$
Controls n:21		1.35 $\pm$ 0.32	0.21 0.02	2.8 0.7

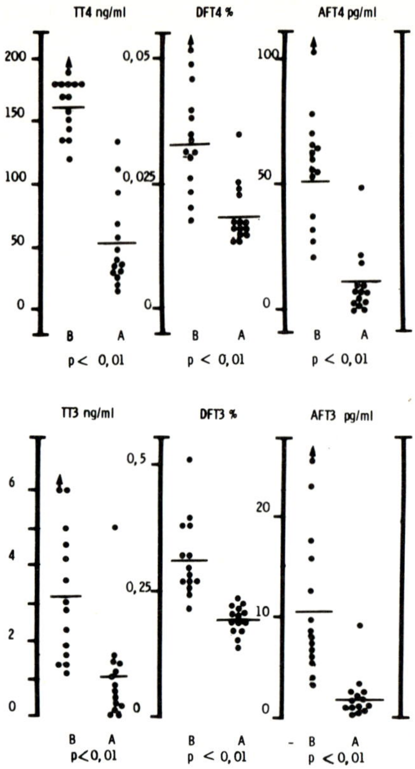

Fig. 5 Total and free thyroid hormones in Graves'disease patients before (B) and after (A) treatment with carbimazole.

In the 10 hypothyroid individuals treated with thyroxine there was a significant rise ($p < 0.01$) in TT4, TT3, DFT3, AFT4, AFT3 and ($p < 0.02$) DFT4 after one month of treatment (fig. 6)

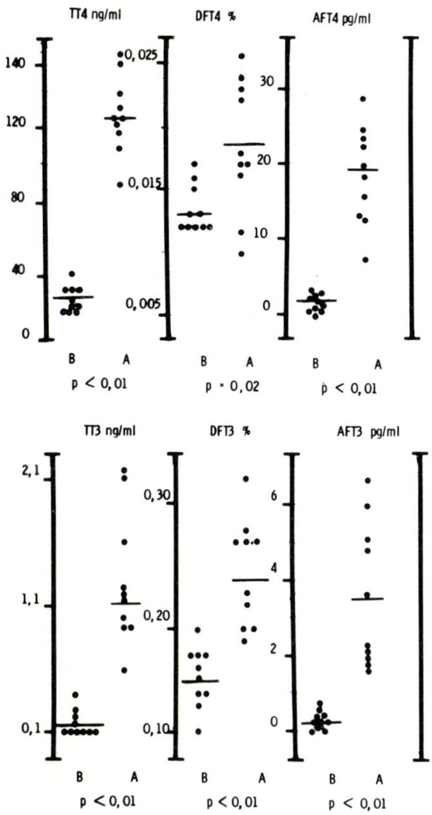

Fig. 6 Total and free thyroid hormones in hypothyroid patients before(B) and after (A) treatment with LT4.

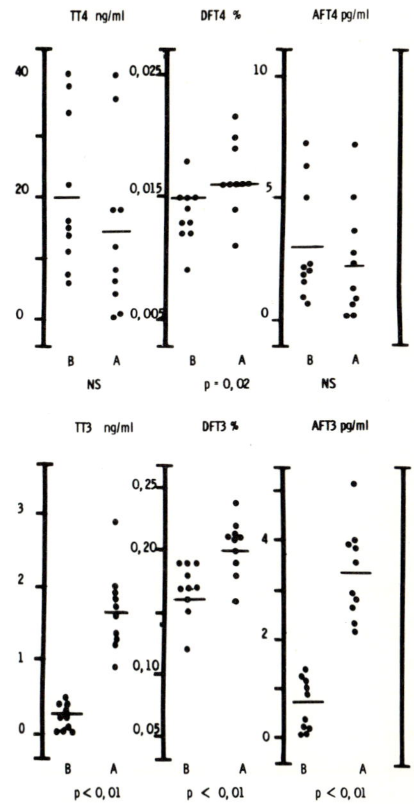

Fig. 7 Total and free thyroid hormones in hypothyroid patients before (B) and after (A) treatment with LT3.

During treatment with LT3, TT3, DFT3 and AFT3 rose significantly ($p < 0.01$) while TT4 and AFT4 did not vary (fig. 7). DFT4, on the other hand, increased under the influence of LT3 treatment ($p < 0.02$).

DISCUSSION

Reproducibility in equilibrium dialysis depends critically upon the maintenance of certain conditions. These include the dialysis period, membrane quality, pH and molarity of solutions, incubation temperature, concentration of merthiolate added and above all, purity of the tracer. The latter was a major source of variation avoided by recent measurements of free thyroid hormones by radioimmunoassay of the dialysate[6]. Variations in technique explain differences between laboratories. Our own results show a high level of reproducibility with variances of 8.5 % for DFT4 and 7.5 % for DFT3.

The in vitro enrichment experiments show a clear relationship between DFT4/DFT3 and the concentration of cold T4 added. The increment in dialysable fraction was greatest when the TBG binding capacity was lowest. The results corroborate the finding of a higher proportion of free hormone in hyperthyroid than in euthyroid individuals with the same serum T4[2]. Enrichment with LT3 up to 5 ng/ml concentration modified neither DFT4/DFT3 nor the percentage hormone bound to TBG. These agree with the results of Naumann et al[13] that in vitro DFT3 depends more on the concentration of TT4 than on TT3, a fact which could explain the paradoxical absence of a raised DFT3 in certain cases of T3 thyrotoxicosis[14].

We noted in vivo an inverse exponential relationship between both DFT4/DFT3 and the concentration of TBG ; an inverse relationship between the proportion of free hormone and transport capacity of the binding proteins has already been reported[15]. Four individuals were situated well outwith this exponential. These all had very high levels of TT4 and TT3, suggesting that the unusually high DFT4/DFT3 levels were due to saturation of protein binding sites.

The discriminant value of free thyroid hormones (AFT4 and AFT3) was not superior to that of TT4 and TT3 in hyper and hypothyroidism. Arango et al[16] and more recently Yeo[17] who used direct radioimmunoassay came to the same conclusion. Again, Evered[18] underlined the inferiority of free hormone compared with total hormone measurement in the diagnosis of thyroid disorders.

The measurement of AFT4 and AFT3 corrects the elevation of TT4 and TT3 encountered in pregnancy and in women on the contraceptive pill. While diminished free hormone levels have been reported during the third trimester of pregnancy[19] most authors find them to be physiologic [16-20]. We found AFT3 to be significantly lower than controls ($p < 0{,}05$) while AFT4 was the same in pregnant women.

AFT4 and AFT3 were normal in patients with normal TT4 and TT3 whose TRH response was abnormal. It is probable that such anomalies in the TRH test are due to minor deviations of thyroid hormones from the optimum for the individual which remain, nevertheless, within the normal limits for a group.

Normal TT3 levels in patients with hot nodules were accompanied by significantly raised AFT3 which could explain their lack of response to TRH. This observation may be linked to the increased turnover of ^{125}I T3 noted in certain such patients[21].

The fall in both free and total hormone levels noted three months after the introduction of carbimazole may be explained by the association of a fall in hormone secretion and a rise in the binding capacity of TBPA in the hypothyroid state[9]. However the more interesting observation was the rise in DFT4 during the treatment of hypothyroidism with LT3, a phenomenon which was all the more striking because TT4 did not change. The same did not occur in vitro following enrichment of serum pools with T3. The rise in DFT4 in vivo could be due to a reduction in T4 binding capacity of the carrier proteins consequent upon long-term LT3 treatment.

CONCLUSION

Dialysable fractions of thyroid hormones show an inverse relationship with TBG levels in plasma best described by an exponential function. DFT3, in vitro, and probably in vivo, depends more on TT4 than on TT3 concentrations. Free thyroid hormones offer a lower discriminant value than total hormone measurement in the diagnosis of typical or sub clinical hyper- or hypothyroidism. However, the increment of AFT3 in euthyroid patients with hot nodules may give an explanation of their blunted TRH response. The main interest for free thyroid hormones lies in the assessment of thyroid function in patients with anomalies of thyroxine binding proteins.

BIBLIOGRAPHIE

1. Robbins J. and Rall J.E. - 1960 - Physiol. Rev. 40 (Suppl. 4) 415-465.
2. Sterling K. and Hegedus A. 1962 - J. Clin. Invest. 41 - 1031-1040
3. Sterling K. and Brenner M.A. - 1966 - J. Clin. Invest. 45 - 153-163.
4. Oppenheimer J.H. and Surks M.E. - 1964 - J. Clin. Endocr. 24, 785-793.
5. Ingbar et al - 1965 - J. Clin. Invest. 44, 1679-1689.
6. Ellis S.M. and Ekins R.P. - 1975 - Radioimmunoassay in clinical Biochemistry (C.A. Pasternak ed.) pp 187-194. Heyden London.
7. Weeke J. and Orskow H. 1975 - Scand J. Clin. Lab. Invest. 35, 237-244.
8. Romelli P.B. and Pennisi F. - 1977 - Convegno su "RIA 77 Recenti progressi in radioimmunologia clinica" Brescia March 1977.
9. Jaffiol C. et al - 1977 - Horm. Metab. Res. 9 - 73-81.
10. Jaffiol C. and Baldet L. - 1974 - In la Thyroïde tome III (Zara ed.) pp. 188-216 - L'expansion Scientifique Paris.
11. Romeder J.M. - 1973. In Methodes et programmes d'analyse discriminante. Dunod Ed.
12. Schwartz D. - 1965 - In Methodes statistiques à l'usage des médecins et des biologistes - Flammarion ed.
13. Nauman J.A. et al - 1967 - J. Clin. Invest. 46 - 1346-1355
14. Baldet L. et al - 1974 - Ann. Endocr. 35 - 263-264.
15. Inada M. and Sterling K. - 1967 J. Clin. Invest. 46 - 1442-1450.
16. Arango et al - 1968 - Mayo Clinic. Proc. 43 - 503.
17. Yeo P.P.B. et al- 1977 - Clin. Endocrinol. 6 - 159-165.
18. Evered D. - Unpublished data.
19. Avruskin T.W. et al - 1976 C.S. Ann. J. Med. Sci. 271 - 309.
20. Osathanondh R. et al 1976 - J. Clin. Endocr. - 42 - 98.
21. Mirouze J. et al 1975 - Ann. Endocr. 36, 173-174.

Radioimmunology 1979, Ch. A. Bizollon, editor.

CLINICAL INTEREST OF DIRECT RADIO-IMMUNOLOGICAL DETERMINATION OF FREE THYROID HORMONE PLASMA LEVELS (FT3, FT4)

J.L. CODACCIONI*, P. CARAYON**, E. CASTANAS*, M. GUIBOUT***

* Service d'Endocrinologie et des Maladies du Métabolisme, Hôpital de la Conception, F 13385 Marseille Cedex 4

** Laboratoire des Hormones Protéiques, Faculté de Médecine, Marseille

*** Clinique Endocrinologique, Hôpital de la Timone, Marseille

INTRODUCTION

3, 5, 3' triiodothyronine (T3) and thyroxine (T4) are present in human plasma in either the free (FT3 and FT4) or protein-bound form. The physiologic importance of the free fraction of thyroid hormones has been recognized for quite some time[1-2]. Additionally, it has been clearly demonstrated that plasma FT3 and FT4 levels are better correlated to clinical thyroid status than are the circulating total T3 and T4[3-10]. Although it is widely accepted that measurement of the free plasma hormones would be the best method for evaluating thyroid function, the technical complexity involved in such measurements has impeded their use as routine prodecures.

Older indirect methods were very tedious : hormone tracer methods[3] followed by dialysis[3-4], gel filtration[5-6], ultrafiltration or electrophoresis[7], or charcoal absorption[8] have been proposed. Recently a direct technique was proposed[9-10], consisting in dialysis of the serum followed by radioimmunoassay of the FT3 and FT4 in the dialysats. This approach, which eliminates most of the difficulties inherent to the indirect techniques of measurement[3-8], was adapted to routine situations by Romelli and Pennisi[11] : free hormone fractions, separated from those bound to proteins using column chromatography, were measured by radioimmunoassay.

The aim of this study was to evaluate the clinical significance of free thyroid hormone levels by studying the values detected in normal subjects and in patients with disturbed thyroid function. These new diagnostic tests were compared to others designed to evaluate thyroid function, i.e. measurement of TSH, total T3 and T4 and the free thyroxine index (FTI). This comparison was done in order to determine the usefulness of FT3 and FT4 measurements in the assessment of thyroid function.

MATERIAL AND METHODS

Subjects. Studies were performed on 169 subjects, 18 to 70 years old, presenting various clinical status. Normals (n = 45) were volunteers from the medical staff or healthy subjects examined for athletic reasons. Hyperthyroid (n = 42) and hypothyroid (n = 51) patients were selected on the basis of the usually admitted clinical and laboratory criteria ; none of them was under thyroid treatment. Furthermore women under oral contraceptives (n = 31) were studied.

The conditional probability of hyper- or hypothyroidism (clinical indexes) was calculated from the clinical signs presented by the patients according to Overall et al.[12] and Winkler et al.[13] and using Bayes'formula.

Hormone assays. Plasma TSH and T3 were determined by previously described radioimmunological procedures[14-15]. Serum T4 was assayed by a competitive protein binding method and T3-uptake test was achieved by a resin absorption method (Tetrasorb and Triosorb from Abbott Laboratory). Plasma FT3 and FT4 concentrations were determined by column chromatography and radioimmunoassay method according to Romelli and Pennisi[11].

Statistical Analysis. In order to account for the homogeneity of variance and normal distribution assumptions, the following transformation of data was applied :

$$X = \frac{\log x - \log x_{min}}{\log x_{max} - \log x_{min}}$$

where x is the observed hormone level, x_{min} and x_{max} the least detectable and the greatest measurable concentrations respectively ; in practice, regarding the radioimmunoassay, x_{min} and x_{max} values were obtained from the lower and upper limit of the standard curve. This transformation succeeds in homogeneizing the variances of all groups studied and in normalizing the distribution of the normal subjects, regardless of the hormone measurement considered. But, this transformation failed to normalize the distribution of hyper- and hypothyroid patients. Consequently, the confidence intervals of the mean of these two populations was not determinable. Nevertheless, the number of individuals in each group ($n > 40$) is sufficient to allow further statistical analysis.

The Student's t-test as well as the analysis of variance and covariance (linear regression analysis) were performed as usual[16]. The misclassification procedure was performed by the computation of the normal range ($m \pm 2$ SD) from the normal population. The multivariate statistical analysis (linear discriminant analysis) was performed according to Anderson[17]. This kind of statistical investigation leads to : calculating the most potent subset of variables, from a given group, which can discriminate between two or more populations. The selection procedure takes into consideration the distance obtained between the centers of each pair of populations specified by the set of variables used ; classifying an individual in one of two or more multivariate normal populations. The criteria of classification used was the distance between the mean vectors of the groups, premultiplied by the total variance covariance matrix.

All calculations were performed using a Hewlett-Packard HP 30 Desk-Top Calculator.

RESULTS

In the normal subjects the 95% confidence limits for FT3 measurement was 2.4 - 4.9 pg/ml plasma and that for FT4 measurement was 5.8 - 18.2 pg/ml plasma ; the 99% confidence limit was 2.0 - 5.9 and 4.3 - 24.2 pg/ml plasma for FT3 and FT4 measurement, respectively (Table 1). FT3 levels detected in hyper- or hypothyroid patients consistently fell outside the 95% confidence interval corresponding to the normal value range. On the other hand, FT4 levels in hypothyroid patients overlapped those in normal subjects (Table 1). In women under oral contraceptives FT3 ranged from 2.7 - 4.1 pg/ml and FT4 from 5.7 - 15.9 pg/ml showing that no case displayed values outside the 95% confidence interval of normal levels.

TABLE 1

FREE THYROID HORMONE PLASMA CONCENTRATIONS IN VARIOUS THYROID STATES (pg/ml)

	Hyperthyroids (n = 42)		Normal (n = 45)		Hypothyroids (n = 51)	
	FT3	FT4	FT3	FT4	FT3	FT4
Mean	21.0	52.9	3.5	10.2	1.0	1.7
Calculated range (m ± 2SD)			2.4-4.9	5.8-18.2		
Observed range	9.3-50	22.3-94.7	2.3-4.9	5.5-21.9	0.5-2.3	0.5-6.3

The normal ranges of TSH, T3, T4 and FTI were calculated in the same way as those of FT3 and FT4, i.e. using the data transformation described in material and methods. With respect of hyper- or hypothyroid patients displaying values within the 95% confidence interval of the corresponding normal levels (Table 2), the number of hyperthyroid patients misclassified as normal was zero in the case of FT3 and FT4 measurements, low with respect to T3 and FTI determinations (1 and 3 cases respectively) and rather high when the T4 level was used (11 cases). Misclassification of hypothyroid patients as normal did not occur when FT3 was measured, was low in the case of FT4 (1 case) and elevated in the case of T3, FTI and T4 (6,6 and 11 cases respectively).

TABLE 2

MISCLASSIFICATION OF HYPER- AND HYPOTHYROID PATIENTS

	Hyperthyroid Patients (n = 42)	Hypothyroid Patients (n = 51)	Overall Misclassification (n = 93)
FT3	0*	0	0
FT4	0	2.0	1.1
T3	2.4	11.8	7.5
FTI	7.1	11.8	9.7
T4	26.2	21.6	17.2
TSH	92.9	0	41.2

* : Per cent of patients with hormone level in the 95% confidencs limits of normal mean.

If the TSH level is excluded (of no interest in hyperthyroidism, but of major significance in hypothyroidism), our results seem to indicade that measurement of FT3 and FT4 leads to better distinction between normal status and thyroid dysfunction when compared to the other tests analyzed.

The laboratory data and calculated indexes of clinical diagnosis were found to be highly correlated ($p < 0.001$). Table 3 shows that the correlation between the clinical probability of hyperthyroidism and hormone levels decreases in the following order : FT3, FT4, FTI, T3, T4, with TSH displaying the poorest correlation. In the case of hypothyroidism the rank order was different since TSH levels were more highly correlated to clinical probability than the FT4 and FTI values, followed in decreasing order by FT3, T4 and T3 levels.

TABLE 3

CORRELATION BETWEEN CLINICAL DIAGNOSIS INDEXES* AND PLASMA HORMONE MEASUREMENTS**

	Hyperthyroidism Index	Hypothyroidism Index
FT3	0.814***	- 0.512
FT4	0.796	- 0.533
FTI	0.788	- 0.523
T3	0.784	- 0.467
T4	0.776	- 0.502
TSH	- 0.465	0.742

* Calculated from J.E. Overall et al, JAMA 183 : 307 (1963)
** Clinical indexes and plasma hormone levels were determined on normals (n = 45), hypothyroid (n = 51) and hyperthyroid patients (n = 42)
*** Coefficient of correlation

The relative diagnostic capacity of the hormone measurements was further studied by discriminant analysis (Figure 1). When each variable was examined separately we found that only FT3 levels in the case of hyperthyroidism, and TSH values in hypothyroidism, were able to significantly ($p < 2.5\%$) distinguish between normal and pathological status. When pairs of variables were analyzed FT3 coupled with either FT4 or FTI were of the most diagnostic value in cases of hyperthyroidism as compared to pairing FT4 with T3 and FTI with T3. In hypothyroidism TSH coupled with FT4 displayed greater diagnostic ability than TSH-FTI. Finally, when variables were grouped by 3, the association of TSH-FT3-FT4 displayed an error probability almost identical to than obtained when all variables were taken together. Association of TSH-FTI-T3 compared to TSH-FT3-FT4 demonstrated a very clear diagnostic superiority in the latter group when hyperthyroidism was involved ($p < 2.5\%$ vs. $p < 5\%$), whereas the difference between the 2 groups was less pronounced in hypothyroidism ($p < 2.5\%$ for both groups of 3 variables).

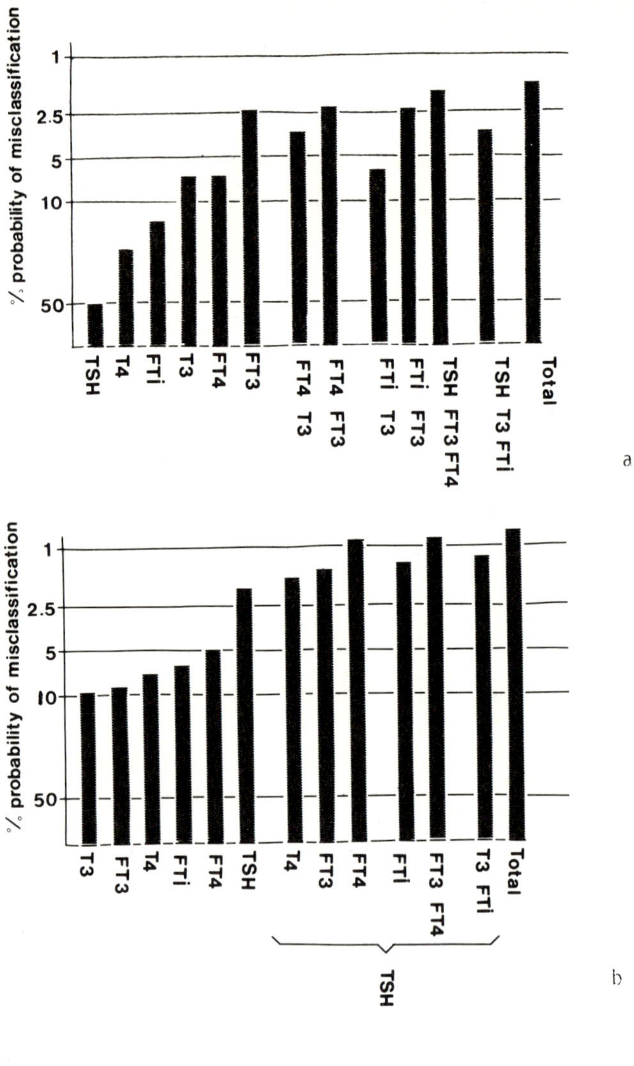

Fig. 1. Relative probability for hyper- (a) or and hypothyroid (b) patients to be misclassified as normal condisering different clusters of hormone determinations. Discriminant analysis was performed as indicated under methods.

Another point to be examined involves the eventual benefit of adding free hormone measurements to those commonly used in thyroid evaluation. Figure 2 shows that supplementing FTI and T3 with measurement of FT3 leads to better discriminant in hyperthyroidism. However, in both hypo- and hyperthyroidism even the probability of misclassification is reduced when free hormones are associated with other tests, the same error level is roughly attended as that found when TSH, FT3 and FT4 measurements are exclusively taken into account.

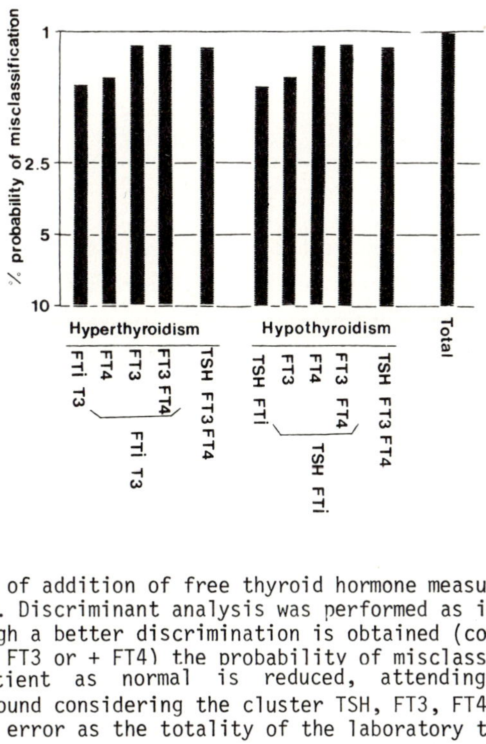

Fig. 2. Effect of addition of free thyroid hormone measurements to other available tests. Discriminant analysis was performed as indicated under methods. Although a better discrimination is obtained (compare total and routine tests + FT3 or + FT4) the probability of misclassification of a thyrotathic patient as normal is reduced, attending roughly the same level as that found considering the cluster TSH, FT3, FT4. This late provides almost the same error as the totality of the laboratory tests taking together.

Results obtained in the comparative study of diagnostic ability of the different hormone measurements are summarized in Table 4.

TABLE 4

RELATIVE DIAGNOSTIC POTENCY OF HORMONE LEVEL MEASUREMENTS

		Hyperthyroidism	Hypothyroidism
UNIVARIATE ANALYSIS	Misclassification of Hyper- and hypothyroid patients	FT3 >FT4 = T3 >FTI	TSH >FT4 = FT3 >FTI
	Analysis of variance followed by t-test	FT3 >FT4 >T3 >FTI	TSH >FT4 >FTI > T4
	Correlation between clinical indexes and hormone levels	FT3 >FT4 >FTI >T3	TSH >FT4 >FTI >FT3
MULTIVARIATE ANALYSIS	Bivariate discriminant analysis	(FT3-FT4) >(FTI-T3)	(TSH-FT4) >(TSH-FTI)
	Trivariate discriminant analysis	(FT3,FT4,TSH) > (FTI-T3-TSH)	(TSH-FT4-FT3) > (TSH-FTI-T3)

DISCUSSION

As previously described[18] the method for FT3 and FT4 determinations matched well with the requirements of routine clinical laboratory : the sensitivity (least detectable concentrations of FT3 and FT4) was respectively 0.43 and 0.55 pg/ml ; cross-reactivity was always less than 0.3% at the exception of Triac 30% with the anti-T3 antisera ; the reproductibility (between-assay variability) was 11.2 for FT3 and 12.6 for FT4.

The normal ranges found in this study were 2.4-4.9 pg/ml and 5.8-18.2 pg/ml for FT3 and FT4, respectively. These evaluations in 45 normal subjects fit well with assays performed on 31 women under oral contraceptives. In the case of FT4 measurement the normal values obtained are practically identical to those published by authors using RIA of the free hormon fraction[11, 19]. On the other hand, our normal values are lower than those reported by workers using indirect measurement techniques[4, 8], as previously pointed out by Ekins[19]. In the case of FT3 measurement, the observed mean value is slightly lower than that described by authors using either the same technique of measurement of free fractions after dialysis : 5.1[11], 5.0[18], 5.2[10], and 6.5 pg/ml[20]. This slight difference may be related to technical considerations (measurement in plasma, freeze-thawing) or variations in selection of normal subjects.

Our results showed that measurement of FT3 and FT4 led to better discrimination between normal status and hyperthyroidism. In the case of hypothyroidism, coupling of TSH and FT4 determinations showed the most significant diagnostic ability. It was also demonstrated that supplementing commonly performed thyroid tests with measurement of the free hormone fractions was of only poor diagnostic importance. This point leads to discuss the eventual position of FT3 and FT4 measurement in the battery of thyroid function tests. Regarding use of these tests the commonly accepted approach is as follows : in suspected hyperthyroidism FTI is measured and if doubt persists T3 should be ascertained ; when hypothyroidism is suspected TSH and FTI are generally advised. Since the advent of free hormone measurements, the following approach is feasible : FT3 and FT4 should be ascertained in suspected hyperthyroidism whereas TSH and FT4 should be measured when suspecting hypothyroidism. The relative difficulty in measuring FT3 and FT4 as compared to ascertaining FTI and T3 would be compensated by the increased diagnostic discrimination using the former.

Another point in favor of the free thyroid hormone measurements is the cost/benefit ratio : indeed, FT4 determination is more discriminant than FTI, for a price ratio 1/2 i.e. 1 test in the case of FT4 in contrast with two (T4 and T3 uptake test) in the case of FTI. On the other hand for the same price equivalent as FTI (2 tests) the measurement of FT3 and FT4, much more discriminative than the former, permits the evaluation of the active circulating concentrations of both thyroid hormones which, are not always correlated in altered thyroid status. Such a modification in the longstanding laboratory approach to thyroid disease requires further studies of the diagnostic ability of free hormone measurements and that results obtained by different workers be similar.

ACKNOWLEDGMENTS

We thank Pr. G.Kaphan, (Laboratoire des Isotopes, Hôpital de la Conception, Marseille), Pr. H. Roux, Pr. J.P. Bisset, Dr. F. Roux (Service Central de Médecine Nucléaire, Hôpital de la Timone, Marseille) for having carried out the T4 and T3-uptake measurements.

We thank Dr E. Goldstein for preparation of the English manuscript.

The secretariat assistance of Nicole Ghirardi and Marie-Christine Vaillant was greatly appreciated.

REFERENCES

1. Recant, L. and Riggs, D.S. (1952) Thyroid function in nephrosis, J. Clin. Invest. 31, 789.

2. Robins, J. and Rall, J.E. (1957) The interaction of thyroid hormones and proteins in biological fluids, Recent Progr. Hormone Res. 12, 161.

3. Christensen, L.K. (1959) A method for the determination of free non-protein bound thyroxine in serum, Scand. J. Clin. Lab. Invest. 11, 326.

4. Sterling, K. and Hegedus, A. (1962) Measurement of free thyroxine concentrations in human serum, J. Clin. Invest. 41, 1031.

5. Cavalieri, R.R., Castle, J.N. and Searle, G.L. (1969) A simplified method for estimation free thyroxine fraction in serum. J. Nucl. Med. 10, 565.

6. Lee, N.D., Henry, R.J. and Golub, O.J. (1964) Determination of the free thyroxine content of serum. J. Clin. Endocrinol. Metab. 24, 486.

7. Schussler, G.C. and Plager, J.E. (1967) Effect of preliminary purification of I-131 thyroxine, on the determination of the free thyroxine in serum, J. Clin. Endocrinol. Metab. 27, 242.

8. Kumagai, L.F., Jubiz, W. and Jessop, L.D. (1967) A simple and rapid method for determining free thyroxine by charcoal adsorption, Clin. Res. 15, 124.

9. Ellis, S. and Ekins, R. (1973) The direct measurement by radioimmunoassay of the free thyroid hormone concentrations in serum. Acta Endocrinologica (Kbh)) 106, Suppl. 177.

10. Weeke, J. and Örskov, H. (1975) Ultrasensitive radioimmunoassay for direct determination of free triiodothyronine concentration in serum, Scand. J. Clin. Lab. Invest. 35, 237.

11. Romelli, P.B. and Pennisi, F. (1977) A simple and precise method for measurement of free T3 and free T4 in serum, Convegno su "RIA 77. Recenti progressi in radioimmunologica clinica". Brescia, March.

12. Overall, J.E., Williams, K.M. and Williams, C.M. (1963) Conditional probability program for diagnosis of thyroid function. J. Am. Med. Assn. 183, 307.

13. Winkler, C., Reichertz, P. and Kloss, G. (1967) Computer diagnosis of thyroid diseases. Comparison of incidence data and considerations on the problem of data-collection, Am. J. Clin. Sci. 253, 27.

14. Jacquet, Ph., Franchimont, P., Rinaldi, J.P., Sianty, J.M. (1972) Le dosage radioimmunologique de hTSH plasmatique. Résultats chez le sujet normal et en pathologie, Ann. Endocrinol. 33, 305.

15. Carayon, P., Jaquet, Ph., Codaccioni, J.L., and Vague, J. (1974) Dosage radioimmunologique simultané de la thyroxine et de la triiodothyronine. Techniques et applications cliniques, Ann. Endocrinol. 35, 275.

16. Armitage, P. (1974) Statistical methods in medical research, 3rd Printing. Blackweel Scientific Publication, London.

17. Anderson, T.W. (1958) An introduction to multivariate statistical analysis, J. Willey, N. York.

18. Carayon, P., Castanas, E., Guibout, M. and Codaccioni, J.L. (1978) Assessment and clinical significance of free thyroid hormone radioimmunoassays. International Symposium on Free Thyroid Hormones, Venice December 11-12, Excerpta Medica Publ. Amsterdam (in press).

19. Ekins, R. (1977) Radioimmunoassay of free thyroid hormones in serum, Congress RIA 1977 "Recent Progress in Clinical Radioimmunology" Brescia, March.

20. Yeo, P.P.B., Lewis, M. and Evered, D.C. (1977) Radioimmunoassay of free thyroid hormone concentrations in the investigation of thyroid disease, Clin. Endocrinol. 6, 159.

Radioimmunology 1979, Ch. A. Bizollon, editor.

VALUE OF THYROID HORMONE ASSESSMENT DURING STIMULATION AND SUPPRESSION TESTS

J.L. LATAPIE, D. DUCASSOU, G. LEFORT, M.J. LANET ; Hôpital du Haut-Lévèque
33604 PESSAC.

INTRODUCTION

In the past, the investigation of the functional activity of the thyroïd gland has utilized mainly the uptake of radioactive isotopes of Iodine. With the development of thyroïd hormone assays and the oncoming of thyrotropin - releasing hormone (TRH) test, such tests as the TSH stimulation test (Querido) and the T3 suppression test (Werner) have somewhat lost their value. Such dynamic tests assessing the functional activity of the thyroïd with the use of thyroïd hormones assays as indicator are not of common practice.

What does not have at one's disposal in this field ?

The suppression of T4 by T3 as proposed by Stein and Nicolof in 1971 and by Duick (1) in 1975 : when 100 g of T3 is given daily, the serum levels of T4 decrease regulary to a minimum value within 3 weeks. This procedure has not become a routine investigation probably because of its duration and also because of the large doses of T3 required.

Hormonal stimulation by TSH : the simplest procedure as describeb by VAN HERLE and CHOPRA (2) consists of a 10 I.U. injection of TSH wich induces at the 8th hour a 100 % increase of T3 (132 ± 6 ng/100 ml) and (264 ± 46 ng/100 ml) and a 60 % rise in T4 values (7.5 ± 0.9 g and 11.4 ± 1.4 g).

The most interesting test however, appears to be the measurement of T3 coupled with the TRH stimulation test.

From a theoretical point of view, the response yields information on the hypothalamus - pituitary - thyroïd axis. From a practical point of view, it answers the demanding criteria one is entitled to expect from such an investigation : a simple, rapide, convenient, easily repeated and low costly procedure. After Shenk in 1972, then Loos and Rotenbuchner, because of the inter relationship between the T3 delta and the TSH delta, Squire and Gimlett (3) proposed the test as a routine diagnostic investigation.

Our study concerning 307 cases, covers the period extending from January 77 to April 78.

MATERIALS AND METHOD

The 307 subjects are divided in the following way :

- Control group : 22 normal subjects without the least clinical evidence of disease and who were not receiving any therapy ;
- Euthyroīd patients : 62 cases aged 16 to 70 having come to the clinic for complaints independant of the thyroīd field (excess weight 20 % of the theoretical weight, anxiety neurosis, non organic weakness and fatigability, male intertility with idiopathic oligo spermia) ;
- Hyperthyroīd patients : 69 cases of which 33 were in active phase and 36 clinically cured after treatment with I 131 ;
- TOXIC adenomas : 36 cases with or without signs of thyrotoxicosis ;
- Hypothyroidism : 33 patients, excluding thoses cases of historical mexoedema where the clinical diagnosis leaves no doubt and for which the TRH test obvioully has no interest ;
- Treated hypothyroīdism : 7 cases, the investigation was performed when clinically a normal metabolic state had been obtained ;
- Non secreting pituitary tumors ; 37 (adenomas, craniopharyngiomas) ;
- Simple goitre : 10 cases with a normal thyroīd function ;
- Simple goitre treated with triiodothyronine : 15 cases ;
- Finally, 25 patients suffering from various diseases of which 5 isolated exophtalmos, 7 cases of depression receiving antidepressant drugs, 4 constitutional dwarfisms, 3 anorexia nervosae, 4 isolated hyperprolactinisms, 1 adrenocortical insufficiency, 1 adrenocortical hyperfunction.

The TRH test was performed with an I.V. injection of 200 g and began between 8 and 8.30 a;m; after a night's fast.

Blood samples were taken for the assy of TSH at the following times : - 10 min. 0 min, 10, 20, 30, 60, 90, 120, 180. For the T3, T4, RT3U, 2 blood samples were taken at the times 0 min and 180 min. All the assays were done in duplicate.

Different radioimmunoassay kits were used : T3 (Lepetit), TSH (Pharmacia), T4 (Saclay), RT3U (Amersham).

RESULTS

1) Normal subjects.

The values obtained for the control group with respect to the euthyroid patients were not significantly different ; the delta TSH (mean + 2 SD) being set between 3 and 20 microg. Whereas for the delta T3 it was difficult to define a normal range because of the considerable standard deviation. The delta T3 was therefore considered negative when the increase was less than 10 % of the basal value, the maximum normal rise being arbitrarily fixed at 60 % (mean + 1 SD).

NORMAL SUBJECTS

(No = 84)

	MEAN ± SD	95 % Confidence limits
T4	7.75 ± 1.56 μg/dl	4.5 - 11 μg/dl
T3	122 ± 27 ng/dl	70 - 180 ng/dl
RT3U	102 ± 7.25	88 - 118

NORMAL SUBJECTS

	Δ TSH Max μ U/dl)	Δ T3 1) ng/dl 2) % of increase
Controls	11.6 ± 4.2	1) 39.3 ± 18 2) 34.5 ± 18 %
Euthyroid subjects	11.3 ± 4.6	1) 36.8 ± 22.8 2) 32.9 ± 22.3 %

There was no correlation (linear, parabolic or exponential) between the maximum TSH and the delta T3 whether expressed in absolute values or percent increase.

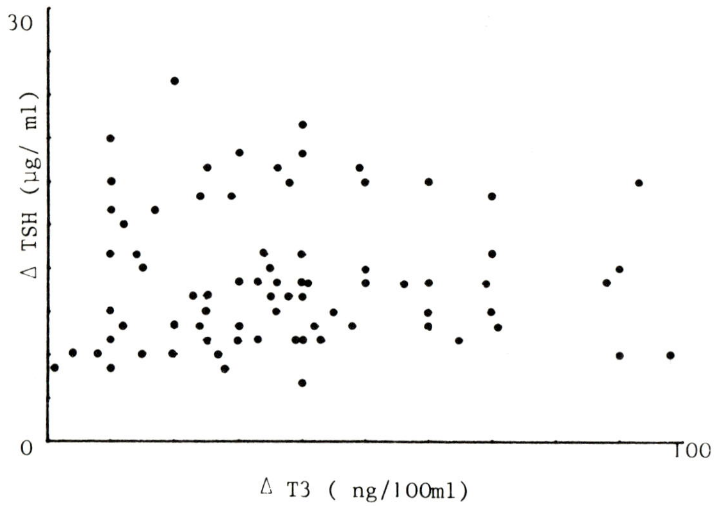

Fig. 3. T3 increment at t = 180 min after Bolus TRH Versus maximal increment of TSH during the same test, in 84 euthyroïd subjects. No significant correlation.

There was no correlation either, between the delta T3 and the basic values of T3 T4 and ITL.

The correlation between T3 and the total cumulative response loci of TSH values during the TRH test was also negative (R = 0.01).

Out of the 84 cases, 10 times there was no reponse in terms of T3 whereas the TSH delta was normal (5 obese, 3 neurovegetative disorders, 2 control subjects). On the other hand in one case a delta TSH of 1.5 was accompanied by a surprisingly high response of T3 of above 80 % ; all the other hormonal parameters were normal in these cases.

2) Active hyperthyroïdism

In all the cases the delta TSH was null and the delta T3 either null or negative. In 4 cases there was an isolated rise in T4 levels and in another 4 cases an isolated rise in T3 levels.

3) Cured hyperthyroïdism

7 of these cases had hyper TSH responses with normal T3 responses, 2 of

which became hypothyroïd ; of the latter one had a low ITL value whilst the other had low ITL and T3 values.

The 3 cases with a hyper TSH response and no T3 response became hypothyroïd but 2 of these already had low ITL values.

Finally, 2 of the 8 cases where there was no response either in terms of TSH or T3 developed secondary hypothyroïdism with normal hormonal parameters.

All the other patients were still stabilized one year later.

APPARENTLY EUTHYROID PATIENTS AFTER TREATMENT FOR GRAVES DISEASE'
n = 27

	ΔT3 > 60% No subjets	Δ T3 N No subjects	ΔT3 < 10% No subjects
Δ TSH > 20 μU/dl		7 [a]	3 [b]
Δ TSH N	1	3	1
Δ TSH < 3 μU/dl		4	8 [c]

HYPOTHYROIDISM FOLLOWING 131 I THERAPY

	T4< 4.5	RT3U> 118	T3 < 70
a) 2	2	2	1
b) 3	2	2	
c) 2			

4) Toxic adenomas

Twice all the static and dynamic hormonal parameters were normal. In 34 cases there was no TSH increase, correspondingly 26 of these showed no rise in T3 values. 8 times however the delta T3 was normal. On the whole, considering the 36 toxic adenomas, 3 patients only showed an isolated rise in T3, 3 other patients showed an isolated rise in T4 too, and there was a simultaneous rise in both hormones in 13 cases.

T4and T3.

In the population of 17 positive T3 reactions there was a positive correlation (0.72 p, 0.001).

HYPOTHYROIDISM (No = 33)

	ΔT3 > 60 % No subjects	T3 N No subjects	ΔT3 < 10 % No subjects
Δ TSH > 20 μU /dl		17 a	15 b
Δ TSH N			
Δ TSH < 3 μg /dl			1

	T4 < 4.5 μU/dl and RT3U > 118	T3 < 70 ng/dl	T3 and T4 < N	TSH > 12 μU/dl
a	7	2	6	9
b			15	15

6) Treated hypothyroïdism

All the hormonal parameters were normal in 5 out of 7 cases, twice a lowering of thyroïd hormone values was accompanied by a TSH hyper response to TRH stimulation whilst the triiodothyronine values did not vary during any of the tests.

7) Simple goitre

The TSH response were all normal except the one case where a hyper TSH response was followed by a delta T3 of over 80 %.

8) Treated goitre

14 patients receiving 50 to 75 g of T3 failed to respond either in terme of TSH or T3 values. One case showed a simultaneous rise of TSH and T3.

9) Pituitary tumours

The results obtained were quite varied and dependant on the extension of the tumour whether associated with hypopituitarism or not. Although 16 cases had normal biological charecters, 8 times however there was a lack of TSH

HOT NODULES
No = 36

	ΔT3 > 60 % No Subjects	T3 N No Subjects	ΔT3 < 10 % No Subjects
Δ TSH > 20 μU/dl			
Δ TSH : N		2	
Δ TSH < 3 μU /dl		8 a	26 b

	T3 > 180 ng / dl	T4 > 11 μg / dl	T3 and T4 > N
a		2	2
b	3	1	11

5) Hypothyroïdism

We have not included in this study early post radioiodine hypothyroïdism in Graves' disease because they are usually transitory and frequently lack TSH response to TRH stimulation. In very mild cases, the clinical and biological course of the disease confirmed that the hypothyroïd state was definitive and that it gradually worsened as time went by.

32 times out of 33 the TSH values rose above 20 microU., once however, there was no response, this concerned a patient with Graves' disease known for several years already and who had been treated 4 months earlier with radioiodine.

T3 response was paradoxically normal in 17 subjects with an isolated fall in T4 alone in 7 cases, of T3 alone in 2 cases and of both hormones in 6 cases.

The basal value of TSH was above normal 9 times only. In all the 15 cases for which a hyper TSH response was accompanied by a lack of T3 response, there was an increase of TSH above 12 microU. and a simultaneous lowering of both response followed by a normal T3 response (mean 45 %). 6 times the T4 values fall during the test and twice both T3 and T4 decreased. In one case however the delta TSH was not absolutely null but increased from 2 micro U. to 3.5 microU./ml. One may suppose that there was in fact a more important transient increase in between the two samples and that continuous blood sampling would have been preferable.

PITUITARY TUMORS
n = 37

	T3 > 60 % No subjects	T3 = N No subjects	T3 < 10% No subjects
TSH > 20 µU / dl	2 a	3 b	1 c
TSH = N		16 d	3 e
TSH < 3 µU / dl		8 f	4 g

	T4 < 4.5 µg/dl	CLF > 118	T3 < 70 ng/dl	T3 and T4 < N
a	1	1		
d				1
f	6	4		2
g				4

10) Various diseases

It is worth retaining that of 7 patients receiving antidepressant and anxiolitic drugs, 5 had no TSH response whilst T3 reaction was subnormal. Static hormone levels were nevertheless normal.
This type of response is quite similar to that obtained in sellar and suprasellar tumours.

Of the 5 isolated exophtalmos, 4 did not respond in terms of both TSH and T3, there was onlyahigh T3 basal value.

In all the other cases, the delta T3 did not bring any further information than did the static hormonal assays and TSH response to TRH.

CONCLUSIONS

There seems to be a very limited practical interest in the assessment of delta T3 during TRH test.

The individual variations of the responses are so important that the standard deviation, whether expressed in absolute figures or in percent increase from the initial level, is almost equal to half the mean value. This is not surprising as the TSH response itself can vary from a single to a seven fold increment (3 to 20 microU/ml) and that the thyroïd has a variable response potential from one person to another. This is illustrated in the fact that several normal subjects who responded in terms of TSH did not show any change in T3 levels (almost 10 % of the normal cases).

T3 increase after TRH stimulation does not seem to be able to replace the TSH assays as was proposed by Squire and Gimlette. However, T3 assessment may eventually serve as a substitute to TSH assays in the diagnosis of hyperthyroïdism, except for toxic adenomas, with the reserve that other cases confirm this notion.

This technique seems to have a certain prognostic value after radioiodine therapy for hyperthyroïdism. When there is a normal or increased response in TSH with a lack of T3 increment, there seems to be a significant frequency of secondary hypothyroïdism, but we are too near (1 year) to be able to certiffy that the other cases will not have the same course. The fact that T3 does not respond in certain normal subjects makes this idea even more difficult to assert.

Finally, it is worthwile recalling that 14 % of the cases without TSH responses increased their T3 values during the test.

This noteworthy paradox was found in those disorders where there is a hypothalamus - pituitary inertia (cured hyperthyroïdism, hypopituitarism, toxic-adenomas, neuroleptic induced), - which may lead one to believe that TSH recepters increase when the gland is hypo-stimulated.

REFERENCES

1 Duick (D.S.) et al, (1975) J.Clin. Endocr. Metab. 41, 229 - 234

2 Uller (R.P.) et al, (1977) J. Clin. Endocr. Metab. 45, 312 - 318

3 Squire (C.R.) and Gimlette (T.P.D.) (1977) J.Clin. Path. 30, 635 - 637

© 1979 Elsevier/North-Holland Biomedical Press
Radioimmunology 1979, Ch. A. Bizollon, editor.

APPLICATIONS OF THYROGLOBULIN IN MEASUREMENT TO THE FOLLOW-UP OF PATIENTS WITH CARCINOMA OF THE THYROID.

Martin SCHLUMBERGER, Pierre CHARBORD, Paule GARDET, Claude PARMENTIER, Maurice TUBIANA
Laboratoire de Physiopathologie thyroïdienne, Institut de Recherches de Radiobiologie Clinique, Villejuif, France.

The production of iodoproteins by metastases of differentiated thyroid carcinoma was demonstrated by the measurement of serum protein bound Iodine (PBI) and by the presence of labelled PBI after the administration of radio-iodine (1).

In 1967, Roitt and Torrigiani (2) described a radioimmunoassay of thyro-globulin (Tg) in human serum. Later Van Herle (3) simplified the technique and increased its sensitivity. This made its use possible in the follow-up of patients with differentiated thyroid carcinoma. Tg appears to be a useful marker since its level is low or undetectable in cases of complete remission but ele-vated in cases of metastases or of local recurrences (4, 5, 6).

The purpose of thisstudy was both to assess the usefulness of this assay during the follow-up of patients with thyroid carcinoma and also to analyse factors which may influence the level of serum Tg.

METHODS AND PATIENTS

The technique used is that described by Van Herle (3). The antibody was raised in white New Zealand rabbits challenged with Tg provided by A.J.Van Herle. The dilution used was :1:50 000.

Then we purified Tg from the thyroid of a patient with Grave'sdisease which had the same immunoreactivity as the one supplied by A.J. Van Herle.

^{131}I-Tg was obtained by labelling purified Tg according to the method of Greewood, Hunter and Glover. Its specific activity ranged between 60 and 120 μCi/μg which made possible the introduction of less than 10^{-2} ng of tracer per tube. Sucrose density gradient centrifugation showed the predominance of ^{131}I-Tg of 19S variety. The immunoprecipitability was 87 % in the presence of an excess of a specific antibody. 6 to 8 % of the radioactivity added was non specifically bound. In the absence of unlabelled antigen and with the antibody dilution used, 45-60 % of ^{131}I-Tg was bound. The dilution curve could be used between 5 and 80 ng/ml. Sera containing more than 100 ng/ml were diluted and measured again. The overall sensitivity of the system was 2,5 ng/ml.

There was no cross reaction with T_4, L-T_3, RT_3, MIT or DIT concentrations up to 100μg/ml, concentrations which greatly exceed those encountered in thyrotoxic individuals.

The dilution curves of 3 sera from patients with lung or bone metastases of differentiated thyroid carcinoma were parallel with that of the standard Tg preparation. Moreover the 12S, 19S and 27S fractions isolated by sucrose density gradient centrifugation had the same immunoreactivity as purified Tg.

The recovery of the Tg added to a normal serum (10, 20, 40 and 50 ng) ranged from 95 to 105 %. Intra-assay variation was 6.2 % and inter-assay variation 18 % (20 assays) for a sample having a Tg level of 11.5 ng/ml.

Before measurement, all serum samples were tested for the presence of Tg autoantibodies by the tanned red cell agglutination technique (Wellcome Kit). Samples with positive titers were not assayed. The incidence of positivity among patients with differentiated thyroid carcinoma was 5.9 % (11 patients out of 186 tested patients).

Among 51 subjects of both sexes, aged 21-80, without known thyroid disease, the level was 13.9 $\pm$ 6.9 ng/ml ($\overline{m} \pm$ SD). The levels ranged from undetectable values (4 subjects) to 29.5 ng/ml.

TSH was measured with the CEA Kit (normal range 2-6 μU/ml).

Patients

We studied the Tg levels in serum samples from 150 patients with thyroid carcinoma who had already been treated and followed-up at the Institut Gustave-Roussy and for whom the search of Tg autoantibodies had been negative.

RESULTS

1 -Patients without any known metastases or residual tumoral tissue (figure 1)

1a) 30 patients had no residual thyroid tissue after thyroidectomy and a prophylactic administration of Iodine 131. In 17 patients without former detection of areas of ectopic I-131 uptake, Tg levels were $\leq$ 5 ng/ml in 10 patients, between 5 and 9 ng/ml in 6 and equal to 38.5 ng/ml in 1 patient. The average value for these 17 subjects was 7.4 ng/ml.

In 13 patients, scintigraphy performed after the therapeutic application of Iodine 131 had formerly shown the existence of an ectopic cervical zone of uptake. The Tg levels were inferior to 5 ng/ml in only 2 patients and ranged from 7 to 19.5 ng/ml in 11 patients, the average being 12.8 ng/ml which was significantly higher than in the former group ($p < 0.001$). Despite the present absence of any zone of uptake, this suggested the existence of residual tumoral tissue but either in too small quantities or with too low uptake to be detected by scintigraphy.

Figure 1

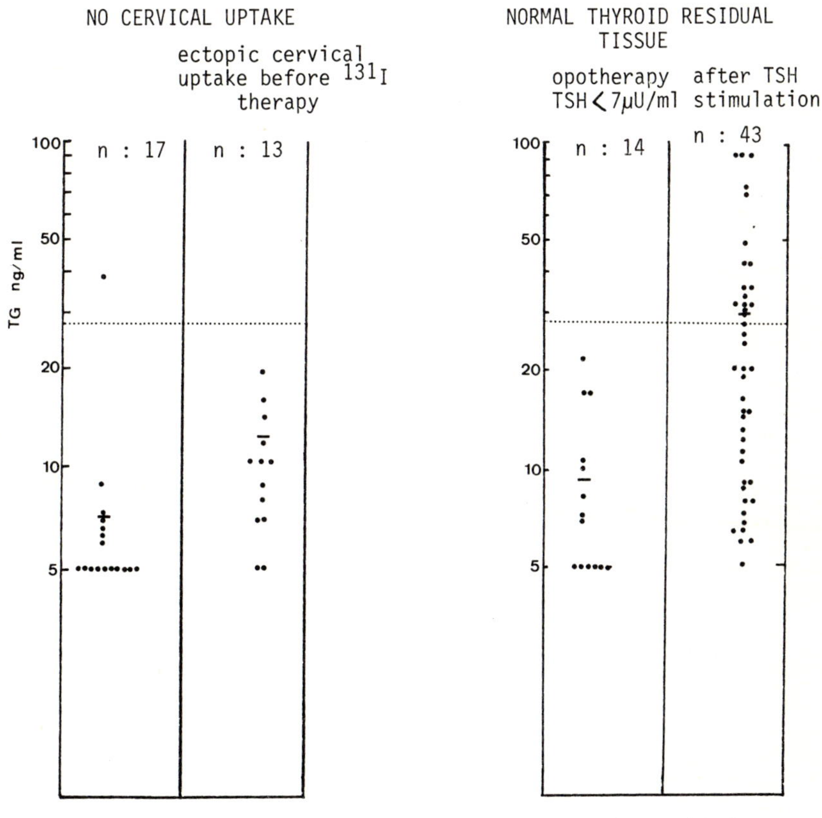

Serum Tg levels in 87 patients without detectable residual tumoral tissue. The upper limit of the normal range is indicated by the interrupted horizontal line.

1b) 57 patients treated by surgery alone had normal thyroid residual tissue without known metastases. In 14 patients under replacement hormonal therapy in suppressive doses (TSH $< 7\,\mu U/ml$), the Tg levels ranged from 5 to 22.5 ng/ml ($\overline{m}$ = 9.3 ng/ml). After stimulation with bTSH (3 x 10 uI , serum drawn on the fourth day) the levels ranged from 5 to 120 ng/ml ($\overline{m}$ = 29 ng/ml). This wide range of values could be due to factors such as the quantity of normal residual thyroid tissue, the intensity of TSH stimulation or the existence of occult tumoral tissue. We did not find any correlation between the Tg level and the radioiodine uptake on the third day.

2- Patients with bone or lung metastases after destruction of normal thyroid tissue (figure 2 and 3).

2a) Metastases with radioiodine uptake (n = 29) (figure 2).

Under hormone administration in suppressive doses, the Tg levels were elevated in all patients and ranged between 34.5 and 750 ng/ml ($\overline{m}$ = 233 ng/ml). After stimulation by bTSH or 7 days after withdrawal of replacement therapy by LT_3, the levels ranged from 81 to 8100 ng/ml for 15 cases whose radioiodine uptake by metastases on the third day was greater than 1 % of the administered activity. When the metastatic uptake was $<$ 1 % (n = 14), the Tg levels ranged from 37 to 280 ng/ml. Thus on the average the Tg levels were higher in the patients with the highest uptakes but there was an overlap between the two groups.

3 patients had had pulmonary miliary metastases formerly shown by scintigraphy and previously treated with several therapeutic I-131 doses. No uptake had been detectable after radioiodine administration for at least two years. Their post TSH stimulation levels were 6 ; 19.5 and 36.5 ng/ml.

2b) Lung or bone metastases of differentiated thyroid carcinoma without radioiodine uptake (n = 7)

Under replacement therapy in suppressive doses, the Tg levels were elevated, ranging from 43 to 220 ng/ml ($\overline{m}$ = 111 ng/ml).

2c) In 3 anaplastic giant cells carcinoma under replacement therapy in suppressive doses, Tg levels were : 7.5 ; 12.5 and 29 ng/ml

2d) In 4 cases of medullary carcinoma with metastases the Tg levels ranged between 11 and 33 ng/ml.

Figure 2

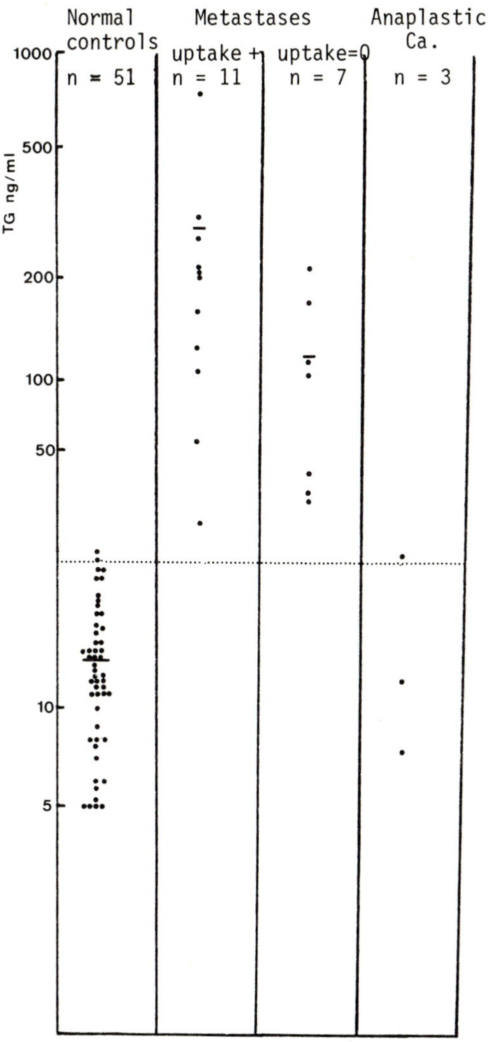

Serum Tg concentrations under replacement therapy in patients with metastases.

Figure 3

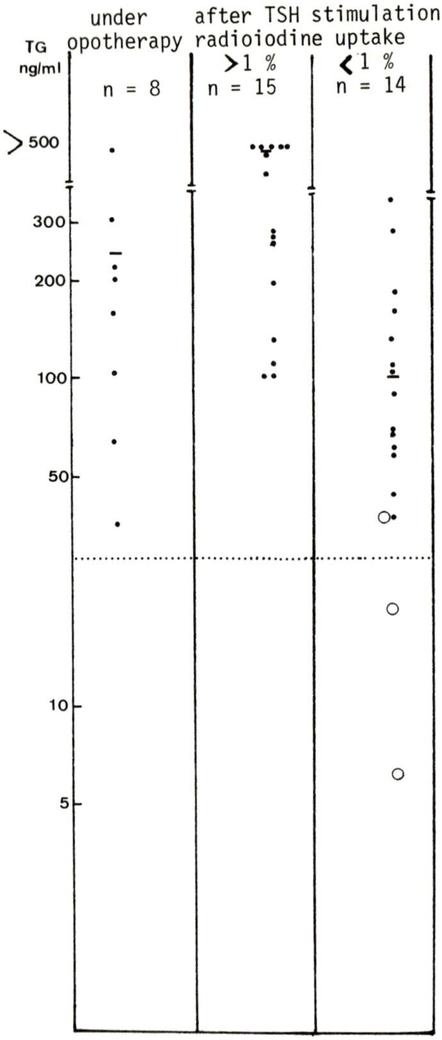

Serum Tg levels in 29 patients with metastases of differentiated thyroid carcinoma. O : treated lung isotopic miliary.

3 -12 patients without metastases but with cervical nodes which occurred after initial treatment were studied (figure 4). In 4 of these patients the surgical control showed that the nodes were free of metastases, their pre-operative levels after stimulation by bTSH were <5 ng/ml for 2 patients and 9.5 and 29 ng/ml for the 2 others. The latter ones had some residual normal thyroid tissue which could explain the observed levels.

In 8 patients whose nodes were involved with cancer the preoperative levels ranged from 13.5 to 260 ng/ml.

Figure 4

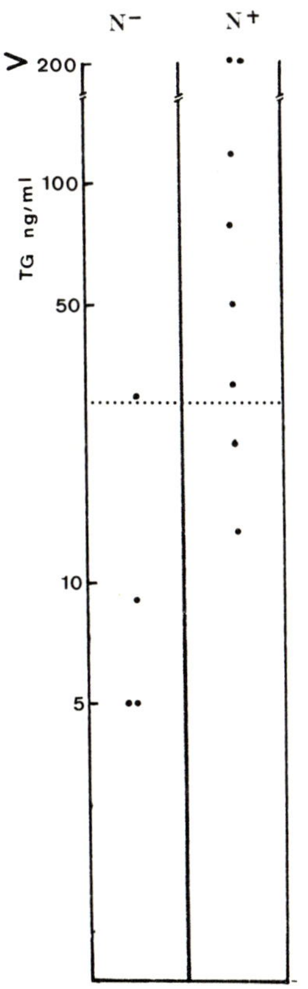

Cervical nodes : surgical control.

4 -Factors which could influence the Tg level.

4a) Bovine TSH (10 UI x 3)

In 1 patient with lung metastases of a papillary carcinoma, after injections of bTSH (10 UI x 3) under replacement therapy, the Tg level increased from 280 to 490 ng/ml 2 days after the third injection. The level remained high during 3 days, then dropped back to its initial value 5 days after the third injection.

4b) Effect of endogeneous TSH (figure 5)

In 4 patients with lung or bone metastases, the increase in Tg level after withdrawal of opotherapy occurred 3 to 8 days after the increase in the TSH level and reached, within 8 to 16 days, a plateau equal to 2.3 to 12 times its initial value.

In 1 patient with lung metastases without radioiodine uptake, the drop of TSH level from 95 to 8 μU/ml under replacement therapy occurred simultaneously with the drop of Tg level from 93 to 45 ng/ml.

Figure 5

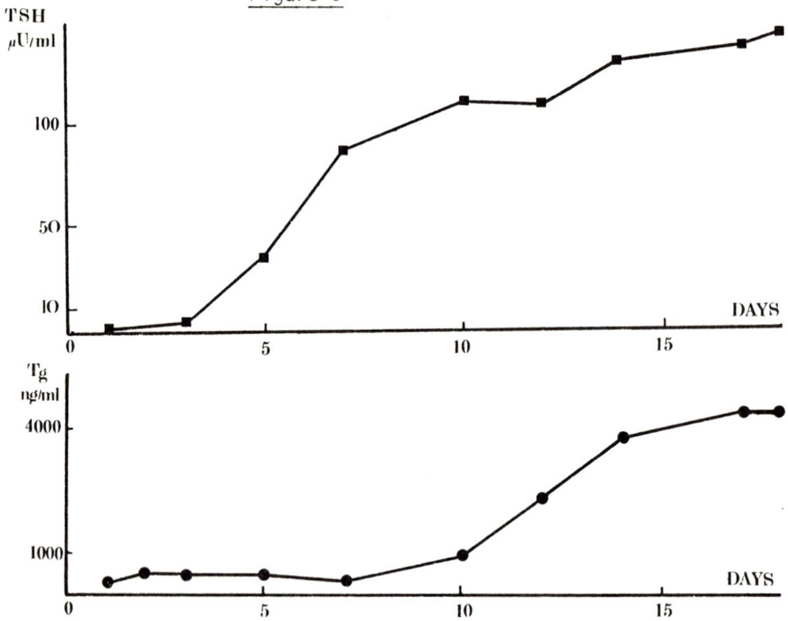

Effect of TSH on serum Tg level in a patient with lung metastases of a papillary carcinoma.
Study after withdrawal of LT_3 on day zero.

However in 1 case of anaplastic giant cells carcinoma relapsing in the neck and the mediastinum, the Tg level during replacement therapy (12.5 ng/ml) was only 16 ng/ml 10 days after withdrawal of replacement therapy. During this period an increase in the cervical and mediastinal tumoral mass was observed.

4c) Effect of Carbimazole

In 1 patient after TSH and Tg plateau level concentrations had been reached, Carbimazole (60 mg per day) was administered during 9 days. The level of LT_3 dropped to undetectable values. No significant variation in the TSH or Tg levels were observed till the tenth day after the end of Carbimazole administration. This finding suggests that there is no direct effect of Carbimazole on the synthesis of Tg or its release in the serum.

4d) Effect of Iodine 131

After the administration of 100 mCi of Iodine 131, it was possible to follow the activity linked to the circulating Tg in 8 patients with metastases of differentiated thyroid carcinoma with radioiodine uptake. In 5 of them no radioactive Tg was found 5 days after the administration of Iodine 131. Ih 3 patients the activity increased as soon as the third day and was still high in 2 patients on the 9th and 17th day of the study. Moreover, in thecases studied, later than five days after the administration of a therapeutic iodine 131 activity, a considerable amount of Tg (figure 6) was found in the serum.

FIGURE 6

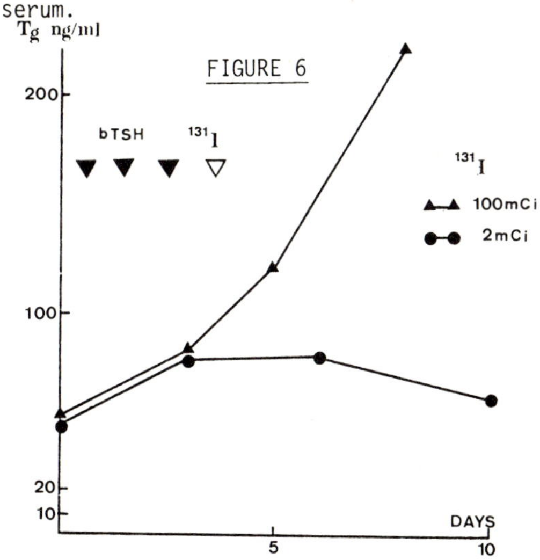

Effect of 131 Iodine on serum Tg level.

DISCUSSION

The significance of Tg measurement in the follow-up of treated carcinoma has already been point out by Van Herle (4, 5) and Logerfo (6). The data presented in this paper confirm this observation.

The serum Tg level was undetectable after complete removal of the thyroid tissue and was found elevated in cases with local recurrences or distant metastases. However during relapses of anaplastic giant cell carcinomas the Tg level remained low.

There seems to be some correlation between the amount of malignant tissue and the serum Tg level. In fact the Tg levels were higher in cases of large metastases easily detected by other investigations (radiology or scintigraphy) and lower when the volume of metastases was small. However the amount of tumor cell mass which can be detected by an increase in Tg level cannot be evaluated. Prospective studies in these patients are being carried out in order to assess the timing of the Tg level increase in comparison to other means of detection, as well as the implications of an early diagnosis of recurrences for the long term course of these patients.

The Tg assay however seems already to be useful in determining the nature of cervical nodes appearing during the follow-up especially when there is no iodine 131 uptake. Present data suggest that an increase should lead to surgery while a low level would indicate further follow-up. It has also been possible to determine the thyroid origin of a pulmonary nodule or of bone abnormalities by Tg measurement, even in absence of radioiodine uptake.

The Tg serum level is influenced by several factors. First, it is higher, on the average, in patients whose carcinome is able to concentrate radioactive iodine. It was already known that serum Tg is not elevated in patients with undifferentiated carcinoma. Our data further show that Tg is less elevated in differentiated carcinoma with a low functional activity than in tumors with greater functional activity, but that it can be elevated even in the absence of any detectable iodine uptake by malignant tissues. In fact there is among our patients a marked contrast between the rare occurrence of T_3 and T_4 secretion by the malignant tissues and the frequent occurrence of elevated amounts of Tg in the sera (7).

Carbimazole does not impact the Tg release by the metastases. This has already been shown during thyrotoxicosis (8). The administration of Iodine 131 activities increased Tg serum level. Our date demonstrate that neoplastic tissues release Tg even in the absence of any stimulation by TSH, however the most interesting finding is that TSH, endogeneous or bovine, causes an increase in serum Tg level. This effect was observed in all patients with metastases of differentiated thyroid carcinoma whether or not they were able to concentrate Iodine 131. This finding suggests the existence of TSH receptors in the cells of those differentiated carcinomas even when they are deprived of any functional activity. On the other hand, no effect of TSH was observed in cases of giant cells anaplastic carcinomas, which is not surprising as in vitro studies have already pointed out that those are unable to synthesize Tg.

These findings further emphasize the importance of relating the Tg level to other parameters, particularly TSH stimulation. In the absence of normal thyroid tissue, an increase in the Tg level appears to be a good marker of a tumoral recurrence and TSH stimulation seems to make this method more sensitive. However when normal thyroid tissue is still present, while an increase in Tg level under replacement therapy suggest a tumoral reccurrence, an increase after stimulation may also be due to normal tissue stimulation.

REFERENCES

1. Robbins, J., Rall, J.E. and Rawson, R.W. (1955) A new serum iodine component in patients with functionnal carcinoma of the thyroid. J. Clin. Endocrinol. Met., 15, 1315-1331

2. Roitt, I.M. and Torrigiani, G. (1967) Identification and estimation of undegraded thyroglobulin in human serum. Endocrinology, 81, 421-429

3. Van Herle, A.J., Uller, R.P., Matthews, N.L. and Brown, J. (1973) Radioimmunoassay for measurement of thyroglobulin in human serum. J. Clin. Invest., 52, 1320-1327

4. Van Herle, A.J. and Uller, R.P. (1975) Elevated serum thyroglobulin, a marker of metastases in differentiated thyroid carcinomas. J. Clin. Invest., 56, 272-277

5. Van Herle, A.J. (1977) Serum thyroglobulin levels in patients with differentiated thyroid carcinomas. Ann. Radiol., 20, 743-745

6. Logerfo, P., Stillman, T., Colacchio, D. and Feind, C. (1977) Serum thyroglobulin and recurrent thyroid cancer. Lancet, 1, 881-882

7. Schlumberger, M., Charbord, P., Fragu, P., Parmentier, C., and Tubiana, M., (1979) Production sérique d'iodoprotéines par le tissu thyroïdien métastatique. Ses relations avec la sécretion hypophysaire de TSH (en préparation).

8. Izumi, M. and Larsen, R.P. (1978) Correlation of sequential changes in serum thyroglobulin triiodothyronine and thyroxine in patients with Grave's disease and subacute thyroiditis. Metabolism, 27, 449-460.

© 1979 Elsevier/North-Holland Biomedical Press
Radioimmunology 1979, Ch. A. Bizollon, editor.

QUALITY CONTROL "IN CONTINUOUS" OF THYROID HORMONES ASSAY : THE ROLE OF THE COMPUTOR AND THE METHOD

Jean C. SAVOIE, Ghias KAWADRY, Françoise A. LEGER and Jean L. BAULIEU
Service Central de Médecine Nucléaire, Hôpital La Pitié, Paris France

The assay of thyroid hormones T4 and T3 in the serum has, over the past few years, become the key to the exploration of the thyroid function. Closely linked with this is the estimation of the free fraction of TBG, the evaluation of the Free Thyroxine Index, assay of TSH. A further problem is set by the generalized use of these measurements : that of the reliability of the results of large series that are frequently repeated. Individual verifications are not entirely satisfactory, whether undertaken in random samples or in control samples checked at regular intervals by a metrology Laboratory. A permanent verification of quality or "in continuous" which involves the use of a computor can alone straight away provide the overall data required to a/ assess the validity of any new series, b/ guarantee the value of every new result. We have developed a means of verification of this type and describe here the structure, advantages, effectiveness and limitations of this method.

1 - THE STRUCTURE of this verification is a programme of calculations of the standard curve and evaluation of variance for each point of the curve and for each measurement of the unknowns. The straightening out of the standard curves for assays of T4 and T3 was obtained by Logit-Log transformation and the best straight line of weighted regression after a maximum of four cycle criterion. The statistical calculations comply with model n°2 of RODBARD's method which takes as variance of the response a linear function of the response. This programme was developed on a SIMIS 3 - INFORMATEK system. The verification includes : binding of the tracer (Bo/T), the origin and slope of the straight line of regression, its correlation coefficient, the values of the weights, the 95 % confidence limits for each point of the standard curve or for each result, the coefficient of variation of the duplicates, the results obtained from pooled reference sera from normal and hyperthyroid subjects. The main data from the verification tests for each series are stocked on recording tapes.

These data can be compared statistically with those from n previous series for interassay comparison.

2 - THE ADVANTAGE of checking quality "in continuous" which we have experimented over the past two years resides in the multiplicity of the criteria kept under observation which have been deliberately substituted for the three criteria for estimating quality, that are just as traditional as they are unsatisfactory, i.e. precision, sensitivity and accuracy.

The following is a critical study of these three criteria.

2-1 - by precision is usually meant the degree of dispersion of a row of measurements on any one sample repeated for example from 6 to 20 times in each series : this precision being expressed by the standard deviation or relative deviation $\sigma/\bar{m}$ also called the coefficient of variation C.V. The coefficient C.V. is calculated both for any given series (intraassay) and for n series (interassay).

In actual fact this notion of precision is somewhat illusory since :

2-1a - it varies with the concentration of the ligand (heteroscedasticity particularly marked in Logit coordinates) and the C.V. is only valid for a narrow zone of concentration corresponding to that of a sample measured n times.

2-1b - it does not take into account the precision of the standard curve.

2-1c - it is at its best an optimistic estimation of the precision of unknown measurements carried out only in duplicate since a large number of repetitions of the control sample cancels out various errors (pipetting, inattention, counting position etc...)

2-1d - it is particularly necessary when devising a new method to establish its efficiency but it becomes ineffective because it is both too costly and time consuming to be integrated into the everyday practice of a routine technique.

2-2 - by sensitivity is meant both the absolute sensitivity i.e. the smallest quantity of detectable hormone and the relative sensitivity in any one given portion of the standard curve, which is maximum when a small increase in the concentration of the ligand corresponds to a large variation of the effect on B/Bo. But the sensitivity of the method which could be improved upon, should in fact, as far as the assay of thyroid hormones is concerned, comply to the objective in view. This objective is to measure as best possible the values that are lower or higher than the normal by situating the intercept B/Bo 50 % at the centre of the normal values, theoretical optimum precision for Logit representation, while allowing a wide margin above and below, necessary for estimating infra or supra normal quantities.

2-3 - by accuracy we usually mean the degree of similarity of a series of measurements deriving from any given sample in comparison to its true value. But even if the number of measurements is high and involves numerous serial examinations, it has yet to be proved that the average value is closer to the true value and it is generally agreed that the notion of "true value" is difficult to define. This is particularly true of polypeptide hormones. But it does not apply so much to the smaller haptenes such as the steroids or drugs and not at all to thyroid hormones. It so happens that for the thyroid hormones it is possible to readjust the imperfect concept of accuracy. This can be done by including within the series several normal controls where the normal values of T4 are known and measurable by independent methods (assay of ^{127}I). Furthermore it is quite feasible to prepare reference samples of exactly known concentration for example from T4 and T3-free sera enriched in accurately known amounts of synthetic T4 and T3 obtained from rigourously controlled solutions by assay of ^{127}I, by spectrophotometry, or by any other reliable method.

3 - THE EFFECTIVENESS of checking quality by continuous assay depends on taking into account numerous factors which condition the quality while conferring a numeric expression to them.

3-1 - With regard to Bo/T it is essential to realize that the radioimmunoassay (RIA) of T4 and T3 without previous extraction is a method of double protein binding. In the case of the unknowns an aliquot of known volume of the serum to be assayed contains an unspecified amout of TBG whose affinity constant is very close to that of the specific antibody. The reagents certainly contain inhibitors of TBG, but Thiomersalate, ANS... etc nevertheless leave a residual

TBG effect. So that the reference curve and unknowns can be measured in the same way, imperative condition for accuracy, only if it is included in the samples of the standard curve a volume of serum "zero" or "T4-T3 free" equal to that of the unknowns and prepared from a pool of normal sera containing a normal average quantity of TBG. Sera from subjects who have undergone total thyroidectomy and who are not submitted to a replacement therapy can also be used. Only under these conditions is Bo/T really representative of the total binding which involves the antibody and part of the TBG. Bo/T is of such great importance in the control of quality - as it is also for the absolute sensitivity of the assay - that in our programme six identical samples of Bo/T were included in every series and their average as well as their standard deviation served to calculate the parameters of RODBARD's method, making it possible to establish the confidence limits for the various points of the standard curve as well as for that of the unknowns.

3-2 - Blank : radio-ligands T4 and T3 should be as pure as possible in order to reduce the blank to a minimum. An increase in the specific activity of the tracer, although desirable, has the disadvantage of causing a radiochemical fragility of the ligand and hence an increase of the blank or "non specific binding" (NSB). The level of NSB is therefore established for each series, and included among the parameters that are used to calculate the confidence limits.

3-3 - Logit representation. The statistical calculations of quality are closely dependent on the transformation used to render the standard curve linear. The respective advantages of Logit, Probit, Arc-sin, polynomial ... transformations have been widely discussed. In practice a definite decision should be made. Most of the RIA methods can be correctly rendered linear by a Logit-Log transformation. For the RIA of T4 and T3 we chose not only the Logit transformation but also methods which can be closely and consistently made linear by Logit-Log. It so happens that among the most rapid methods for estimating T4 and T3, by solid phase methods which facilitate the separation of B and F, we chose that of using antibodies bound covalently to special type glass beads (Corning glass - USA)*, these methods being perfectly well adapted to our purposes. However many other methods are certainly quite as favourable for linear transformation by Logit-Log. The programme for automatic quality control provides, after several cycle criterion, the best adjustment of the reference curve.

3-4 - The weights. Adjustment is made by a weighted regression and the weights of the best adjustment are indicated. The quality of each point of the standard curve is inversely proportional to the value of the corresponding weight. So it is possible to immediately assess the relative precision of each portion of the standard curve. This relative precision is numerically expressed by the 95 % confidence limits for each point of the curve and for each individual result. This precision could not be assessed by averaging C.V.'s and "overall precision" is fundamentally meaningless. Moreover the confidence limits of the different points of the standard curve are purposely drawn out on a graph in which the heteroscedasticity relative to each series stands out clearly.

3-5 - Rho. The overall quality of the adjustment is expressed by the coefficient of correlation of the line of regression "Rho" (or ρ). To size up its value it shoud be emphasized that this coefficient is usually situated in the neighbourhood of 0.995 and that any coefficient lower than 0.990 is considered to indicate a defective series which should in principle be rejected or, in other words, worked out again.

3-6 - B/Bo-50. The intercept B/Bo 50 % is used as major reference of accuracy. The method was devised to situate this intercept at the centre of the normal values i.e. at the theoretical optimum of precision. It was found in practice that this was also an optimum for accuracy and that any appreciable shift of the intercept B/Bo 50 % resulted in a quite appreciable modification of the apparent normal values.

3-7 - Limits of detection. The Logit-Log transformation straightens out validly only the centre of the reference curve. Fundamentally it remains sigmoid. Consequently the utilization of the two extremities of the straight line of the Logit-Log regression is faulty since the extent of the errors due to the exploitation of the extreme limits of the straight line is the ransom of Logit transformation. Automatic assessments normally make use of any of the values situated within these extremes and this should be avoided. Evidently it is certainly possible to calculate the absolute sensitivity of the method and establish the smallest quantity usually detectable. But we felt it was closer to reality to define the utilizable region of the B/Bo interval included between 95 % and 5 %. Below and above these values the method of quality control provides two forbidden zones in which the response is either :

quantity inferior (or superior) to a minimum (or maximum) detectable, a response that is far more utilizable for a clinical interpretation than an illusory figure.

3-8 - Intraassay variation. The establishment of intraassay variation has already been mentioned and is based on the measurements of 6 different points of Bo/T. What is important in the practical estimation of thyroid hormones is to define the interval in which the normal values are situated for any one given series. Nothing of this type has been provided for in the traditional method of control of precision and accuracy. We have been obliged to innovate. Four normal sera, very well known as they derived from male members of the Department, were measured in duplicate and, from these eight values, the average value and standard deviation (σ) were established and the limits of the normal defined arbitrarily by $\left[\text{average} - 2\,\sigma \text{ and average} + 2\,\sigma\right]$.

3-9 - Interassay variation. It seemed to us that it might be useful to situate the interassay comparison at different levels of the scale since, as has already been mentioned above, the precision established for any one portion of the scale is not transposable to the other portions. At the least possible cost it was necessary to have a monitor of the characteristic zones of hypo- normo- and hyperthyroidism. A comparison was made of two pools of normal sera, as well as two pools of sera from hyperthyroid patients together with their dilutions by a third. These values were compared to those of n previous series (approximately ten) by a special programme that utilizes for this comparison only the previous series known to be statistically acceptable. At the end of this comparison the series is accepted only if the overal interassay reference parameters are situated within the 95 % confidence limits.

3-10 - Proportionality. A one to nine dilution of two hyperthyroid sera have been included. In Logit-Log coordinates it is easy to appreciate the parallelism of the 3 dilutions (1-1/3-1/9) with the straight line representing the standard curve thus providing this control of quality with the suitable criteria of identity and proportionality of the results.

3-11 - Recuperation. At least for the assay of T3 it seemed expedient to provide some additional support of accuracy because an independent assay is not possible by measurement of ^{127}I. Verification of the good recovery of two calibrated doses of T3 added to normal sera was made thus testing three different points of the scale both with regard to accuracy and proportionality.

3-12 - The stability of the methods of assaying T4 and T3 is one of our most current preoccupations, whereas on the contrary the tendency of instability is by far the most serious weakness of RIA. The interassay control has been devised so as to immediately assess stability, shift or a sudden deviation by giving the average $\pm$ 2 standard deviations of the principal parameters : Bo/T, blank, Rho, slope of the line of regression, its value at the origin, the intercepts B/Bo 80 % - 50 % - 20 %, two normal sera, two hyperthyroid sera.

3-13 - Technician. This is probably one of the most important factors in the control of quality at least for the efficient functioning of the Laboratory and for the fiability of the results. No computor system is able to detect an error of technique of infinite variety, the outcome of which would be an error in the same direction and of the same magnitude affecting the result of each one of the duplicates of an unknown serum. In such a circumstance only the lack of concordance with the clinical context enables one to prevent an error of diagnosis otherwise unavoidable. There is no possible check for a group of technicians - for the thousands of precision pipettings they are likely to do - that can avoid a momentary lack of attention or thoughtlessness or the neglect of air bubbles coming through the tip of automatic pipettes. Each series is labelled with the name of the technician responsible. The programme of automatic control has not included so far a mark concerning the technician who undertook the series, a factor which could be included but which would be both useless and undesirable. On the other hand it has been proved that Laboratory technicians are not equal as to their performance and quality of work.

3-14 - Management of errors. The general programme has been devised to take account of the management of errors in radioactivity measurements as supplied by the changers.

Some errors are taken into account automatically. An example of this would be broken tubes so that in the result one of the duplicates would be correct and the other one nil. In such a circumstance the programme does not calculate the average between the good value within the duplicate and that which gives a result nil but only takes into account the result that is positive. This is the case also for the coefficients of variation between duplicates equal or superior to a programmed threshold (20 or 30 % of the C.V.'s) since the printed results always include the C.V.'s and only if the latter exceeds the threshold, the print includes the word : warning.

The programme has also provided for the correction of every conceivable error before allowing the statistical calculation to be undertaken. It is essential to be able to correct a value known to be false in one of the duplicates of any given point of the standard curve which the programme is devised not to correct or suppress as apposed to an automatic correction of the duplicates of the unknowns. On the other hand the facility available to a technician to correct a known error comprises a risk of camouflage.

4 - THE LIMITATIONS of the control of quality.

4-1 - Time. The verifications described above in fact take a few minutes from the time of reading the punched tape of the Teletype coupled to the gamma sample changers up to the emission of all the data in figures on a rapid electrostatic printing machine. The endpoint of these verifications is achieved by the sorting out of this mass of data. Experience is rapidly acquired and the indispensable human assessment itself only takes a few minutes. It is then simple to validate or reject any new series before its exploitation which in practice consists in allowing the personalized edition of each result, an edition monitored by the computor which, being of fairly long duration, is favourably effected automatically at night when the working day is over.

4-2 - Defects. The control of quality by continuous assay has revealed punctual instabilities or more or less regular shifts according to time signifying defects which otherwise would most often remain unsuspected. The verification is confined to pointing out these eventual defects - a result that is already precious and a reliable aid - but up until now does not suggest an interpretation.

4-3 - Quality. The role of those responsible is however not only to control quality but primarily to ensure it day after day. This means that it is necessary to try to find the methodological, congenital or temporary causes of the defects observed. This then is the object of further verifications released by this control of quality but would be of an entirely different type. In outline these verifications of laboratory work would include : buffer solutions, sera that are "hormone free" and that are used in the standard curve, and in particular dilutions of cold T4 and T3, that have become unstable during, or as a result of, storing, justifying a strict control by spectrophotometry or ^{127}I measurement. Up until now we have not been able to assess any correlation between an anomaly revealed by computor control and a type of defect attributable to methodology. We hope eventually to achieve this although the problems to be solved would be to be able to distinguish the factors attributable to the two main causes of error : daily variations in the method which have probably an apprehendible internal logic, and haphasard idiosyncrasies which are dependent on the worries and fatigue of the technicians.

4-4 - Utility of coupled assays of T4 and T3. Experience has shown that for example each progress achieved in the methodology for T4 helps to solve similar problems for T3 and vice versa. This may only be true because the two methods comprise numerous points in common (same buffer solutions, the same binding of the antibody on solid support, same smallness in size of the ligand etc...).

TO CONCLUDE, the verification of quality by continuous assay of T4 and T3 was found to be useful in discovering deficiencies but insufficient to detect causes thus indicating the necessity of the strict control of working methods and their perfect execution. This constitutes a typical example of the present individual roles of the computor and the method.

ACKNOWLEDGMENTS

We are indepted to Mr M. MATHIOT, Director of the Service d'Etudes et de Traitement de l'Information (S.E.T.I.), Administration de l'Assistance Publique â Paris, for his understanding of our problems and his help for providing the necessary hardware.

This study would not have been possible without the aid from Mr M. SAUCE, General Director of INFORMATEK Co, France, which supported the software developments.

We wish to express our thanks to our technicians : Z. Hantour, B. Antoine, A. Le Hen, M. Pujo, L. Patalin and also to Mrs B. Lacas for her secretarial assistance.

REFERENCES

1. Fanton, H. and Bizollon, C.A. (1976) Automatisation dans la gestion des données, le calcul et l'analyse des résultats. *In :* Acquisitions Récentes en Radioimmunologie, Compte-Rendus du IIIe Colloque International de Radioimmunologie de Lyon, C.A. Bizollon et al Editors, Lyon, France, pp. 499-509.

2. Rodbard, D. (1974) Statistical quality control and routine data processing for radioimmunoassay and immunoradiometric assay. Clin. Chem., 20, 1255-1270.

3. Rodbard, D. and Hutt, D.M. (1974) Statistical analysis of radioimmunoassays and immunoradiometric (labeled antibody) assays : A generalized, weighted, iterative, least-squares method for logistic curve fitting. *In :* Symposium on RIA and Related Procedures, International Atomic Energy Agency, Vienna. New York, Unipub, p. 165.

4. Samols, E. and Barrows, G.H. (1978) Automated data processing and Radioassays. Sem. Nucl. Med., 8, 163-179.

5. Stahl, T.J. (1975) Radioimmunoassay and the hormones of thyroid function. Sem. Nucl. Med., 5, 221-246.

Radioimmunology 1979, Ch. A. Bizollon, editor.

A RADIOIMMUNOASSAY FOR SERUM THYROGLOBULIN : RESULTS IN NORMAL SUBJECTS AND IN THYROID DISEASE.

C. ARDIET, H. BORNET, H. FAVRET, B. CLAUSTRAT, J-O. PEYRIN, M. MAYER, B. LAHNECHE.
ISOTOPES LAB., CENTRE LEON BERARD, 69373 LYON CEDEX 2 FRANCE

INTRODUCTION

In an early work[1] Roitt and Torrigiani showed by radioimmunoassay (RIA) that human thyroglobulin (hTg) was measurable in the serum of normal individuals. Then, Van Herle et al[2] developed a more sensitive RIA for hTg and studied its clinical applications ; they emphasized the importance of this determination in the follow-up of subjects with differentiated thyroid carcinoma[3]. We report here our results using an hTg RIA in normal subjects and in subjects with thyroid disorders.

MATERIALS AND METHODS

Radioimmunoassay : hTg was extracted from a non-toxic goiter by saline buffer phosphate pH 7.4, then purified by gel-filtration through Ultrogel AC 34, then Sepharose CL 4B. The purity of hTg was checked by analytical ultracentrifugation (single peak at 18.6 S) and polyacrylamide gel electrophoresis yielding only one band. The iodine content was 0.05 %. The purified hTg was then used as immunogen and as standard, the concentration of which being determined from $E^{1\%}_{280\ nm,\ 1\ cm} = 10.0$ after Schneider[4].

Antisera anti hTg were raised in rabbits by multi-injections of immunogen emulsified with Freund's complete adjuvant, followed by booster immunization one month later, and bleeding after one week ; our usual antiserum works at a final concentration of 3.10^{-5}.

Tracer hTg was labelled with 125 I by the Chloramine-T method[5] purified on a G-50 Sephadex column.

RIA procedure consisted in a 3 days preincubation stage at 4°C of standard hTg (up to 300 ng/ml in EDTA phosphate buffer) or unknown sera with the antiserum dilution, the protein content being equalized either with EDTA phosphate buffer or with fetal calf serum. The tracer hTg was added to all tubes and after 24 hours of incubation the centrifugation of labelled complex was performed after a second incubation overnight with the second antibody system. This procedure was validated by : lack of cross reactions with T_3 and T_4 ; close parallelism of standard curve and dilution curves of elevated (hyperthyroid) sera ; our usual sensitivity is 2.5 ng/ml.

PATIENTS : Normal sera (n = 116) were obtained from the local blood bank, laboratory staff, and euthyroid subjects.

Non-malignant thyroid disorders involved four groups : 9 haematoceles, 9 toxic adenomas, 32 non-toxic goiters and 49 cold nodules. In all patients the diagnosis was assessed by thyroid scan and usual clinical and laboratory data.

Differentiated thyroid carcinomas were separated in a non-metastatic group (n =30) and a metastatic group (n = 10) on the bases of total-body scan with 131 I, roentgenographic and clinical data. All non metastatic patients but one underwent a partial thyroidectomy ; total surgery was followed by radioiodine in the metastatic group. Sera were sampled under substitutive therapy or immediately after its cessation. All sera were tested for the presence of anti hTg autoantibodies ; positive sera are not included in the following results.

RESULTS

Normal levels ranged from 0 to 50 ng/ml with a mean of 13 ng/ml. 85 per cent of the control sera showed a level below 20 ng/ml ; 9 out of the 116 had undetectable or nil levels.

Non malignant thyroid diseases are presented in fig.1. The four groups exhibit a mean hTg level higher than the control group, i.e : haematoceles : 129 ng/ml, toxic adenomas : 38 ng/ml, non-toxic goiters : 69 ng/ml, cold nodules : 75 ng/ml. There is in all groups an important overlap with normal levels. The most elevated level, 1350 ng/ml, is a kystic nodule.

hTg levels in differentiated thyroid carcinomas are presented in fig2. A striking difference exists between the non-metastatic and the metastatic group. All samples but one in the group without documentated metastases are in the normal range. At the opposite, 8/10 of the patients with documented metastases have abnormal levels, up to 1450 ng/ml, under substitutive therapy. In these patients, the circulating hTg is linked to the presence of metastatic effusion since total thyroidectomy had been previously performed. In our metastatic patients, 2 of them bearing medullary carcinoma(not shown in the figure) had low-ranged hTg levels as previously described by Van Herle and Uller[3].

During the follow-up of non-metastatic differentiated carcinomas (fig.3) after partial surgery and under hormonal substitutive therapy, the lack of recurrence or metastatic effusion is correlated with normal levels of hTg. In these cases, the circulatinghTg is very likely released by the thyroid remnant.

We have not yet observed the shift of hTg level preceding clinical or paraclinical proofs of recurrence or metastases as others[6]. However, some of our patients treated with radioiodine did show a decrease in their level, showing at least in part a positive response to the treatment.

DISCUSSION

From a methodological point of view, our double-antibody disequilibrium procedure satisfyes the usual criteria of specificity, its sensitivity being sufficient for usual clinical purposes. A relatively few number of double-antibody RIA's has been described at present ; they are strikingly different in their normal ranges. Our normal values are somewhat higher than those reported by Van Herle et al[2] and Pezzino et al[7] but closer to those observed by Bodlaender et al[8], Lo Gerfo et al[9], Schneider et al[10]. This difference could be due to geographic differences since the french group of Schlumberger et al. (This symposium) demonstrated a normal mean of about 13 ng/ml, which is very close to our own. The difference observed could also be due to methodologic differences. One must emphasize here on the lack of an international standard of human thyroglobulin, and on the very critical point of obtaining an equivalence of the protein content between standards and samples. Much animal species are not satifactory in this respect ; in our opinion, human hTg free serum would be the best, but is not easily available.

From the clinical point of view, hTg RIA demonstrates an impor-

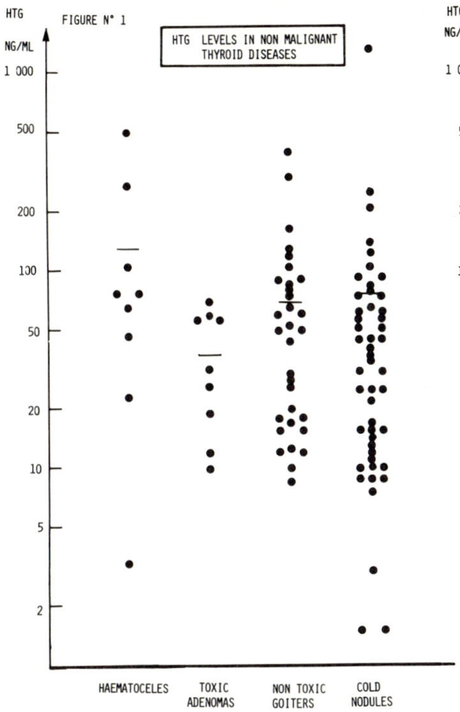

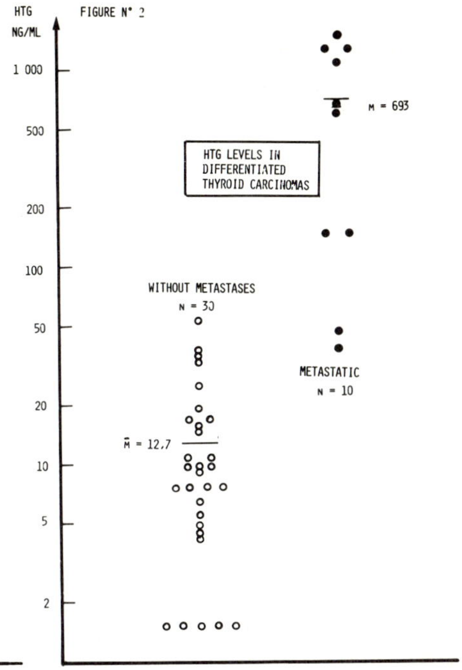

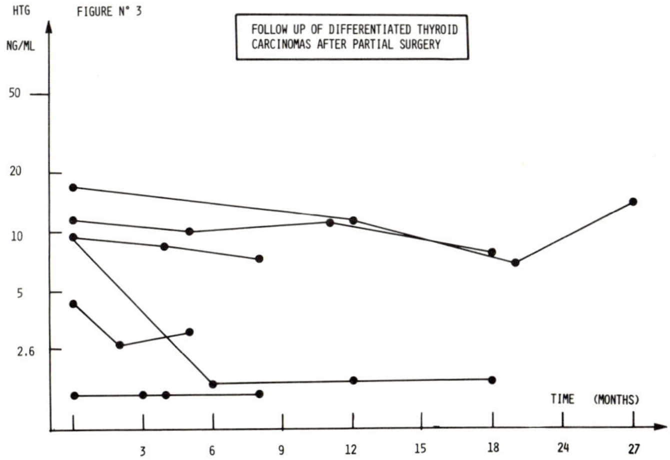

Fig.1: hTg levels in non-malignant thyroid diseases.
Fig.2: hTg levels in differentiated thyroid carcinomas.
Fig.3: hTg during follow-up of non-metastatic differentiated thyroid carcinomas after partial surgery.

tant overlap between the levels found in various non-malignant thyroid diseases and the levels of normal individuals. This overlap is also found between these different pathological conditions, including carcinoma. These facts exclude the feasibility of diagnosis or differential diagnosis of thyroid disease, by means of hTg RIA.

The difference observed here between the metastatic and the non-metastatic groups of our patients, however, indicate the usefulness of the measurement of thyroglobulin to diagnose the recurrence of the disease or the development of metastases, in the cases of differentiated thyroid carcinomas following partial or total surgery.

ACKNOWLEDGMENTS

We wish to thank Mrs Gebuhrer (C.T.S., Beynost) for the gift of check sera, and the secretarial assistance of Mrs Potzwa and the Service d'Iconographie.

REFERENCES

1 ROITT I.M., TORRIGIANI G. (1967) Endocrinology 81, 421.

2 VAN HERLE A.J., et al. (1973) J. Clin. Invest. 52, 1320.

3 VAN HERLE A.J., ULLER R.P. (1975) J. Clin. Invest. 56 272.

4 SCHNEIDER A.B., PERVOS R. (1978) J. Clin. Endocr. Metab. 47, 126.

5 HUNTER W.H., GREENWOOD F.G. (1962) Nature 194, 495.

6 VAN HERLE A.J. (1977) Ann. Radiol. 20, 743.

7 PEZZINO V., et al. (1977) Eur. J. Clin. Invest. 7, 503.

8 BODLAENDER P., et al. (1978) clin. Chem. 24, 267.

9 LO GERFO P., et al.(1977) Lancet i, 881.

10 SCHNEIDER A.B., et al.(1977) Ann. Inter. Med. 86, 29.

Radioimmunology 1979, Ch. A. Bizollon, editor.

SERUM THYROGLOBULIN AS A MARKER FOR METASTATIC SPREAD IN THYROID DIFFERENTIATED CARCINOMA

M. EBER, J.C. GROB, G. OTT, J. ABECASSIS, B. MOYSES, G. METHLIN
Centre Paul Strauss, 3 rue de la Porte de l'Hôpital, 67085 Strasbourg (France)

The presence of thyroglobulin (Tg) in normal subjects was described in 1967 by ROITT and TORRIGIANI[1]. More recently VAN HERLE[2] showed the interest of its determination in thyroid pathology, and in particular in cases of thyroid carcinomas[2]. However, in their hands, the radioimmunoassay failed to detect Tg in the presence of anti-Tg auto-antibodies. We have developed a solid phase immunoradiometric assay which is not sensitive to the presence of such auto-antibodies[3]. A purified anti-Tg antibody labelled with ^{125}Iodine was used. We report the results of measurements of Tg levels in sera of patients who have undergone total thyroidectomy for differentiated thyroid carcinomas. We have also looked for a possible correlation between serum Tg concentrations and the volume and number of the metastases.

PATIENTS AND METHODS

92 patients have been subjected to a total thyroidectomy for a differentiated thyroid carcinoma. They were divided into 4 subgroups, according to the extent of metastases.

Group I : 60 patients without any metastases
Group II : 8 patients with one metastasis
Group III : 14 patients with less than 5 bone and/or lung metastases
Group IV : 10 patients with multiple bone and/or lung metastases.

Serum Tg assay. Tg was extracted from normal thyroid tissue and purified by chromatography on Sepharose 6B and Sephadex G200 (Pharmacia, France).

Anti-Tg antiserum was raised in New-Zeeland rabbits by 4 subcutaneous injections of 1 mg of purified Tg emulsified in 1 ml of Freund's adjuvant.

The purification of the anti-Tg antibodies was performed by affinity chromatography on a Sepharose-Tg immunoadsorbent (Sepharose 4B CNBr activated). Purified anti-Tg antibodies were iodinated by the chloramine T method of HUNTER and GREENWOOD[4].

The Tg assay consists in 3 steps :

Anti-Tg antibodies were adsorbed on the inner wall of polystyrene plastic tubes by incubation of a 1/2000 dilution of the whole antiserum.

100 µl of the patients' sera were incubated in polystyrene tubes coated with anti-Tg antibodies for 18 hours at 20°C. The reaction was terminated by 2 washes with phosphate buffered saline (PBS).

The tubes were then incubated with 100 µl of ^{125}I-labelled antibodies (≠ 0.1 µCi) for 4 to 18 hours at 20°C followed by 3 washes with PBS.

The radioactivity of the tubes was measured in an automatic well type gamma counter (Ultrogamma II, LKB). The amount of Tg in the sera of the patients was estimated by reference to a standard curve established in the same way by using dilutions of known amounts of purified Tg.

RESULTS

Validation of the Tg assay and normal values.

The sensitivity of the assay was 2,5 ng/ml. The non specific binding measured in the absence of Tg wass less than 1 % of the total radioactivity.

Reproducibility within and between experiments was respectively 5-9 % and 7-12 %.

The specificity was checked by measuring Tg concentrations on serial dilutions of a serum containing a high concentration of Tg.

The interference of auto-anti-Tg antibodies was verified by performing a recovery test using a serum containing a high titre of auto-anti-Tg antibodies (1/250000 measured by inhibition of hemagglutination).

The normal values were measured in 60 normal controls. 70 % of the normal values were between 0 and 15 ng/ml. In 12 % of the controls no serum Tg was detectable.

Results in differentiated carcinomas.

The results of serum Tg in patients with metastases of differen-

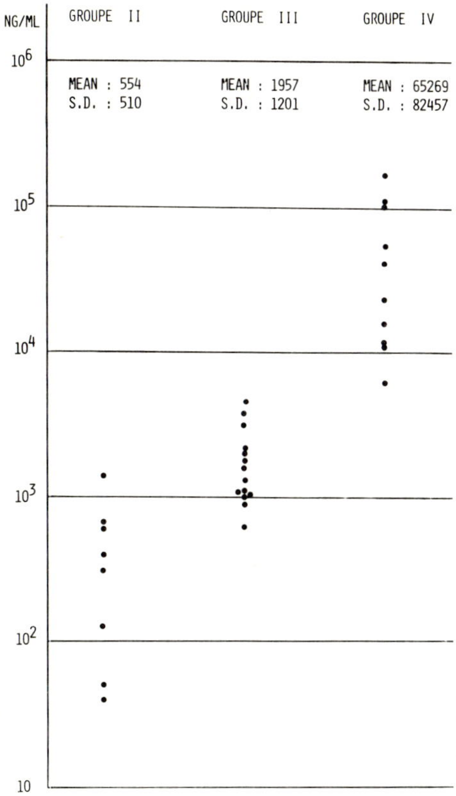

FIG.1. SERUM Tg LEVELS IN PATIENTS WITH METASTASES OF DIFFERENTIATED THYROID CARCINOMAS

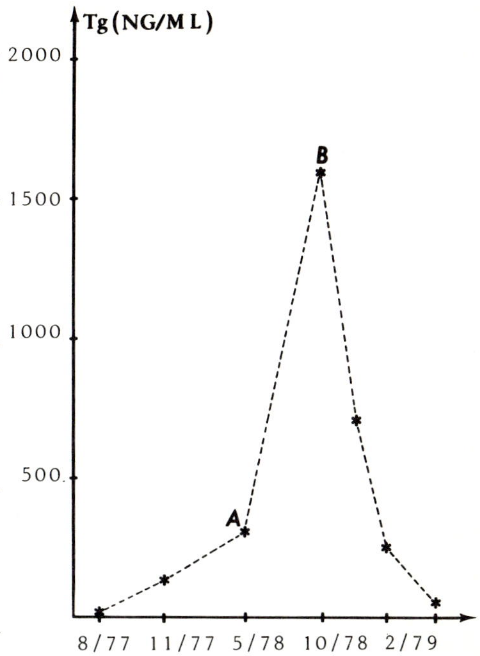

FIG.2.FOLLOW UP STUDY OF A PATIENT WITH DIFFERENTIATED THYROID CARCINOMA (thyroidectomized in february 1977)

A:Lung metastases treated by ^{131}I
B:Lung and bone metastases.
^{60}Co therapy (5600 rads)

tiated carcinomas after thyroidectomy are illustrated Fig. 1.

The 60 patients without documented metastases had low Tg levels, with a mean value of 15 ng/ml. In 39 cases, no serum Tg could be detected.

DISCUSSION

The immunoradiometric assay for serum Tg provides a sensitive and reproducible determination of this protein, with a very low non specific binding. In addition, as pointed out by IKEKUBO[5], anti-Tg auto-antibodies did not significatly interfere with the assay.

The presence of high Tg in patients with metastases of differentiated thyroid carcinomas was described by VAN HERLE[2].The present results suggest a direct relationship between the serum Tg concentration and the metastatic extent. This relation is further supported by the follow-up study, illustrated in Fig. 2. In this patient, a progressive increase of the serum Tg concentration occured simultaneously with an increase in the number and the size of lung metastases, and the apparition of bone metastases. After an external ^{60}Co irradiation (5600 r), a progressive decrease of serum Tg could be observed.

Serum Tg secretion did not seem to be related to the uptake of ^{131}Iodine by the metastases, since we have observed high Tg values in patients with multiple metastases without any uptake of ^{131}Iodine. In remains to be determined what is the minimal size of metastatic tissue resulting in a measurable increase of serum Tg. It was recently suggested[6,7] that the secreted Tg might differ from normal Tg by molecular weight and carbohydrate content, but with a similar antigenicity.

Although it is difficult to assess the metastatic extent, serum Tg seems to be a reliable index of metastatic growth in patients with differentiated thyroid carcinoma who have undergone total thyroidectomy. In addition serum Tg determination may be helpful in the aetiologic diagnosis of bone or lung metastases of unknown origin.

REFERENCES

1. Roitt I.M., Torrigiani G. (1967), Endocrinology, 81, pp.421-429.
2. Van Herle A.J., Uller R.P. (1975), J. Clin. Invest., 56, pp.272-277.
3. Van Herle A.J., Uller R.P., Matthews N.L., Brown J. (1973), J. Clin. Invest., 52, pp. 1320-1327.
4. Hunter W.M., Greenwood F.C. (1962), Nature, 194, pp. 495-496.
5. Ikekubo K., Konishi J., Morita R., Mori T., Hamada S., Torizuka K. (1974), Recent Adv. Nucl. Med., Proc. World Congress of Nucl. Med. 1 st, pp. 846-848.
6. Lo Gerfo P., Colacchio T., Colacchio D., Feind C. (1978), Cancer 42, pp. 164-166.
7. Monaco F., Andreoli M., (1977), Ann. Radiol., 20, pp. 735-738.

Radioimmunology 1979, Ch. A. Bizollon, editor.

STRATEGY FOR THYROID FUNCTION TESTS IN THYROID SECRETION DISORDERS

R. MORNEX, M. FOURNIER, F. PERRIN, A. BODSON
Service d'Endocrinologie et Maladies de la Nutrition
Hôpital de l'Antiquaille, 1 rue de l'Antiquaille, 69005 Lyon (France)

Nowadays a lot of thyroid function tests has been proposed for the diagnosis of thyroid secretion disorders. These tests are in general specific, sensitive and reliable. It is impossible to use all of them in the different situations. The strategy depends upon the clinical problem which must be solved. The comparison of the respective efficacity of the different tests is founded on a physiopathological approach and on large clinical experience.

METHODS FOR STUDYING A BIOLOGICAL TEST

These methods are no peculiar for thyroid problems and they do not need large comments. The successive steps are as follows :

- determination of intra and inter assays variations,
- study of the normality of the control values,
- selection of the normal and abnormal populations. The last one must be defined by the mean of an *independent* parameter,
- determination of the "normal range". The arithmetic mean of the studied normal sample ± 2 SD gives the limits in which falls 95 % of the normal population ; the mean ± 3 SD gives the limits in which falls 99.3 % of the normal population. Any value found out of these limits may be considered as abnormal with a risk respectively of 5 % or 0.7 %. In that way one evaluates the risk of misclassifying a normal value but not an abnormal value. The same procedure can be done with an abnormal sample. The value which minimizes the risk of missclassifying (either as normal or as abnormal) is located half way between the mean of the two samples. A calculation of the risk can be easily evaluated[1]. However in general for the routinal tests the evaluation of the normal range is done on the normal population. Britton et al.[2] use the 5 "decision-aiding ranges" : normal, definitely high, definitely low, borderline raised and borderline low.

To *compare the respective discriminant* value of each test one must use of all of them on the same blood samples drawn on the abnormal population previously defined. The most interesting cases are not the highly abnormal cases but on the contrary the borderline cases.

Five methods are in general used to compare the discriminant values.

a) The graphical expression of the results may illustrate how many patients could be misclassified by one or another test.

b) The correlation between two tests may be highly significant despite one test give a correct classification and the other one an uncorrect classification (fig. 1)

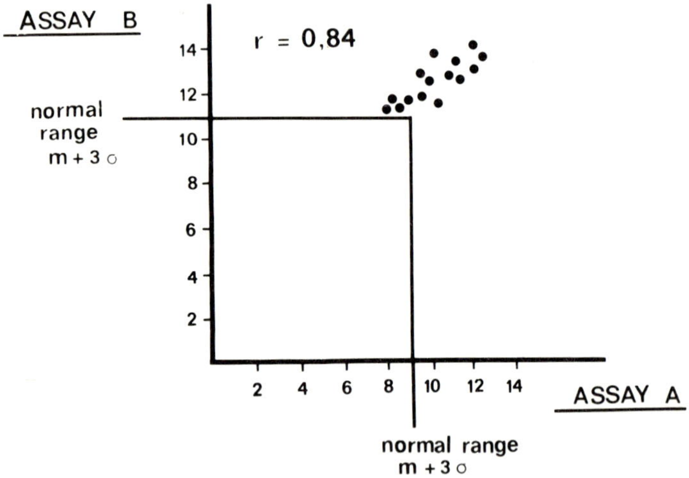

Fig. 1. This figure has been artificially drawn. Despite a rather good correlation (r = 0.84), 4 out of the 16 values are classified as abnormal with assay B and as normal with assay A.

c) Comparison of the means. The test which gives the best discrimination between a normal and an abnormal population having normal distributions and equal variances, on basis of samples drawn from each population, is the test which gives the maximum value to the variable t, which is computed in Student t test when comparing the mean of the two samples[1].

Another way of calculation is to compare for each test the distance between the values of abnormal population and the mean of the normal population in term of standard deviation of the mean. The final comparison is done between the "écarts réduits"[3].

d) The discriminant functions[4]. If several tests are available for each individual the previous procedure is generalized by the discriminant analysis of Fisher. It consists to define a discriminant function which is a linear combination of the results of the tests. The allocation procedure being to assign to one population the individuals having positive discriminant function values and to the other these having negative values. Here again, the discriminant function is chosen in such a way as to minimize the risk of misclassification. Logically the tests which have the highest discriminant values should be first taken in account in the discriminant function, and should produce the most important decrease of the risk of misclassification[1]. This procedure requires in general middle size computer facilities. The most important criticism is that the classification of respective discriminant values does not take in account the physiopathological significance of each of them.

STRATEGY IN THYROID SECRETION DISORDERS

We will limit our attention to 4 clinical problems which are the most frequent in practice.

1 - Toxic adenoma. Toxic adenomas represent in Europe about the fifth of the thyrotoxic patients. It is characterized by mild clinical expression and in 1/3 of the cases by normal concentration of thyroid hormones. The *scintiscan* is the only one test able to give the correct diagnosis. It must be used in every thyroid nodule. The measurement of serum thyroid hormones is interesting at a second step for further information before the treatment.

2 - Graves disease. In the majority of the cases both thyroxine (T^4) and triiodothyronine (T^3) are oversecreted. For a long period only indirect methods measuring Plasma Protein Bound Iodine were available. The development of direct measurement of the hormones with radiocompetition or radioimmunoassays makes the measurement of PBI completely obsolete[5]. If the measurement of total hormonal concentration is an improvement, it does not give a perfect approach of the problem since only the *free fraction* of these hormones is active. Thus the investigations must take in account the concentration of the thyroxine binding globulin (TBG). To study these free fractions one may use two different

groups of techniques :

- direct system : circulating level's determination by equilibrium dialysis (heavy and complicated for user), or radioimmunoassay after fraction's separation on a Sephadex-column recently commercialized in a "kit" (apparently easier to manipulate but with a reliability not still completely demonstrated),

- indirect system in which the free fractions are calculated either after determination of TBG concentration or after appreciation of TBG binding sites by T^3 resin uptake test.

The determination of the strategy for the diagnosis of Graves' disease needs an answer to the following questions :

- what is the best method to appreciate the free fractions of the hormones ?
- do we need to measure T^4 and T^3 ?
- if not, what is the most efficient ?
- do we improve our diagnostic possibilities using the complete set of tests ?
- what is the interest of the isotopic explorations ?

a) To answer the first question , we studied 2 groups of patients refered as suspected of having a Graves' disease and in which the routinal tests gave borderline values. They have been separated according to the results of T^3 suppression test into 2 groups :

group I : euthyroid suppressible (12 patients)
group II : thyrotoxic non suppressible (9 patients)
and compared to a control group of 14 subjects.

The euthyroid group has been reexaminated after one year to check the stability of the thyroid secretion.

On the serum of these patients the following assays have been done :

T^4 by radiocompetition (Tetrasorb ^{R} - Abbott)
T^3 resin uptake (Triosorb ^{R} - Abbott)
T^3 by radioimmunoassay (personal antibodies)
FT^4 by chromatography + radioimmunoassay (FT^3 - FT^4 ^{R} Lepetit)
FT^3 by chromatography + radioimmunoassay (FT^3 - FT^4 ^{R} Lepetit)
TBG : by radioimmunoassay (TBG RIA-GNOST ^{R} Behring)

Free Thyroxine Index (FTI) has been calculated according to the formula :

$$\frac{T^4\ (\mu g/100\ ml) \times T^3\ \text{resin uptake}}{100}$$

The results are indicated on the table I.

TABLE I

VALUES OBTAINED IN NORMAL SUBJECTS, IN GROUP I (SUPPRESSIBLE) AND GROUP II (NON SUPPRESSIBLE) MEAN ± SD

	F T I	T4/TBG	T3 RI ng/100 ml	FT3 pg/ml	FT4 pg/ml
Normal subjects n = 14	2.5 ± 0.3	5 ± 1.2	99.5 ± 21	5.5 ± 1.8	14 ± 3
Group I n = 12	2.2 ± 0.8 n.s.	4.9 ± 1.3 n.s.	110 ± 27 n.s.	5.4 ± 1.9 n.s.	17 ± 5 n.s.
Group II n = 9	2.8 ± 0.6 n.s.	6.2 ± 1.4 n.s.	191 ± 78 $p < 0.01$	9.7 ± 5.6 $p < 0.05$	25 ± 8.6 $p < 0.05$

The individual values appear on the fig. 2 and 3 and the calculation of the respective discriminant values has been conducted by the comparison of the t values and of the "écarts réduits" (vide supra). The only one significant difference ($p < 0.05$) is between T^4/TBG and FT^4 in group II.

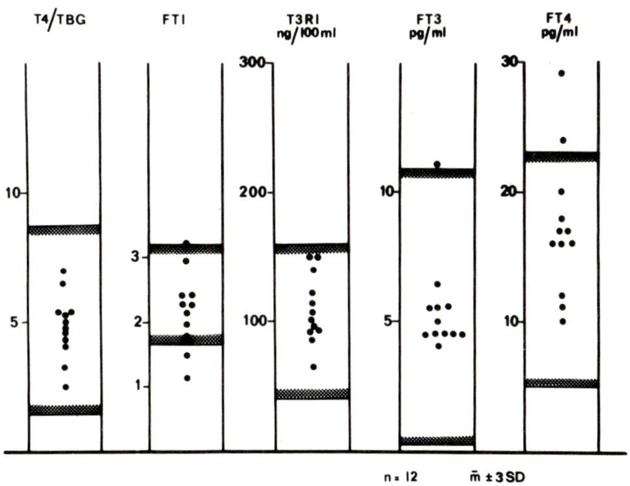

Fig. 2. Results of T^4/TBG, FTI, T^3RI, FT^3 and FT^4 in group I (euthyroid suppressible).

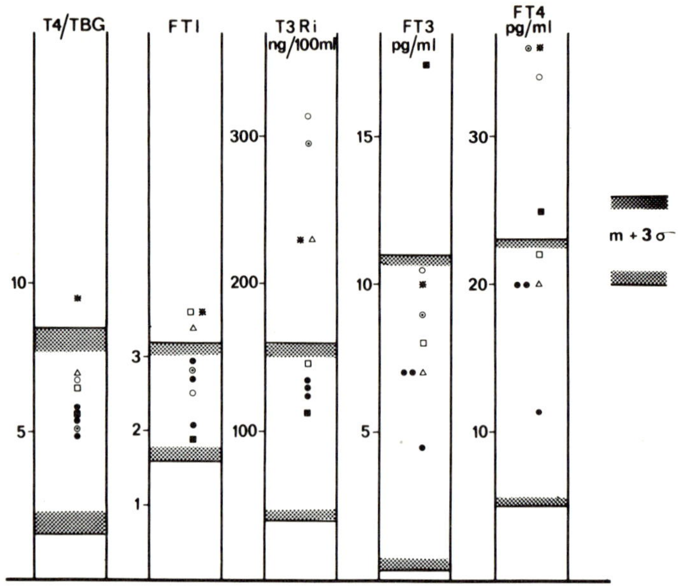

Fig. 3. Results of T^4/TBG, FTI, T^3RI, FT^3 and FT^4 in group II (hyperthyroid non suppressible).

Our conclusions were :

- FT^3 was not more significant that total T^3,
- T^4/TBG was less significant than FT^4 and FTI,
- FT^4 classified correctly 4 patients of group II vs 3 with FTI however 2 patients of group I were misclassified with FT^4 and not with FTI.

Thus if we consider that the method of determination of FT^4 is more sophisticated than the method of determination of FTI we conclude that FTI remains the most useful to appreciate the free fraction of T^4.

b) In a previous study[6] we have shown that the simultaneous measurement of FTI and T^3classifies correctly 99 % of the patients with Graves' disease. With FTI alone this score is 95 % and with T^3 alone it is 92 %. Fragu et al.[7] suggest to do first FTI and T^3 if a doubt subsists. The problem is a practical one and the economy could be cancelled by the difficulties to keep the serum or to recall the patient.

Finally *our strategy* for the diagnosis of Graves' disease depends upon the intensity of the clinical suspicion :

- if the clinical suspicion is strong we ask both FTI and T^3,
- if the clinical suspicion is slight we ask only *one test to eliminate* hyperthyroidism with a minimum of risk.

c) For this last problem the discussion remains open between FTI and T^3 and it seems that there is no strong difference between these tests. We suggest to measure FTI.

d) In our series only 4 patients of group II were well classified with 2 tests and for the others the complete set would not have improve the score. Thus it is clear that for 99 % of the patients 2 tests are sufficient. If the discussion remains the problem needs another way to be solved.

e) Measurement of radioiodine uptake is the first step of a *T^3 suppression test*. This test remains the corner stone of the diagnosis of Graves' disease.

TRH test might be clearly conclusive when the increase of TSH is in the limits of the normal. This rules out the presence of hyperthyroidism[8]. However an absent TSH response to TRH does not prove the reality of clinical hyperthyroidism. This test might be used facing the exceptional suspicion of TSH secreting adenoma.

The measurement of *thyroid stimulating antibodies* is reserved to physiopathological exploration or to the suspicion of hyperophthalmic Graves' disease.

3 - Thyroid insufficiency. Considering only primary hypothyroidism the general opinion[9] is that the *best discriminant test* is the *measurement of serum TSH*. Our results (fig. 4) illustrate this point.

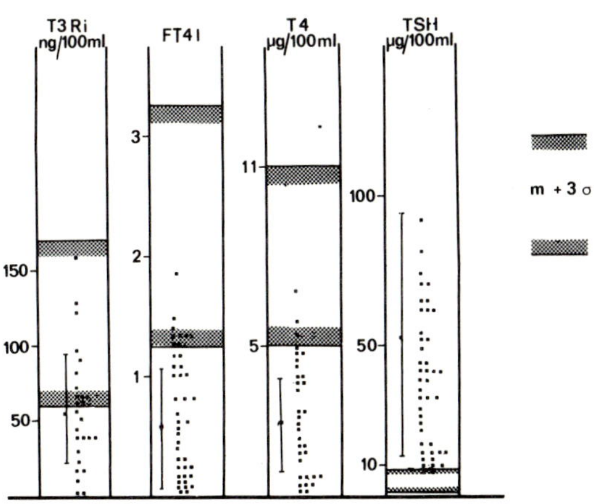

Fig. 4. Values of TSH (RIA), total T^4 (Tetrasorb ^{R}), total T^3 (personal RIA) and FTI $\left(\frac{T^4 \times T^3 \text{ resin uptake}}{100}\right)$ in 42 cases of primary hypothyroidism.

It is clear that T^3 is not a good parameter. Moreover it is wellknown that in some circumstances T^3 may be low despite a normal thyroid secretion.

Surprisingly enough total T^4 seems to be a better parameter than FTI. It is admitted that the TBG concentration is increased in myxoedema[10] ; thus the correction with T^3 resin uptake would improve the discrimination between normal and hypothyroid patients. Nevertheless this discussion seems unuseful since the TSH assay separates very clearly normal and hypothyroid populations.

4 - Follow up of treated Graves' disease. During the follow up after surgical or isotopic treatment the patients may develop :

- euthyroidism,
- borderline remaining hyperthyroidism,
- borderline hypothyroidism,
- definite hypothyroidism.

At least the classification of the patient in one of these categories needs measurement of FTI, T^3 and TSH. However in the borderline hypothyroidism the increase of TSH is sometimes not very clear and it is more evident after TRH stimulation. Thus to simplify the system we do in each of these treated patients every year or every two years simultaneously FTI + T^3 + TRH test.

SUMMARY

The multiplication of the available methods to study the thyroid secretion needs to do a choice and to establish a strategy. The methods for studying a biological test implicates various statistical approaches. They must be tested on normal and abnormal populations defined in an independent way.

The strategy in thyroid secretion disorders depends upon the clinical problem to be solved, and in general one or two tests are sufficient : toxic adenomas = scintiscan, Graves' disease = FTI + T^3, primary hypothyroidism = TSH. Only the follow up of treated Graves' disease needs the association of FTI + T^3 + TRH test.

REFERENCES

1. Dagnelie, P. (1975) Analyse statistique à plusieurs variables, Presse Agronomique de Gembloux, Gembloux, (Belgique), pp. 307-326

2. Britton, K.E., Quinn, V., Brown, B.L. and Ekins, R.P. (1975) Brit. Med. J., 3, 350-352.

3. Schwartz, D. (1963) Méthodes statistiques à l'usage des médecins et des biologistes, Ed. Médicales Flammarion, Paris, pp. 1-288.

4. Fragu, P., Thouin, A., Bazin, J.-P. and Tubiana, M. (1972) Ann. Endocrinol. (Paris), 33, 5-22.

5. Vallée, G., Fandard, J., Morin, M. and Nouchy, J. (1976) Path. Biol., 24, 483-496.

6. Orgiazzi, J., Fournier, M., Magnon-Pujo, B., Quintana, J. and Mornex, R. (1978) Ann. Endocrinol. (Paris), 39, 67-68.

7. Fragu, P., Alperovitch, A., Gardet, P., Charbord, P., Parmentier, C. and Tubiana, M. (1978) Symposium on free thyroid hormones, Venise. Excerpta Medica, Amsterdam.

8. Kaplan, M.M. and Utiger, R.D. (1978) Clin. Endocrinol. Metab., 7, 97-113.

9. Vagenakis, A.G. and Braverman, L.E. (1976) Ann. Intern. Med., 84, 607-608.

10. Hesch, R.-D., Gatz, J., McIntosh, C.H.S., Janzen, J. and Hehrmann, R. (1976) Clin. Chim. Acta, 70, 33-42.

HORMONES REGULATING CALCIUM AND PHOSPHATE HOMEOSTASIS

Radioimmunology 1979, Ch. A. Bizollon, editor.

DEVELOPMENT AND CLINICAL APPLICATION OF A RADIOIMMUNOASSAY FOR CIRCULATING 1,25 & 25,26-DIHYDROXYCHOLECALCIFEROL IN MAN

J.L.H. O'Riordan, G.N. Hendy, L.J. Fraher, S.E. Papapoulos, L.M. Sandler and T.L. Clemens.
Middlesex Hospital, London W.1. England

Vitamin D is metabolised by the liver to 25-OH D which can then undergo further hydroxylation at positions 1,24 and 26 by the kidney and other tissues. With advances in assay methodology it is now possible to measure vitamin D and its metabolites in man. These measurements have been crucial in increasing our knowledge of the role of the vitamin in the control of mineral metabolism. Recent interest is centred on the development of improved assays for 1,25-dihydroxycholecalciferol (1,25-$(OH)_2D_3$) the hormonal form of the vitamin. Because radioimmunoassays have been successful when applied to the measurement of steroid hormones it seemed reasonable to use this approach to assay 1,25-$(OH)_2D_3$. These techniques have now been developed and applied to clinical studies (1.2.3.).

A pre-requisite for a radioimmunoassay for 1,25-$(OH)_2D_3$ was a reactive derivative which could be coupled to a protein. This metabolite differs structurally from 25-OHD_3 and other dihydroxy vitamin D_3 metabolites by having a 1αhydroxy group. In order to expose the A ring in the hapten, 1,25-$(OH)_2D_3$-25-hemisuccinate was prepared (Fig. 1.). This compound was then coupled to bovine serum albumin by the mixed acid anhydride method. U.V. analysis of the conjugate indicated that the reaction had coupled approximately 20 moles of hapten per mole of bovine serum albumin.

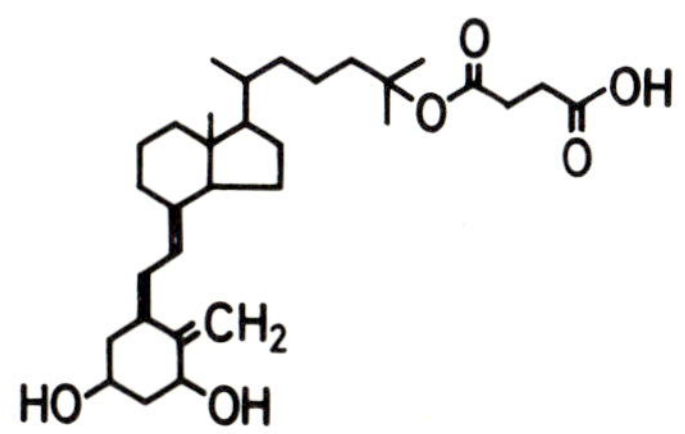

Fig. 1. Structure of 1,25-$(OH)_2D_3$-25-hemisuccinate. This design allowed linkage to protein through the side chain and thus exposure of the A ring of the hapten.

Rabbits and sheep were immunized with this conjugate and in both species antisera of high affinity for 1,25-$(OH)_2D_3$ were produced. Antisera were tested for binding of ^{3}H 1,25-$(OH)_2D_3$ in a barbital acetate buffer pH 8.6; dextran-coated charcoal was employed for phase separation after a 24hr incubation at 4^oC. Since vitamin D binding protein (DBP) - an α globulin which binds 25-OHD_3 and to a lesser extent 1,25-$(OH)_2D_3$ - is present in serum, it was important to establish that the binding of ^{3}H 1,25-$(OH)_2D_3$ was due to an immune fraction of the serum rather than to DBP. Therefore antisera were assessed for reactivity after treatment with rivanol (6,9 diamino-2-ethoxyacridine lactate). This compound is known to precipitate α globulins and to some extent β globulins from serum whereas gammaglobulins remain soluble (4). Fig. 2 shows that prior treatment of antiserum (R7) with 0.4% rivanol effectively precipitated DBP as indicated by greatly reduced binding of ^{3}H 25-OHD_3 (left panel) but did not alter binding of ^{3}H 1,25-$(OH)_2D_3$ (right panel).

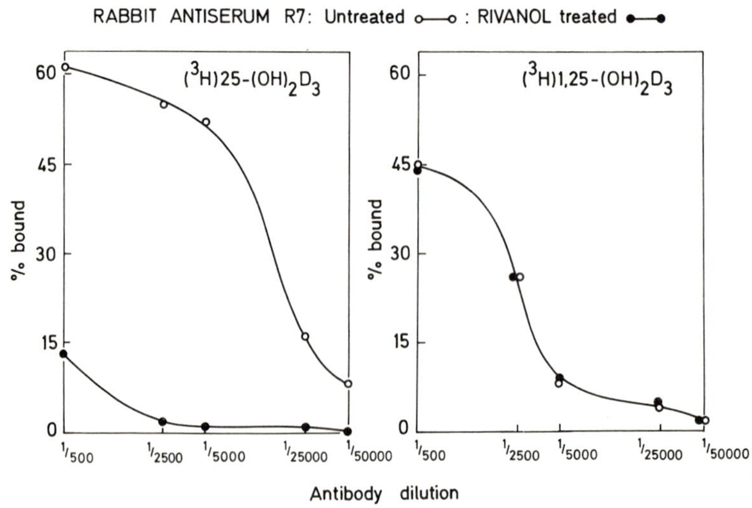

Fig. 2. Binding of ^{3}H 25-OHD_3 (left panel) & ^{3}H 1,25$(OH)_2D_3$ (right panel) by antiserum R_7 before (○) and after (●) treatment of serum with rivanol (0.4%). This treatment precipitated the vitamin D binding protein (DBP).

Antisera produced so far also react with other hydroxylated vitamin D_3 metabolites. From initial studies using the rabbit antiserum (R_7) at a dilution of 1:1000, 1,25 -$(OH)_2D_3$ was found to be 40 fold more reactive than 25-OHD_3 and 24,25-$(OH)_2D_3$. In addition, the displacement curves for these metabolites were not parallel to that of 1,25-$(OH)_2D_3$ (Fig. 3. left panel). However, when crossreactivity was assessed after rivanol precipitation of DBP, the reactivity of 25-OHD_3 and 24,25-$(OH)_2D_3$ was only about 2-4 fold less compared with 1,25-$(OH)_2D_3$ and all three displacement curves were parallel (Fig. 3. right panel).

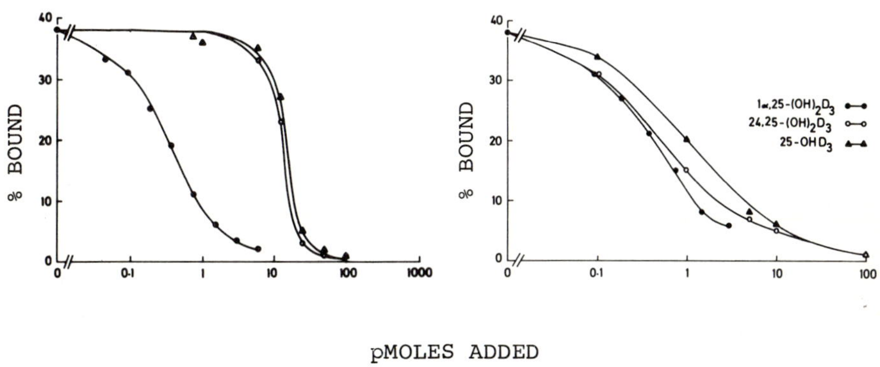

Fig. 3. Reactivity of 1,25-$(OH)_2D_3$ (●), 25-OHD_3 (▲) and 24,25-$(OH)_2D_3$ (○) with antiserum R_7 (1:1000) before (left panel) and after (right panel) treatment. ^3H 1,25-$(OH)_2D_3$ was used as tracer throughout.

Conversely, it has been possible to demonstrate that when antisera of high titre are used, the selectivity for 1,25-$(OH)_2D_3$ could be enhanced by adding DBP in the form of non-immune serum, to the incubation mixture. For example, an antiserum produced in a sheep (02282) has high affinity for 1,25-$(OH)_2D_3$ and may be used at a dilution of 1:50,000. At this dilution 25-OHD_3 is about two fold less reactive than 1,25-$(OH)_2D_3$ (Fig. 4. left panel). However, the reactivity of 25-OHD_3 with this antiserum could be decreased by about 20 fold by adding non-immune sheep serum (1:500) to the incubation mixture (Fig. 4. right panel). Therefore these studies demonstrate that the reactivity of vitamin D metabolites with these antisera is affected by the presence of vitamin D binding protein (DBP). This was most apparent using low titre antisera, ie. when the concentration of DBP was high. Since DBP preferentially binds 25-OHD_3, 24,25-$(OH)_2D_3$ and 25,26-$(OH)_2D_3$ and is less reactive with 1,25-$(OH)_2D_3$ it could conceivably be used in assay to increase the selectivity for the 1,25-$(OH)_2D_3$.

Antiserum 02282 was selected for further development because of its high affinity for 1,25-$(OH)_2D_3$ (Ka=5.0 x 10^9 L/M) and for its high titre. With the aid of a computer optimizing program (5) the antiserum concentration and mass of labelled ligand were adjusted to give an assay of maximum sensitivity.

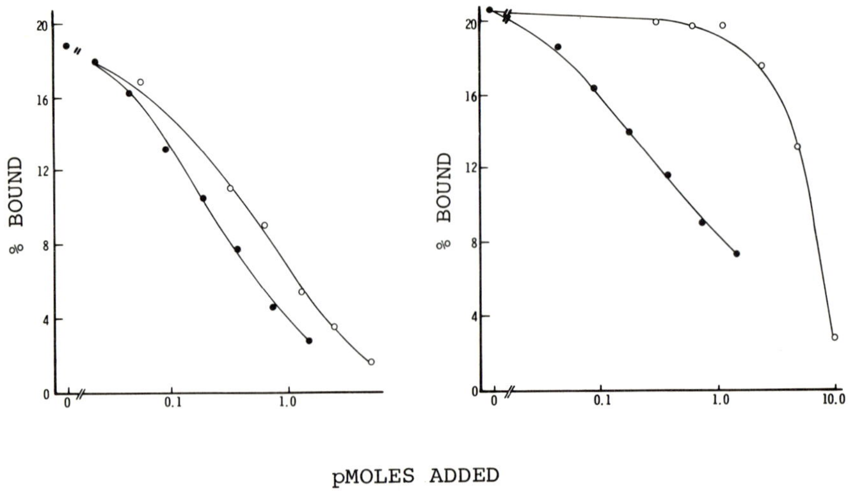

Fig. 4. Reactivity of 1,25-$(OH)_2D_3$ (●) & 25-OHD_3 (○) with sheep antiserum 02282 (1:50,000) either alone (left panel) or in the presence of non-immune sheep serum (1:500) (right panel). ^{3}H 1,25-$(OH)_2D_3$ was used as tracer throughout.

By computer optimization it was found that the most sensitive calibration curve was obtained with an antiserum concentration which gave 20 per cent binding of tracer. Under these conditions the limit of detection is 10 pg per tube. Pre-incubation of antiserum with unlabelled ligand for 1 to 3 days before addition of tracer resulted in only a marginal increase in sensitivity.

Although this antiserum is more selective for 1,25-$(OH)_2D_3$ than for other vitamin D metabolites (3) the fact that 25-OHD_3 and 24,25-$(OH)_2D_3$ circulate in greater concentrations (250 fold and 25 fold higher respectively) necessitates purification of the hormone from serum prior to assay. This is achieved by extraction of serum (5-10ml) with dichloromethane followed by chromatography first on Sephadex LH20 and then on high pressure liquid chromatography (HPLC). A short (8 x 0.8cm) LH20 column (Fig.5) developed with a solvent system of hexane: chloroform: methanol (9:1:1.2) effectively separates 1,25-$(OH)_2D_3$ from both 25-OHD_3 and 1,24,25-$(OH)_3D_3$. In this system, 24,25-$(OH)_2D_3$ is partially resolved and 25,26-$(OH)_2D_3$ migrates with 1,25-$(OH)_2D_3$.

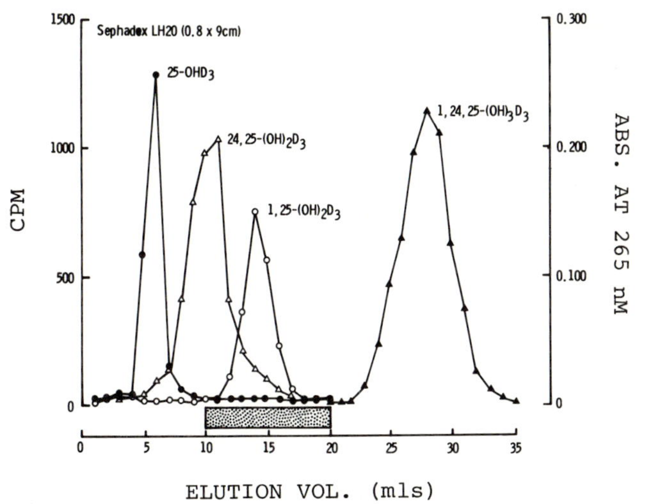

Fig. 5. Elution profile of vitamin D_3 metabolites chromatographed on a Sephadex LH20 (8 x 0.8cm) with a solvent system of Hexane: Chloroform: Methanol (9:1:1.2). The stippled area denotes the elution volume collected for HPLC. The first three peaks represent elution of radioactive compounds and the fourth is measured by absorbance at 265nM.

Final purification by HPLC resolves 1,25-$(OH)_2D_3$ for assay (Fig.6). Recovery is monitored by assessing the loss of a small amount of tritiated 1,25-$(OH)_2D_3$ added to the initial sample and averages 67%.

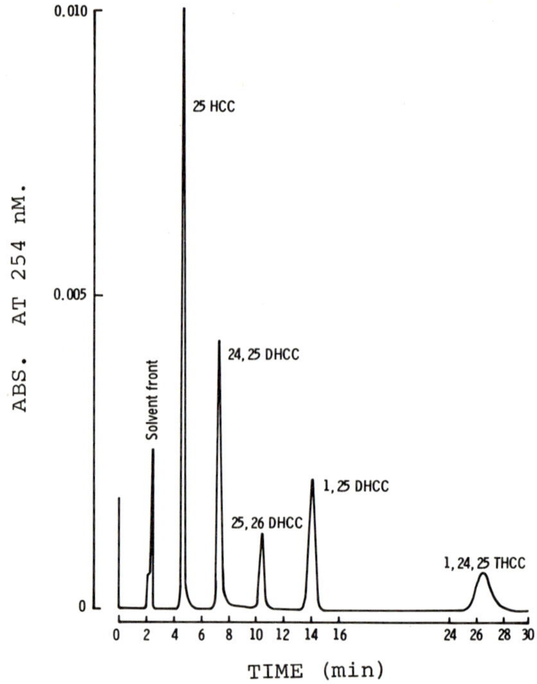

Fig. 6. Separation of a mixture of synthetic vitamin D_3 metabolites by HPLC on a Zorbax-Sil (6.5mmi.d. X 25cm) column eluted with hexane: isopropanol (85:15) with a flow rate of 2ml/min.

A number of experiments were carried out to determine the efficiency of the purification procedure. When serum extracts were spiked with tritiated metabolites and then chromatographed in the usual manner, the carryover of 25-OHD_3 24,25-$(OH)_2D_3$ and 25,26 $(OH)_2D_3$ into the final 1,25-$(OH)_2D_3$ fraction was less than 0.007%, 0.18% and 0.6% of their initial concentrations respectively. Thus 25,26-$(OH)_2D_3$ although not resolved by LH20 chromatography, is effectively removed by HPLC as can be seen in Fig.7. Consequently, the contribution of these metabolites to the final serum 1,25-$(OH)_2D_3$ concentration is negligable.

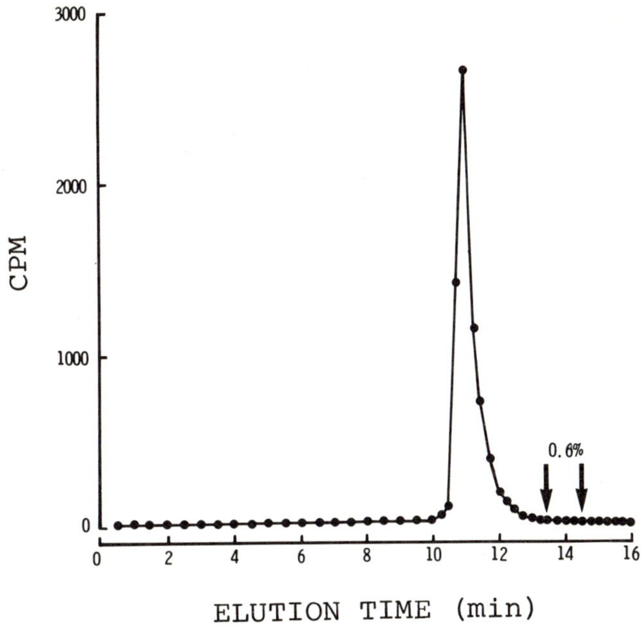

Fig.7. HPLC of post-LH20 serum sample spiked with tritiated 25,26-$(OH)_2D_3$. Column and conditions are identical to those on Fig.6. Arrows indicate the region collected for assay.

Variability of the method was evaluated by purifying and assaying aliquots of the same serum pool. The co-efficient of variation within assays was 9% and between assays was 14%. The addition of a 10 fold excess of 25-OHD_3 or 24,25-$(OH)_2D_3$ to serum samples prior to extraction and chromatography did not effect the measured concentration of 1,25-$(OH)_2D_3$ for this serum pool. By radioimmunoassay, the mean circulating concentration of 1,25-$(OH)_2D_3$ in healthy adults was 41 ± 2.5pg/ml with a range of 22 to 59pg/ml. This mean value is comparable with normal values recently reported for U.S. subjects using competetive receptor binding assays (6,7). No 1,25-$(OH)_2D_3$ could be detected (<5pg/ml) in serum from anephric subjects and the concentration was low or undetectable in serum from patients with severe chronic renal failure. As the kidney is the sole site of production of the 1,25-$(OH)_2D_3$ these findings further validate the method.

In five patients with vitamin D deficiency and histologically proven osteomalacia 1,25-$(OH)_2D_3$ concentrations were found to be below the lower limit of the normal range and were from <5 to 21pg/ml. The 25- OH D_3 concentrations in these patients were also low and ranged between <0.8 and 2.6ng/ml (normal range = 3-30ng/ml). The response of such patients to treatment with synthetic 1,25-$(OH)_2D_3$ (0.5µg twice a day) was characterised by increases in serum 1,25-$(OH)_2D_3$ concentrations between 50-90pg/ml, marked symptomatic improvement, and healing of bone disease.

To gain more information about the kinetics of exogenously administered 1,25-$(OH)_2D_3$, healthy subjects were given 2 µg orally and their serum 1,25-$(OH)_2D_3$ concentration monitored thereafter (Fig.8.). The absorption was shown to be rapid, the concentration reaching a peak within 3 hrs. Disappearance of the exogenous hormone was also rapid with the concentration falling to basal levels by 24hrs.

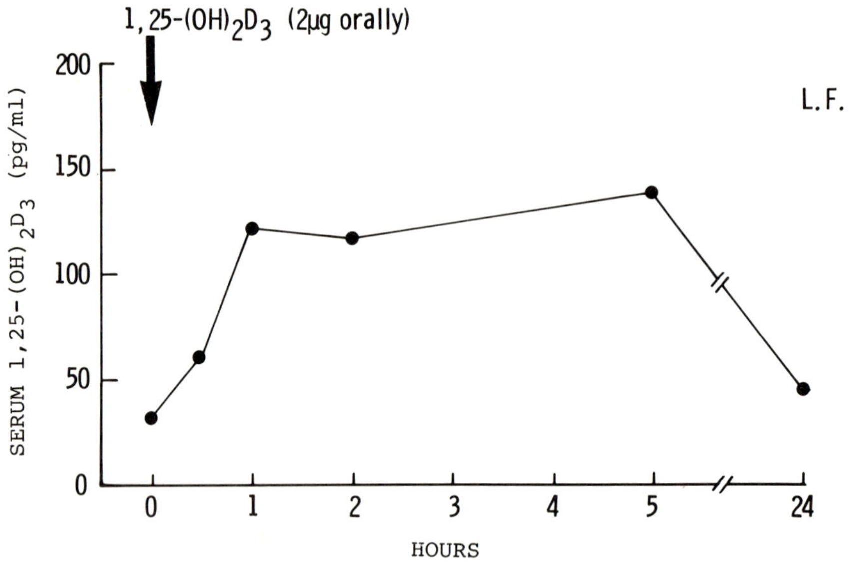

Fig. 8. Circulating 1,25-$(OH)_2D_3$ concentrations in a healthy subject given 2µg synthetic 1,25-$(OH)_2D_3$ by mouth.

In contrast, preliminary studies in patients with severe renal impairment show that the disappearance of exogenous 1,25-$(OH)_2D_3$ from the circulation is delayed pointing to the possible importance of the kidney in the excretion or further metabolism of this compound. These observations are very helpful in the clinical management of such patients and with the selection of a therapeutic approach.

Recently, the radioimmunoassay has been used to elucidate the pathogenesis of the development of hypercalcaemia in a patient with sarcoidosis (2). In this patient (RD) the serum 1,25-$(OH)_2D_3$ concentration was found strikingly elevated (140pg/ml) during a spontaneous hypercalcaemic episode. These changes occured as the results of small rises in serum 25-OHD_3 concentration which were entirely within the normal range (Fig.9).

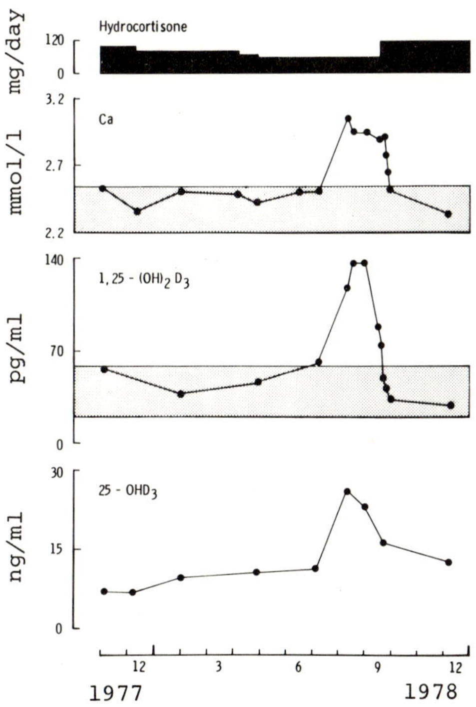

Fig. 9. The changes in serum 25-OHD_3 1,25-$(OH)_2D_3$ and calcium concentrations in a patient (RD) with sarcoidosis during a spontaneous episode of hypercalcaemia. (Reproduced with permission from Papapoulos et al. 1979).

This picture could be mimicked in the same patient and in another sarcoid patient by administration of a low dose (3000 units daily) of vitamin D_3 for 8 days. Thus, in these patients inappropriately high 1,25-$(OH)_2D_3$ concentrations are responsible for their apparent hypersensitivity to vitamin D.

Although the importance of $1,25\text{-}(OH)_2D_3$ as a calcium regulating hormone is well documented, the physiological significance of other hydroxylated vitamin D metabolites in man such as $24,25\text{-}(OH)_2D_3$ and $25,26\text{-}(OH)_2D_3$ is not clear. Taking advantage of the crossreactivity of $25,26\text{-}(OH)_2D_3$ it has been possible to adapt the assay and purification scheme to allow measurement of this metabolite in serum. In this assay, ^3H $1,25\text{-}(OH)_2D_3$ is used as labelled ligand and synthetic $25,26\text{-}(OH)_2D_3$ as unlabelled ligand. Tritiated $25,26\text{-}(OH)_2D_3$, generated biologically, is used to monitor losses during purification. In normal subjects (n=18) the mean $25,26\text{-}(OH)_2D_3$ concentration was 244pg/ml and ranged from 62pg to 423 pg/ml. Seven anephric patients had concentrations ranging from 43pg to 190pg/ml (mean 107pg/ml) which suggests extra-renal production of $25,26\text{-}(OH)_2D_3$ in man.

Clearly, the radioimmunoassay is proving to be a versatile tool in the clinical study of the production and disposition of the hydroxylated vitamin D metabolites. This technique has a distinct practical advantage over existing radio receptor assays in that antibodies provide a continuous supply of stable binding reagent whereas radio receptor assays require preparation of intestinal binding protein from vitamin D deficient chickens. Moreover, with the radioimmunoassay approach there is considerable potential for further development. For example, by immunizing more animals with the same or different immunogens it may be possible to produce antisera with even higher affinity and with greatest structural specificity. These possibilities are now being investigated.

ACKNOWLEDGEMENTS

Financial support of the Wellcome Trust is gratefully acknowledged.

REFERENCES

1. Clemens, T.L., Hendy, G.N., Graham, R.F., Baggiolini, E.G. Uskokovic M.R. and O'Riordan, J.L.H. (1978). Clin.Sci.Mol.Med., 54,329

2. Papapoulos, S.E., Clemens, T.L., Fraher, L.J., Lewin, I.G., Sandler, L.M. and O'Riordan J.L.H. (1979) Lancet, I, 627

3. Clemens, T.L., Hendy, G.N., Papapoulos, S.E., Fraher, J.L., Care, A.D. and O'Riordan. J.L.H., (1979) Clin. Endocrinol. In press.

4. Saifer, A. and Lipkin, L.E. (1959) Proc. Soc. Exp. Biol. Med., 102,220

5. Albano, J.D.M., Ekins, R.P., Maritz, G. and Turner, R.C. (1972) Acta Endocrinol. 70, 487

6. Bilezikian, J.P., Canfield, R.E., Jacobs, T.P., Polay J.S., D'Adamo, A.P., Eisman, J.A. and De Luca, H .F. (1978) N. Engl. J. Med., 299,437

7. Caldas, A.E., Gray, R.W. and Lemann, J. (1978). J. Lab.Clin.Med. 91, 840

Radioimmunology 1979, Ch. A. Bizollon, editor.

A STUDY OF IMMUNOREACTIVE CALCITONIN (iCT) IN HUMAN SERUM USING DIFFERENT ANTISERA AND ASSAY PROCEDURES

G. HEYNEN, C. FIORE, J. KOVARIK, J. KANIS, G. LUISETTO, S. GASPAR, P. FRANCHIMONT
Radioimmunoassay Laboratory, University of Liège, C.H.U. B23, Sart Tilman, Liège 1 (Belgium)

INTRODUCTION

A ten fold difference in absolute values of serum levels of iCT have been reported in the litterature[1-7]. Such a difference may be ascribed to the immunochemical heterogeneity of CT and the different specificities of antisera[8-9], but other causes may include technical aspect of assay procedure.

This study examines the possible causes of such a discrepancy in absolute levels of serum iCT by comparing the values of the serum concentration of iCT obtained by using 5 different antisera raised against human synthetic CT.

MATERIALS AND METHODS

Antisera used in this study were obtained in our laboratory (He) or kindly provided by L. DEFTOS (LJ_1), the WELLCOME Laboratories (W), the Institut National des Radioéléments (IRE) and obtained from a commercial kit, immunonuclear (MN) (further in the text, parantheses refer to the corresponding antiserum).

These antisera are used at the final dilution as indicated in table 1, in a 10 day incubation procedure which include 6 days of preincubation of antiserum and unlabelled hormone before the addition of the tracer for the last 4 days. This will be refered further in the text by PIP (preincubation procedure), as opposed to the incubation procedure, when labelled, unlabelled CT and antiserum are incubated simultaneously. The general feature of our radioimmunoassay (RIA), using antiserum He_1, reported previously in detail[4], utilizes equilibrium conditions during a four day period of incubation.

Synthetic human (h) CT is used as tracer and standard, and activated charcoal is used as separation technique. The amount of serum never exceed 100 ul in a total volume of 500 ul.

Serum samples were obtained from normal individuals, and also from patients suffering from various diseases, chronic renal failure, transplanted patients, Paget's disease of bone and osteoporotics.

RESULTS

Table 1 shows the main features of the assays performed with the different antisera in PIP and also with antiserum He without preincubation. The highest value of binding of labelled CT to the antibody in the absence of unlabelled CT is observed with antiserum He. The best sensitive assays and the lowest ID_{50} values are those obtained by using LJ_1 and He in PIP.

TABLE 1

MAIN FEATURES OF CT ASSAYS

	LJ_1	W	IRE	MN	He(IP)[§]	He
Final dilution of antiserum	6.10^{-5}	5.10^{-4}	10^{-5}	a	25.10^{-4}	25.10^{-4}
$\frac{B}{T}$ x 100[b]	15	12.5	25	20	29	29
Sensitivity (picograms)	0.4	1	4	30	6	0.4
ID_{50} (pg)[c]	4.2	14	34	130	100	4.3

[a] Dilution used as proposed by immunonuclear.
[b] Percentage of labelled CT bound to antibody in the absence of unlabelled CT.
[c] Quantity of CT decreasing the $\frac{Bx}{Bo}$ x 100 value to 50 %.
[§] IP denotes incubation procedure (4 days), whereas a preincubation of 6 days prior to the addition of the tracer was used for all the other cases.

Table 2 shows the correlation coefficient of values of iCT obtained in human serum using the different antisera.

TABLE 2

RESULTS AND COMPARISON OF SERUM iCT LEVELS

	LJ_1	W	IRE	MN	He(PIP)	HeIP
Mean iCT levels pg/ml (SEM)	20 ± 2	13 ± 2	125 ± 13	388 ± 20	20 ± 2	475 ± 65[a] 357 ± 58[b]
Mean Bx/Bo x 100	68[a]	84	74[a]	86[a]	68[b]	69[a] 74.5[b]
r (Vs He IP)*	.78[a]	.65	.40[a]	.26[a]	.78[b]	-
n	80[a]	36	80[a]	80[a]	265[b]	-
p	<0.001	<0.001	<0.001	<0.05	<0.001	-

[a] Refers to the same badge of 80 different sera.
[b] Refers to the same badge of 234 different sera.
* Correlation coefficient calculated for the values obtained in preincubation with the corresponding antibody versus the values obtained with He antiserum in incubation assay.

A typical standard curve of CT assay using antiserum He in PIP is shown in figure 1. No displacement of the tracer can be obtained with parathyroid hormone (PTH), FSH, LH, TSH, ACTH, β endorphin, leu- and met-enkephalin, whereas a complete cross reaction is obtained with multiple dilution of human sera containing high levels of iCT.

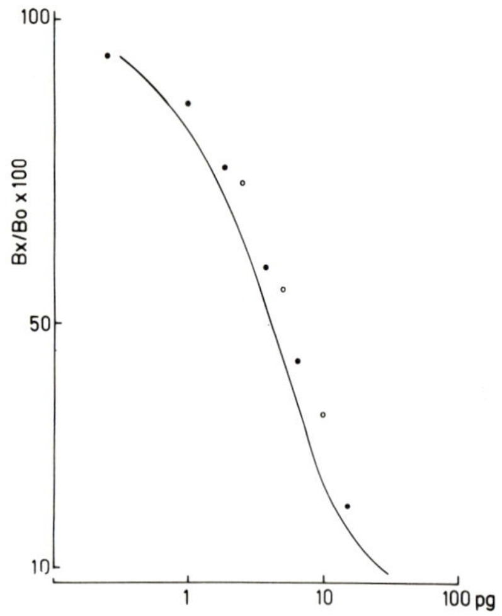

Fig. 1 Standard curve of human CT using antiserum He in a preincubation system. Several dilutions of sera from a patient suffering from primary hyperparathyroidism (O) and chronic renal failure (O).

Figure 2 shows the highly significant realtionship between the $\frac{Bx}{Bo}$ x 100 value of 265 human sera in incubation and the value in preincubation.

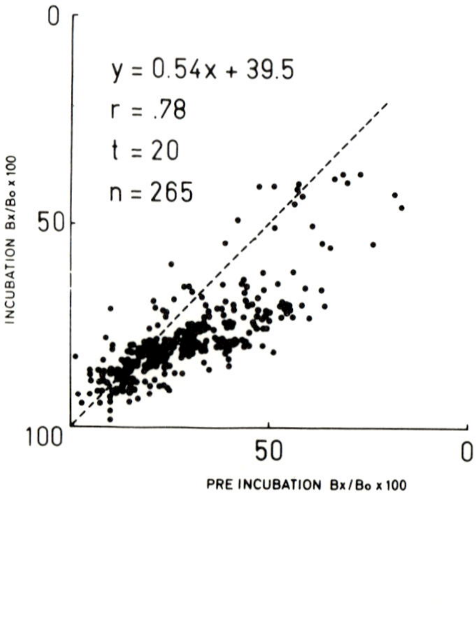

Figure 3 shows the effects of preincubation on CT levels in 77 sera of patients with and without impairement of renal function. With PIP preincubation method, absolute levels of iCT are 10 to 20 times lower than the levels obtained by using the incubation procedure. However, it should be noted again that there is a significant relationship between the values obtained by both methods.

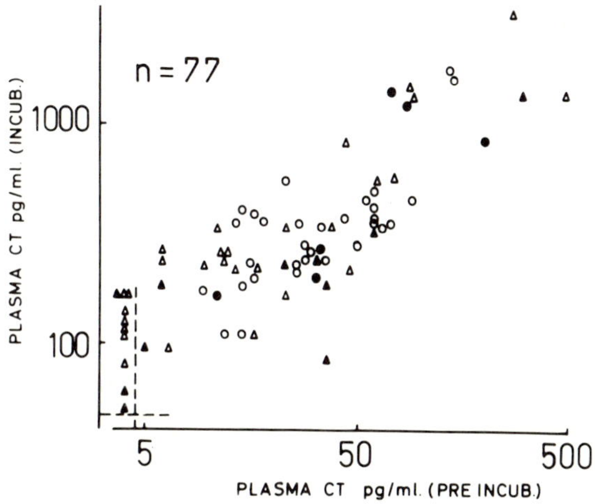

Fig. 3 Effects of preincubation on calcitonin levels, in 77 sera from patients with normal renal function (Δ), normal renal function and transplanted (▲), and patients suffering from chronic renal failure with (O) or without (●) dialysis treatment.

DISCUSSION

The ten fold difference in absolute values of immunoreactive CT concentration in human serum reported by different laboratories has been the subject of conflicting points of view regarding the physiological importance of this hormone in man.

It has generally been suggested that the highest values of serum iCT[10], as we also reported[4], might be due to non specific interference by the serum. However, control studies of specificity were extensively and carefully performed in the presence of human serum to exclude such a possibility. The presence of non specific substances significantly interfering with the assay has never been shown to exist in chromatographic experiments on Sephadex columns[11] or in fractions of serum obtained by preparative isotachophoresis[12]. Furthermore, the clinical relevance of our assay has been well documented. For instance, serum levels of iCT appropriately changed when the concentration of serum calcium was varied[4], and there are now several evidences supporting that endogenous iCT levels, as measured by this assay, is conversely related to the level of bone turn-over in renal osteodystrophy[13-14]. Non specific interference might thus not have been the major reason for this discrepancy in the absolute levels of serum iCT and we investigated more throughly other causes. For that purpose, a comparison was made between the serum iCT levels and the standard curve obtained by using different available antisera raised against human synthetic CT. Results show that, despite a substantial difference in the sensitivity of the standard curves, there is a positive relationship between the values of serum iCT levels, obtained by using He antiserum in incubation procedure and the values obtained by using the other antisera in preincubation assays. The relationship was, however, non significant with antiserum MN, which has the lowest sensitivity.

As the major difference was the use of non equilibrium conditions for all antisera except He, we then decided to compare the main features of CT radioimmunoassay by using antiserum He in preincubation versus incubation assays. The results show that, by using preincubation assay, the absolute sensitivity is increased by a factor of $\simeq$ 15 (from 6 pg to 0.4 pg), and is similar to the sensitivity obtained by using antiserum LJ_1[15]. Moreover, despite a ten to twenty fold difference, absolute levels of serum iCT obtained by both method are highly significantly correlated (Fig. 3).

The absolute amount of tracer bound to the antibody in the absence of unlabelled CT (Bo value) is the same in preincubation and incubation assays. However, the mean Bx/Bo x 100 of 265 human sera is significantly lower (68 % $\pm$ 1) in preincubation assay than in incubation assay (76 % $\pm$ 0.8)($p < 0.001$) and the regression line is significantly different from the line of equivalence (Fig. 2)($p < 0.01$).

Thus, the relative capacity of serum to inhibit the specific binding of labelled CT to antibody is greater in preincubation than in incubation assay, but to a much lesser extent than expected from the comparison of absolute levels.

The reason for such a discrepancy is unknown. One might think of a modification of conformational architecture of the molecule of CT during the 6 days period of preincubation with enhanced affinity for the antibody. Such a possibility can be excluded since the standard curve and the sensibility of the assay are the same with freshly prepared solution of CT and with a solution prepared 6 days before the incubation (not shown).

The possible influence of disease on the relationship between preincubation and "incubation" iCT levels was also assessed by comparing the results of serum iCT levels in patients with normal renal function and those obtained in patients with impaired renal function. By inspection of figure 3, it can be seen that this relationship is the same, independently of renal function.

Another possibility is that serum immunoreactive CT has a greater affinity for the antibody than labelled synthetic CT.

Finally, the specificity using antiserum He in a preincubation assay has been established on the basis of immunochemical similarity between serum iCT and synthetic CT (Fig. 2).

CONCLUSIONS

From these results, it is concluded that several causes might explain the difference in absolute levels of CT in human serum. Besides differences in sensitivity and immunochemical specificity of the antisera[8,9,14], it appears that method of assay is another important cause, the values of hCT being greater in equilibrium assays than in non equilibrium assays. It is also obvious that despite all the differences between preincubation and incubation assays with antiserum He, the overall clinical relevance of both methods are quite similar.

REFERENCES

1. Tashjian, A.H., Howland, B.G., Melvin, D.E.W. and Hill, C.S. (1970), New. Engl. J. Med., 283, 890

2. Moukhtar, M., Julienne, A., Tharaud, D., Taboulet, J. and Michaud, G. (1973), Comptes Rendus Acad. Sci. (Paris),

3. Samaan, N.A., Hill, C.S., Beceiro, J.R. and Schultz, P.N. (1973), J. Lab. Clin. Med., 81, 671

4. Heynen, G. and Franchimont, P. (1974), Europ. J. Clin. Invest., 4, 213

5. Silva, O.L., Snider, R.H. and Becker, K.L. (1974), Clin. Chem., 20, 337

6. Parthemore, J.G., Bronzert, D. and Deftos, L.J. (1975), J. Clin. Invest., 56, 835

7. Hillyard, C.J., Cooke, J.C., Coombes, R.C., Evans, I.M.A. and MacIntyre, I. (1977), Clin. Endocrinol., 6, 291

8. Julienne, A., Calmettes, C., Raulais, D., Michaud, G. and Moukhtar, M.S. (1978), In Endocrinology of Calcium Metabolism, D.H. Copp and R.V. Talmage, ICS 421, Excerpta Medica, Amsterdam-Oxford, pp. 55-63

9. Becker, K.L., Snider, R.H., Silva, O.L. and Moore, Ch.S. (1978), Acta Endocrinologica, 89, 89

10. Samaan, N.A.C., Hill, C.S., Beceiro, J.R. and Schultz, P.N. (1973), J. Lab. Clin. Med., 81, 671

11. Heynen, G. and Franchimont, P. (1975), Path. Biol., 23, 815

12. Heynen, G., Gaspar, S., Gysen, Ph. and Franchimont, P., unpublished data

13. Heynen, G., Kanis, J.A., Oliver, D.O., Ledingham, J.G.G. and Russell, R.G.G. (1976), Lancet, 2, 1322

14. Kanis, J.A., Earnshaw, M., Heynen, G., Ledingham, J.G.G., Oliver, D.O., Russell, R.G.G., Franchimont, P. and Gaspar, S. (1977), New Engl. J. Med., 269, 1073

© 1979 Elsevier/North-Holland Biomedical Press
Radioimmunology 1979, Ch. A. Bizollon, editor.

COMPARISON OF TWO N-TERMINAL RADIOIMMUNOASSAYS FOR THE PARATHYRIN, BREWER OR NIALL SEQUENCES.

C. DESPLAN, A. JULLIENNE, M.S. MOUKHTAR, P. RIVAILLE, D. RAULAIS, B. BOCCART & G. MILHAUD.
U. 113 INSERM, C.H.U. Saint-Antoine, 27 rue de Chaligny, 75012 PARIS FRANCE

INTRODUCTION

N-terminal sequence of human parathyrin (1-34 h PTH) is still controversial as three residues (positions 22, 28 and 30)[1-4] are not unequivocally elucidated. Recently the complete amino-acid sequence of h PTH has been reported[5].

Immunological studies involving the two proposed sequences, 1-34 hPTH Brewer sequence (1-34 hPTHB) or Niall sequence (1-34 hPTHN) have been performed but have yielded conflicting results : Fisher et Al.[11], using antibodies raised against extracted hPTH or 1-34 hPTHB showed a completecross reaction between synthetic 1-34 hPTHB and 1-84 hPTH extracted from adenomas.

Segre and Potts[12], using several heterologous antisera (anti bovine PTH bPTH) showed that 1-34 hPTH N displaced 1-34 hPTH^{125}I in an identical manner that 1-84 hPTH ; with 1-34 hPTHB low or no displacement was observed. Hendy et Al.[13], Visser et Al.[14] obtained similar results.

Previous studies have shown that a homologous assay for the 1-34 hPTHN could be used to establish a sensitive radioimmunoassay (RIA) for hPTH [15] . In the present report we have studied the cross reaction of hPTH extracted from adenoma tissue or normal plasma in two immunochemical systems homologous for the two proposed sequences. Our aim was to establish if the high cross reaction we had observed between extracted hPTH and the 1-34 hPTHN was due to common sequences between the two molecules.

MATERIAL AND METHODS

1-34 hPTH Synthesis

The synthesis was performed by the solid phase method of Merrifields[16]. For the Niall sequence[17], the purification was checked by aminoacid analysis and biological activity. For the Brewer sequence the procedure was identical with the exception that aminoacid analysis alone was used to check purification, due to the low biological activity of the peptide. We have also used original synthesis for these peptides[18-19].

hPTH extraction

Parathyroid adenomas was extracted by two differents methods[21-22].
hPTH obtained from parathyroid adenomas culture medium was also used in these studies.

hPTH was extracted from normal human plasma using affinity columns[23] specific for the N-terminal or C-terminal regions of the molecule[24].

Immunochemical studies

Two RIA systems specific for the two sequences were developped. Comparison of each sequence with hPTH extracted from tissues or plasma was carried out using several antibodies specific for one or the other molecule.

RESULTS

hPTH extracted from pathological tissues or normal plasma showed total cross reaction with antibodies specific for 1-34 h PTH N fragment (figures 1-4).

In these systems 1-34 h PTH B showed partial cross reaction and b PTH cross reacted to a low degree.

When the same experiments were performed using the RIA specific for fragment 1-34 h PTH B, h PTH cross reacted only partially and displacement of the 1-34 h PTH B tracer was identical to 1-34 h PTH N.

Radioimmunoassay

A sensitive assay has been developped using an immunochemical system homologous for 1-34 h PTH N. Sensitivity is $<$ 70 pg/ml sufficient to detect 65 % of normal subjects.

Primary or secondary hyperparathyroid subjects show higher levels (0.150 to 3.25 ng ml for primary and 0.3 to 1.75 ng/ml for secondary hyperparathyroidism (figure 9).

DISCUSSION

Our results confirm our previous studies showing that immunochemical system based on the Niall sequence can be used for establishing N-terminal assay for human PTH. Furthermore they indirectly confirm that the sequence proposed by Niall et al. has the greatest homology with the human molecule present in tissue and circulation.

These results further illustrate the exquisite sensitivity of immunological method to detect variations in primary structure of peptide as quite

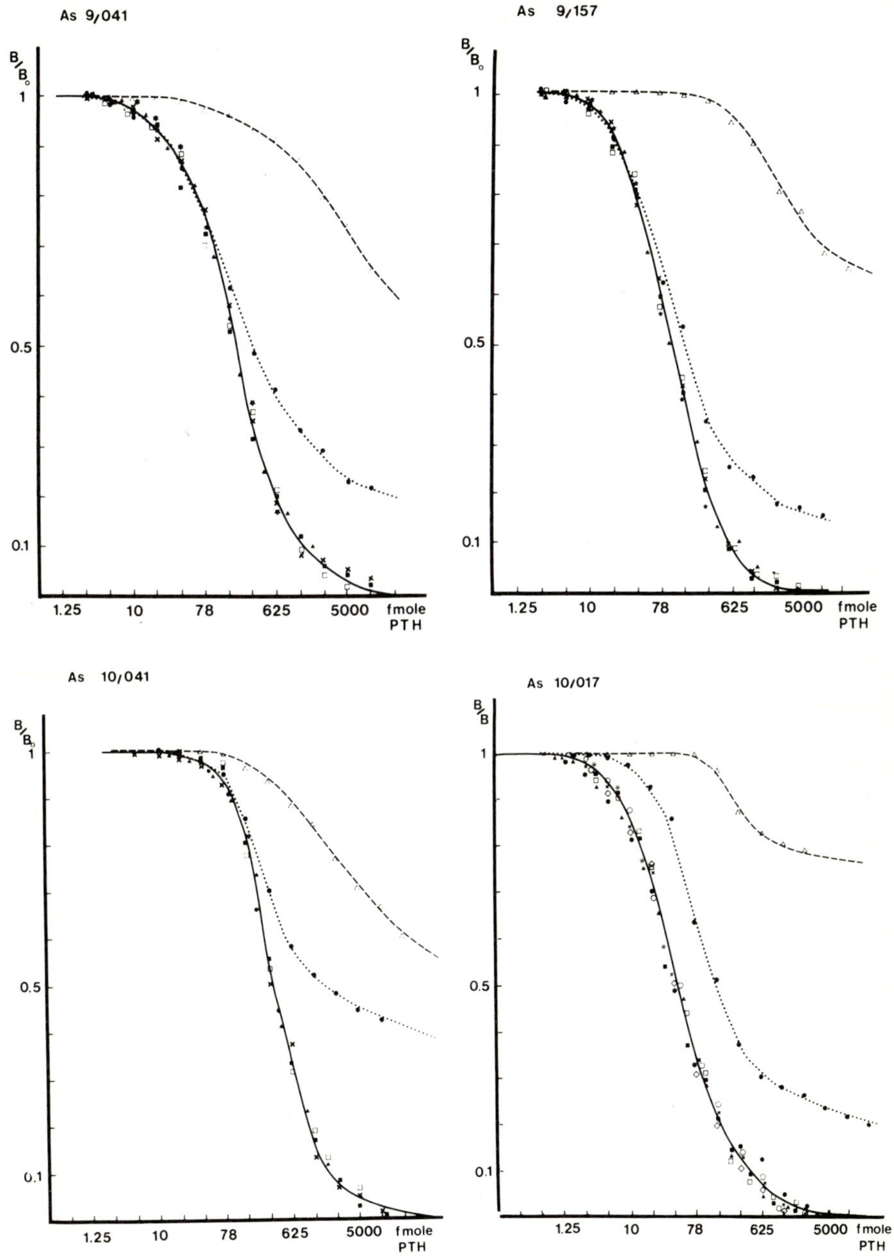

Figures 1-2-3-4 : Displacement of labelled 1-34 hPTH N. by extracted hPTH and by 1-34 hPTH Niall or Brewer sequences in a homologous RIA anti 1-34 hPTH N. Antiserum 9/041 (fig 1) 9/157 (fig 2) 10/041 (fig 3) 10/017 (fig 4).

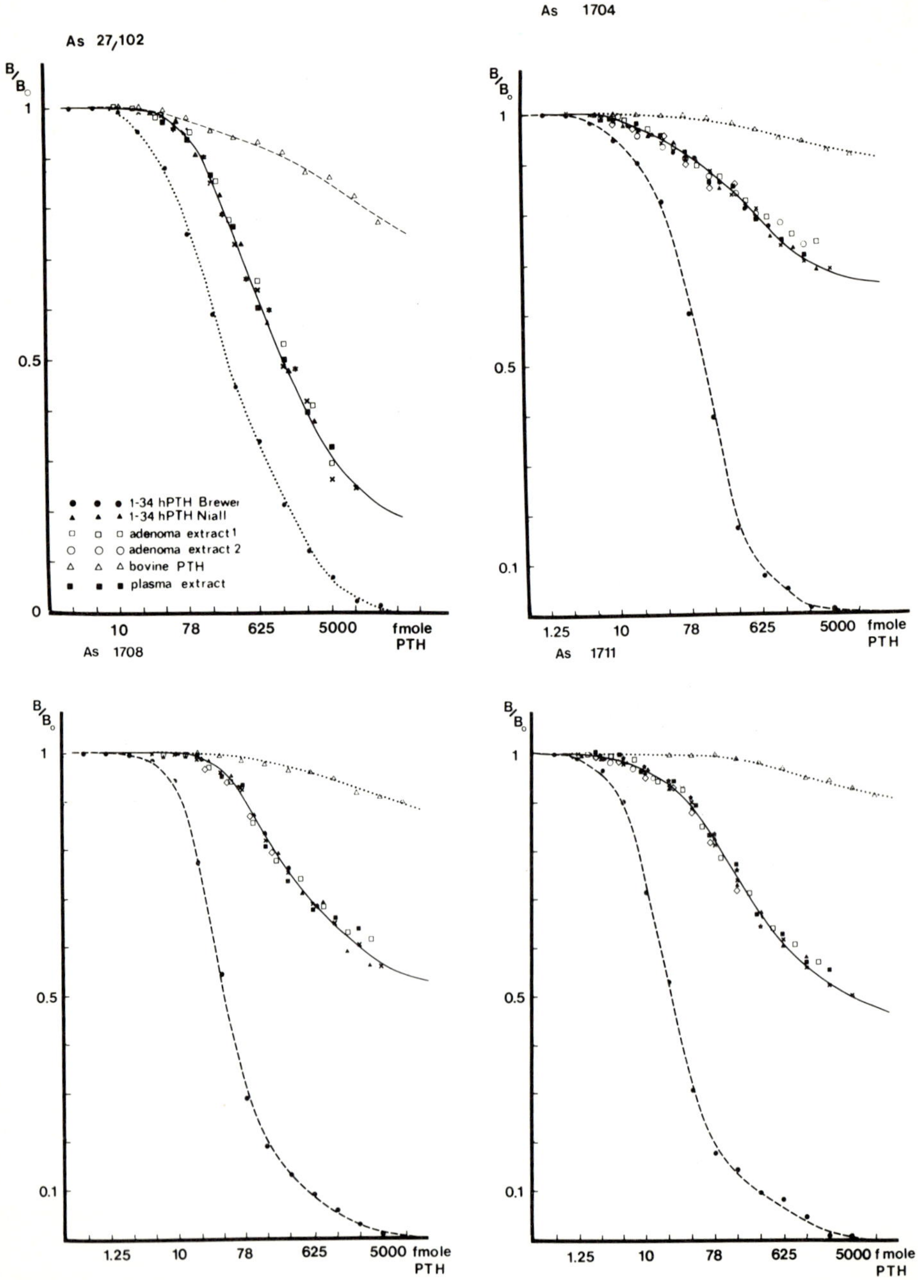

Figures 5-6-7-8 : Displacement of labelled 1-34 hPTHB. by extracted hPTH and by 1-34 hPTH Niall of Brewer seauences in a homologous RIA anti 1-34 hPTHB. Antiserum 27/102 (fig 5), 1704 (fig 6), 1708 (fig 7), 1711 (fig 8).

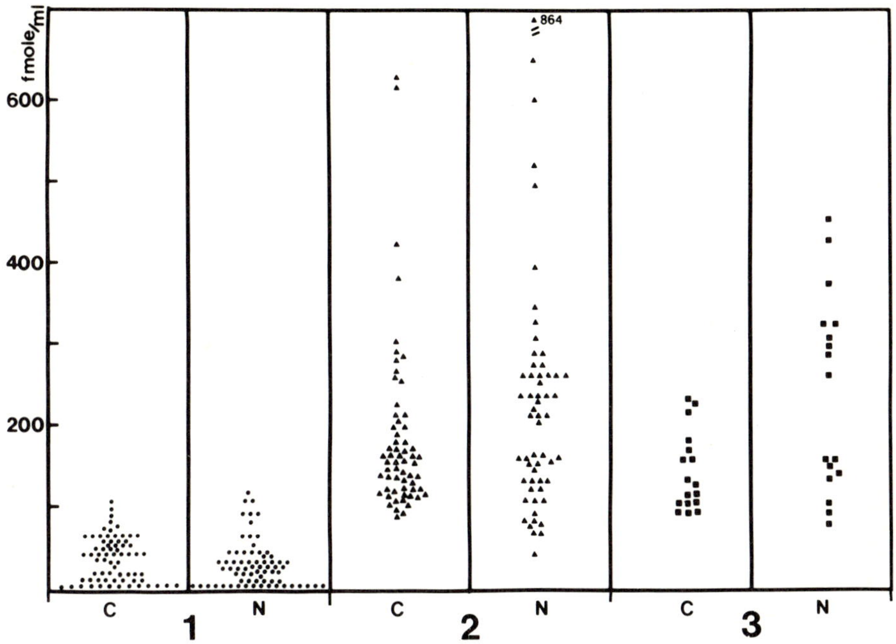

Figure 9 : Estimation of immunoreactive hPTH by carboxy terminal (C) and amino terminal (N) peripheral plasma.
Normal subjects (1), patients with primary hyperparathyroidism (2), and secondary hyperparathyroidism consecutive to renal insufficiency (3). Results are expressed in femtomoles of 1-84 bovine PTH and 1-34 hPTHN.
Measured in fmol/ml (fmol bPTH = 9.5 pg, 1 fmol 1-34 hPTH = 3.8 pg).

different cross reactivity is observed with molecules differing by only three aminoacids residues i.e. a difference smaller than 10 %. Though of course immunochemical studies entail considerable pitfalls due to the limited nature of the antigenic sites, the validity of the conclusion can be considerably increased if several antisera differing in the antigenic sites to which they are directed are used.

ACKNOWLEDGMENTS

We thank Dr Claude ARNAUD for generous gift of antisera anti 1-34 hPTH B (As 1704, 1708, 1711).

REFERENCES

1. Brewer, H.B., Jr., Fairwell, T., Ronan, R., Sizemore, G.W., and Arnaud, C.D. (1972), Proc. Natl. Acad. Sci. U.S.A. 69, 3585.

2. Niall, H.D., Sauer, R., Jacobs, J.W., Keutmann, H.T., Segre, G.V., O'Riordan, J.L.H., Aurbach, G.D., and Potts, J.T., Jr. (1974), Proc. Natl. Acad. Sci. U.S.A. 71, 384.

3. Brewer, H.B., Jr., Ronan, R.Fairwell, T., Rittel, W., and Arnaud, C.D. (1975), in Proceedings of the Fifth Parathyroid Conference, Talmage, R.V., Ed., Amsterdam, Excerpta Medica, P. 23.

4. Keutmann, H.T., Niall, H.D., O'Riordan, J.L.H., and Potts, J.T., Jr. (1975), Biochemistry 14, 1842.

5. Keutmann, H.T., Sauer, M.M., Hendy, G.N., O'Riordan, J.L.H. and Potts, Jt Jr. (1978), Biochemistry 17, 5723.

6. Potts, J.T., Jr., Keutmann, H.T., Niall, H.D., Deftos, L.J., Brewer, H.B., Aurbach, G.D. (1968), in Parathyroid hormone and calcitonin", Talmage, R.V., and Belanger, L.F., 1968, Excerpta Medica.

7. Potts, J.T., Jr. (1976), Clinical Endocrinology, 5, Suppl. 3075.

8. Parsons, J.A., Rafferty, B., Gray, D., Reit, B., Keutmann, H.T., Tregear, G.N., and Potts, J.T. Jr. (1975), in Calcium regulating hormone (ed. Talmage, R.V., Owen, M. and Parsons, J.A.) Excerpta Medica, 33, Amsterdam.

9. Hermann-Erlee, M.P.M., Heersche, J.V.M., Kekkelman, J.W., Gaillard, P.J., Tregear, G.W., Parsons, J.A. and Potts, J.T. Jr. (1976), Endocrin. Res. Commun. 3, 21.

10. Aurbach, G.D., Keutmann, H.T., Niall, H.D., Tregear, G.W., O'Riordan, J.L.H. Marcus, R., Marx, S.J., and Potts, J.T., Jr. (1972), Recent Progress in Horm. Res., 28, 353.

11. Fisher, J.A., Binswanger, U., and Dietrich, F. (1974), M.J. Clin. Invest, 54, 1382.

12. Hendy, G.N., Barling, P.M., and O'Riordan, J.L.H. (1974), Clin. Sci. Mol. Med. 47, 567.

13. Segre, G.V. and Potts, J.T., Jr. (1976), Endocrinology 98, 1294.

14. Visser, T.J., Buurman, C.J., Birkenhager, J.C. (1977, J. Endocrin. 74, 461.

15. Desplan, C., Jullienne, A., Moukhtar, M.S., Milhaud G. (1977), Lancet ii. 198.

16. Merrifield, R.B. (1967), Recent Prog. Horm. Res. 23, 451.

17. Rivaille P., Staub, J.F., Jullienne, A., Raulais, D., Milhaud, G., (1975), in Peptides 1974, Wolman, Y. Ed. Wiley J., New-York.

18. Rivaille, P., Bader, C.A., Monet, J.D., Gaubert, C.H., Moukhtar, M.S., Milhaud, G., (1976), in Peptides 1976, A. Loffet Editions, Editions de l'Université de Bruxelles, 555.

19. Tregear, G.W., Van Rietschoten, J., Greene, E., Niall, H.D., Keutmann, H.T., Parsons, J.A., O'Riordan, J.L.H., and Potts, J.T., Jr. (1974), Hoppe-Seyler's Z. Physiol. Chem. 355, 415.

20. Andreatta, R.H., Hartmann A., Johl A., Kamber, B., Mair, R., Riniker, B., Rittel, W., Sieber, P., (1973), Helv. Chim. Acta, 56, 470.

21. Rasmussen, H., Sze, Y.L., Yound, R., (1964), J. Biol. Chem. 239, 2852.

22. Keutmann, H.T., Barling, P.M., Hendy, G.N., Segre, G.V., Niall, H.D., Aurbach, G.D., Potts, J.T., Jr., and O'Riordan, J.L.H. (1974), Biochemistry 13, 1646.

23. Axen, R., Porath, J. and Ernbach, S., Nature (London), 214, 1302 (1967).

24. Desplan, C., Jullienne, A., Raulais, D., Barlet J.P., Moukhtar, M.S., Milhaud, G. (1978), in Proc. of third congress of IAEA Berlin, 2, 405, IAEA ed. Vienna.

25. Hunter, W.M., Greenwood, F.C. (1962), Nature London, 194, 495.

26. Fiskin, A.M., Cohn, D.V., and Peterson, G.S. (1977), J. Biol. Chem., 252, 8261.

27. Chou, P.Y., Fasmann, G.D. (1974), Biochemistry, 13, 211.

28. Monet, J.D., Bader, C.A., Herbigny, E., Funck-Brentano, J.L. (1978), FEBS Letters, 96, 79.

Radioimmunology 1979, Ch. A. Bizollon, editor.

25 HYDROXY VITAMIN D IN MATERNAL AND CORD SERUM

G. BAUDIN[+], M.H. VERNET[+], F. MONTOYA[++], H. BONNET[++], A. CRASTES DE PAULET[+]
[+]Biochimie A Institut de Biologie, Bd Henri IV - 34000 MONTPELLIER -FRANCE
[++] Service de Néo-Natalogie - Hôpital St Charles - 34000 MONTPELLIER - FRANCE

INTRODUCTION

The mechanism of neonatal hypocalcemia is unclear. Possibility is a defect in the turnover of calcium due to a disturbance in the action of one or more between the three hormones regulating the phosphocalcic metabolism.

In order to clarify this mechanism, we assessed the circulant levels of 25 hydroxycholecalciferol, the known precursor of 1-25 dihydroxycholecalciferol, in maternal and cord blood.

PATIENTS AND METHOD

Method

25 hydroxyvitamin D (25-OH-D) was determined by a modification of the competitive protein binding radioassay described by HADDAD and CHYU[1].This determination is realised in three steps :

1- Vitamin D compounds were extracted with ethanol. After evaporation of the ethanol phase, the extract is dissolved in a sulfuric aether- petroleum aether mixture (1/2, v/v).

2-Separation of vitamin D metabolites was realised by silica-gel chromatography, elution being done with sulfuric aether for 25-OH-D[2].

3-25-OH-D concentration was estimated using transcalciferin obtained from vitamin D depleted rats as binding protein, ^{3}H-25-OH-D3 as tracer and reference 25-OH-D3 as standard.

Patients

78 paired maternal and cord sera were collected within one year and the samples were grouped according to the seasons (three months by three months).

Women delivering at term were selected and those who have taking vitamin D therapy were discarded (age range 20-40 years).

As control , 25-OH-D was determined in non-pregnant age-matched women : blood was collected at different periods of the menstrual cycle ; some of them were taking oral contraceptives : we have found that such medication had non influence on the level of 25-OH-D (unpublished results).

RESULTS

The main value of serum 25-OH-D concentrations of mothers was significantly lower than the main value found in age-matched control women , at all sampling season (Figure 1).

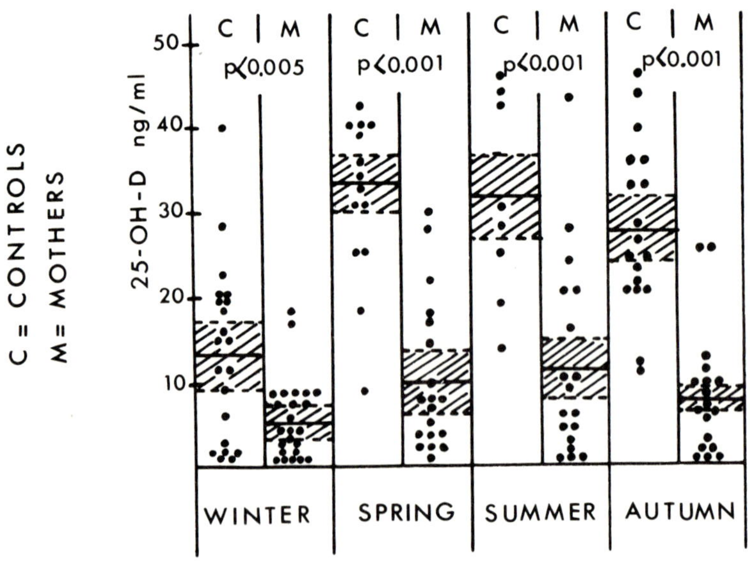

In figure 2 are shown the main levels of 25-OH-D found in maternal and cord blood : fetal concentrations are lower than maternal ones.

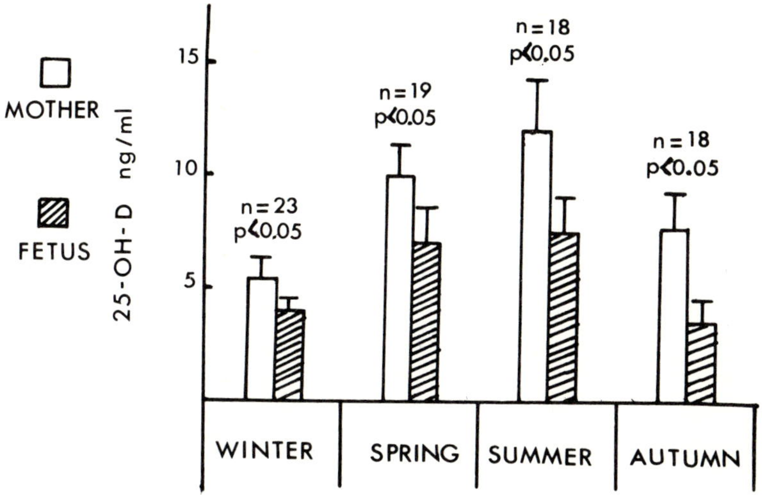

A significant correlation between maternal and cord blood 25-OH-D levels was obtained (figure 3).

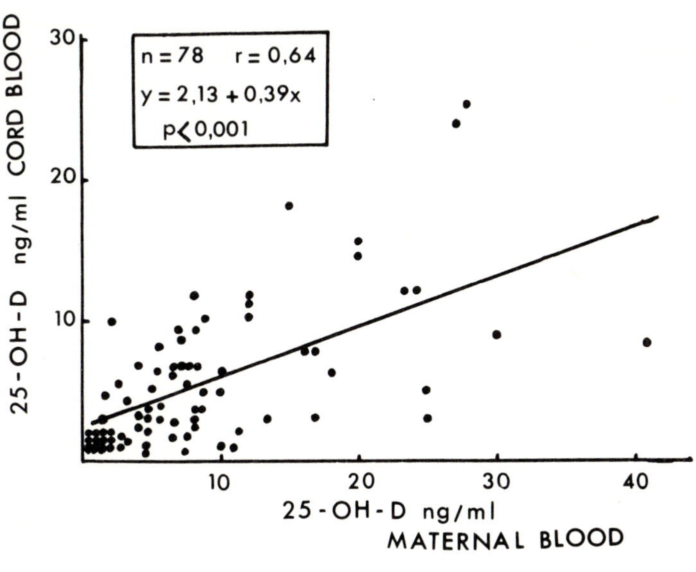

DISCUSSION

These results show that, whatever the season, mothers have lower serum 25-OH-D concentration than non-pregnant age-matched women. In addition, 25-OH-D levels of fetuses were lower than those of mothers and there is a significant correlation between maternal and cord serum 25-OH-D concentrations.

Recently, WEISMAN et al[3] reported similar results in white pregnant women but not in black ones. HILLMAN et al[4] found that 25-OH-D levels was lower in cord blood than in maternal serum ; however, no difference between pregnant and non pregnant women was observed.

It is interesting to note that, in their populations, pregnant women had received systematic multivitamin preparation, containing vitamin D, during gestation.

CONCLUSION

It is no possible, now, to explain this drastic diminution of serum 25-OH-D concentration in mother and fetal blood : we may suppose a diminution of sun exposure at the end of pregnancy, but this hypothesis is very unconvincing, since there is a very high sunlightning by our latitudes.

Not any studied women presented any phosphocalcic trouble : perhaps compensator phenomenons may exist. At any rate, it seems that estrogens increase 1-25 di OH-D synthesis[5].

It would be interesting to perform a complementary study upon serum 25-OH-D concentration along gestation and overall a similar study of 1,25-di OH-D in same subjects.

REFERENCES

1. Haddad J.G.,Chyu K.J. (1971) J. Clin. Endocr., 33,992-995.
2. Graham R.F., Preece M.A., O'Riordan J.L.H. (1977) Calcif. Tiss. Res., 22 suppl., 416-421.
3. Weisman Y., Occhipinti M., Knox G., Reiter E., Root A. (1978) Am.J. Obstet. Gynecol., 130,704-707.
4. Hillman L.S., Slatopolsky E., Haddad J.G. (1978) J. Clin. Endocrinol. Metab., 47,1073-1077.
5. Baksi S.N., Kenny A.D. (1978) Am.J. Physiol., 234 (6), E622-E628.

HORMONES AND REPRODUCTION

Radioimmunology 1979, Ch. A. Bizollon, editor.

ANDROGENS IN WOMEN : METHODOLOGICAL AND PATHOPHYSIOLOGICAL ASPECTS

GUY E. ABRAHAM
50 Penbrand Road - 90274 ROLLING HILLS - CALIFORNIA - U.S.A.

INTRODUCTION

Naturally occurring androgens are C19 steroids capable of stimulating male secondary sex characteristics. In the non-pregnant woman, androgens and their precursors are secreted by the adrenal cortex and the ovary.

In vivo (1) and in vitro (2) experiments strongly suggest that the zona reticularis is the main site of androgen secretion by the adrenal cortex. This zone is controlled by ACTH and other pituitary factor (s) (3). Preliminary data favor prolactin as the pituitary factor responsible for potentiating the effect of ACTH on the zona reticularis (4).

Ovarian androgens originate predominantly from the ovarian stroma (5) under the control of pituitary gonadotrophins, mainly LH (6).

After secretion by the adrenal and the ovary, most androgens are bound to specific plasma proteins (7), which temporarily inactivates them. The 17 β-ol-androgens have a greater biological activity and a greater affinity for these proteins than the corresponding 17-oxo-androgens, resulting in a higher metabolic clearance rate (MCR) of 17-oxo-androgens than the corresponding 17 β-ol-androgens (8). When androgens reach the target tissues, they are further metabolized and sometimes the metabolites are the locally active androgens (9). The skin is capable of converting weak androgens into potent ones. This activity of the skin is significantly higher in hirsute women (10).

The liver is the main site of steroid metabolism, where steroids undergo hydroxylation, reduction, oxydation and conjugation. Conjugated metabolites of steroids are then excreted by the kidney in the urine.

In normal women, Testosterone (T) is estimated to contribute half of the total androgenicity (11). The remaining contribution comes from other androgens such as 5 α-dihydrotestosterone (DHT), Androstenedione (A), dehydroepiandrosterone (DHEA) and its sulfate (DHEA-S), androst-5-ene, 3β, 17β-diol (Δ5-diol) and 5α-androstane-3α-17β-diol (5α-A-diol).

MEASUREMENT OF ANDROGENS

The two most common biological fluids used to asses androgen levels are urine and serum. There are pitfalls in the use of either fluid. Urinary levels of steroids represent integrated levels over a period of time whereas serum level only indicates peripheral levels at that instant. Urinary metabolites may not represent the level of the steroid precursors since there is rarely a unique precursor for each steroid.

Urine

Urinary methods are now considered less reliable and practical than measurement of plasma androgens.

17-ketosteroids. Urinary 17-ketosteroids (17-KS) are only a rough parameter of androgen secretion since they represent the end metabolites of androgens with different biological activity. The available data indicate that the 17-KS represent a mixture of nonspecific chromogens and steroid metabolites of which the precursors are C21 steroids and C19 androgens of adrenal and ovarian origin. Metabolites of 11-oxygenated C21 and C19 steroids compose 10-55 % of the total fractionated 17-KS. The remaining 45-90 % come primarily from the 11-desoxy metabolites of peripheral androgens. The C21 steroids 11-desoxycortisol (CPS) and 17 hydroxyprogesterone (17-OHP) contribute only minimally to the 11-desoxy-17-KS except in the case of congenital adrenal hyperplasia. About one-half of peripheral androgens are excreted as urinary 11-desoxy-17-KS, while the rest are excreted in the feces or in the urine as non-17-KS. Therefore, the androgens with the highest production rate contribute the greatest to urinary androgens in premenopausal nonhirsute women. The production rates calculations are based on serum levels obtained in our laboratory and from clearance rates previously reported. From this table, it can be seen that the major contributors to urinary 17-KS are the weak androgens dehydroepiandrosterone (DHEA) and its sulfate (DHEA-S). The potent androgens, testosterone (T) and dihydrotestosterone (DHT), contribute less than 1 % to the total 17-KS. It is not surprising, therefore, that a poor correlation has been observed between serum T and urinary 17-KS in hirsute patients (24) (25).

Testosterone glucuronide. This urinary metabolite is not a unique metabolite of serum testosterone (26), since peripheral androstenedione contributes significantly to urinary level. Also, a small fraction of peripheral testosterone is excreted as urine testosterone glucuronide.

5α-androstane 3α, 17β-diol glucuronide. This urinary androgen metabolite was postulated to represent a good parameter of peripheral formation of DHT at the target level (27), but this is not generally accepted (28).

Serum

The advent of the technic of radioimmunoassay has made practical and

TABLE 1

MEAN VALUES FOR METABOLIC CLEARANCE RATE (MCR), PLASMA LEVELS AND PRODUCTION RATE OF VARIOUS ANDROGENS IN PREMENOPAUSAL NONHIRSUTE WOMEN*

Androgens	MCR (L Plasma/DA)	Plasma Concentrations (NG/ML)	Production Rate (MG/DA)	Contribution %
DHEA-S	17	1700	28.9	73
DHEA	1500	4.20	6.34	16
A	1900	1.90	3.44	9
Δ5-diol	590	0.75	0.44	1.1
T	830	0.31	0.27	0.7
DHT	210	0.19	0.04	0.1
5α-A-diol	1200	0.02	0.024	0.06

* Modified, by permission, from Maroulis et al (1977) Obstet. Gynecol. 49, 454.

TABLE 2

OVARIAN AND ADRENAL CONTRIBUTION TO PERIPHERAL ANDROGENS (NG/ML)

Steroid	Ovarian Contribution			Adrenal
	F	M	L	Contribution
Testosterone	0.1 (33)	0.3 (60)	0.1 (33)	0.2 (40-66)
Dihydrotestosterone		90.1 (50)		0.1 (50)
Androstenedione	0.5 (45)	1.5 (70)	0.8 (60)	0.6 (30-55)
Dehydroepiandrosterone*		0.8 (20)		3.2 (80)
Androst-5-ene-3β, 17β-diol		0.2 (25)		0.6 (75)
Dehydroepiandrosterone sulfate	80 (4)	200 (10)	80 (4)	2000 (90-96)

* Ovarian contribution not influenced by phase of menstrual cycle.
( ) = percent contribution ; F = early follicular ; M = midcycle ; L = late luteal phase. Modified, by permission, from Abraham (31).

reliable the measurement of low levels of androgen in serum. This approach is now considered more advantageous over urinary measurement. However, because of nycthemeral, diurnal and circadian variations of serum steroid, the timing of serum sampling is critical, and must be consistant. Also, frequent sampling tends to average out these variations and narrow the normal range. The optimization of there variables has not yet been worked out.

Serum DHEA-S can be measured directly in diluted serum (29), but measurement of other androgens requires chromatographic purification (30).

ANDROGENS IN NORMAL WOMEN

In the normal adult women, the adrenal and the ovary contribute a certain amount of androgens capable of stimulating hair growth to a terminal stage on the extremities axilla and pubis. The production rate of the most important weak and potent androgens are shown in table I. The adrenal and ovarian contributions to the peripheral levels of these androgens are depicted in table II. These values were obtained by adrenal suppression studies from normal menstrual cycle (31).

ANDROGENS IN HYPERANDROGENIZED WOMEN

For a comprehensive evaluation of the hyperandrogenized women the peripheral levels of all known androgens should be measured. In addition, the measurement of serum 17-hydroxyprogesterone and 11-desoxy-cortisol would help to ruse out congenital adrenal hyperplasia due to 21-and 11-hydroxylase deficiency (32-33-34-35).

Although ideal, it is obviously not practical nor economical to perform extensive peripheral steroid studies in hirsute patients on a routine basis. However, if a comprehensive evaluation of peripheral steroid levels is performed in a large number of hirsute patients, some guidelines may be derived from such studies about the usefullness of the measurement of individual steroids.

Our experience in this field indicates that :

- Among the stimulation and suppression tests, the dexamethasone (Dex) suppression test, administered for 14 days, gives a reliable index of androgenicity and source of androgen excess.
- The measurements of serum F, DHEA-S, T and DHT before and following 14 days of Dex give adequate evaluation of hyperandrogenism and its source. In cases of ovarian hyperandrogenism, serum A levels may be of value (36-37).
- The measurements of serum DHEA and Δ5-diol are of no practical value in

the initial evaluation of hirsutism.

- The zona reticularis is more sluggish in its response to Dex than the zona fasciculata : only 40 % of hirsute patients suppress adequately DHEA-S after 4 days of Dex, 55 % do so after 7 days and 70 % do so after 14 days. We are at the present using the 14 days suppression test.

- The measurement of 17-OHP and S in the initial evaluation of hirsutism is not warranted. We would favor the measurement of 17-OHP and S only in hirsute patients with adrenal or mixed hyperandrogenism who show recurrence of hirsutism following discontinuation of Dex after 1 year of therapy. The yield of patients with adrenal enzyme defect (11- or 21-hydroxylase defects) would be greater and meanwhile, the treatment is the same in cases of adrenal hyperandrogenism not due to enzyme defect.

CONCLUSION

The advent of steroid radioimmunoassy has made possible measurement of relatively low levels of serum androgens. Since, there has been a shift from urine to serum as the prefered biological fluid to assess androgen levels, because serum levels give a more accurate picture of tissue levels than urinary levels.

The most important serum androgens have been assessed in normal and hyperandrogenized women. It is the opinion of the author that a limited number of androgens, measured before and after adrenal suppression, can give an accurate picture of the hyperandrogenism and its source. The timing and frequency of blood sampling remain to be optimized.

REFERENCES

1. Ofstad J. et al (1969) Acta Endocr. 37, 321.
2. Cameron E.H.D. et al (1969) J. Endocrinol. 45, 215.
3. Mills I.H. et al (1962) The human adrenal cortex, Williams & Wilkins, New-York, pp. 1-204.
4. Boyns A.R. et al (1969) J. Endocr. 45, 215.
5. Savard K. et al (1965) Recent Prog. Horm. Res. 21, 285.
6. Givens J.R. (1976) Adv. Internal Med. 21, 221.
7. Vermeulen A. and Verdonck L. (1968) Steroids 11, 609.
8. Abraham G.E. (1974) Clin. Lab. 4, 999.
9. Price V.H. (1975) Archs Derm. 111, 1496.
10. Thomas J.P. and Oake R.J. (1974) J. Clin. Endocrinol. Metab. 38, 19.
11. Rosenfield R.L. (1973) J. Reprod. Med. 11, 87.

12. Greenblatt R.B. (1963) The hirsute female, Springfield, New-York pp. 1-90.
13. Mahesh V.B. et al (1964) J. Clin. Endocrinol. Metab. 24, 1283.
14. Herrmann W. et al (1960) Fertil. Steril. 11, 74.
15. Goldzieher J.W. and Axelrod L.R. (1962) J. Clin. Endocrinol. Metab. 22, 425.
16. Slaunwhite W.R. et al (1967) J. Clin. Endocrinol. Metab. 27, 663.
17. Loras B. and Migeon C.J. (1966) Steroids 7, 459.
18. Hamburger C. (1958) Acta Endocrinol. 28, 536.
19. Abraham G.E. et al (1969) J. Clin. Invest. 48, 696.
20. Saez M. et al (1972) J. Clin. Invest. 51, 1226.
21. Kirschner M.A. et al (1973) J. Clin. Endocrinol. Metab. 37, 183.
22. Yang D.Y. et al (1967) J. Endocrinol. 38, 307.
23. Gower D.B. (1975) Biochemistry of steroid hormones, Blackwell scientific publications, New-York pp. 1-149.
24. Lloyd C.W. et al (1966) J. Clin. Endocrinol. Metab. 26, 314.
25. Maroulis B.G. et al (1977) Obstet. Gynec. 49, 454.
26. Korenman S.G. and Lipsett M.B. (1964) J. Clin. Invest. 43, 2125.
27. Kutten F. and Mauvais-Jarvis P. (1975) Acta Endocrinol. 79, 164.
28. Doberne Y. and New M.I. (1976) J. Clin. Endocrinol. Metab. 42, 152.
29. Buster E.J. and Abraham G.E. (1972) Analytical Letters 5, 543.
30. Abraham G.E. et al (1975) Clin. Biochem. 8, 374.
31. Abraham G.E. (1974) J. Clin. Endocrinol. Metab. 39, 340.
32. Loriaux D.L. et al (1974) J. Clin. Endocrinol. Metab. 39, 627.
33. Lippe B.B. et al (1975) J. Pediat. 85, 782.
34. Franks R.C. (1975) J. Clin. Endocrinol. Metab. 39, 1099.
35. Riddick D.G. and Hammond C.B. (1975) Obstet. Gynec. 45, 21.
36. Abraham G.E. et al (1976) Obstet. Gynec. 47, 395.
37. Abraham G.E. and Buster J.E. (1976) Obstet. Gynec. 47, 581.

© 1979 Elsevier/North-Holland Biomedical Press
Radioimmunology 1979, Ch. A. Bizollon, editor.

HORMONAL EXPLORATION OF MALE STERILITY

ALEX VERMEULEN, FRANK COMHAIRE & MARC VANDEWEGHE
Department of Endocrinology, University Hospital of Ghent, De Pintelaan, 135,
B-9000 Ghent (Belgium)

The interest in and development of non-surgical andrology in recent years is largely attributable to the stormy development of hormonal methodology. Indeed, although in the vast majority of males consulting for infertility no hormonal abnormalities are found, a minimal hormonal exploration is nevertheless generally required, as the finding of hormonal abnormalities permits to draw important conclusions concerning prognosis and therapeutic possibilities.

The testis is a gland with both an endocrine and an exocrine secretion, the endocrine gland being represented by the Leydig cells, the exocrine gland by the tubuli seminiferi, reflecting the dual interrelated function of the testes, virility and fertility. The Leydig cells are the most important source of androgens of which biologically by far the most active is testosterone, the daily secretion of which in adult males below 50-60 yrs varies between 4 and 10 mg and the peripheral plasma concentration between 280 and 1200 ng/dl.

Whereas testosterone in peripheral plasma is responsible for the general effects of the hormone, in the testis itself testosterone is required for normal spermatogenesis. The concentration required for this effect is much higher than the concentration in peripheral plasma and in tubuli seminiferi the concentration is about 100 times the concentration in plasma. This explains why systemic administration of testosterone does not restore normal spermatogenesis.

Testicular function is under the control of two pituitary hormones, the gonadotropins LH and FSH. Only the Leydig cells and the interstitial fibroblasts that can differentiate into Leydig cells have LH receptors[1] which mediate the stimulatory effect of LH on androgen secretion. FSH, receptors of which are found on the Sertoli cells, is required for initiation of spermatogenesis, especially division of spermatogonia, but once initiated, it seems that spermatogenesis can go on in the absence of FSH, if testosterone is present in appropriate amounts. FSH moreover stimulates the synthesis of an androgen binding protein by the Sertoli cells[2]. A small number of FSH receptors have been found on the Leydig cells[3] which explains that FSH might potentiate the effect of LH.

Pituitary gonadotropin secretion is under the control of the hypothalamus which secretes in the portal system a decapeptide GnRH; this stimulates LH and, to a lesser extent, also FSH secretion; its effects are modulated by the hormonal environment of the patient.

Testicular secretion products inhibit gonadotropin secretion by a negative feed back mechanism. Testosterone inhibits LH secretion, directly at the pituitary and indirectly via GnRH inhibition at the hypothalamic level; there is some evidence that this inhibition is not realized by testosterone itself but that prior local transformation to estradiol in the hypothalamus and to DHT or Adiol, at the pituitary level is required[4].

Although these steroids, via a decreased GnRH secretion, inhibit also FSH secretion, a low molecular protein, inhibin, secreted by the Sertoli cells appears to inhibit selectively FSH secretion at the pituitary level[5] although an action at the hypothalamic level cannot be excluded[6].

The whole system moreover is under the influence of the central nervous system , the stimuli of which are integrated at the hypothalamic level. As to the role of prolactin, there is evidence that at physiological levels it increases LH receptors on the Leydig cells[7], whereas at supraphysiological levels it may inhibit GnRH secretion and eventually decrease the sensitivity of the receptors for LH. Moreover at supraphysiological levels it appears to induce impotence, apparently independent of its effect on the pituitary-gonadal axis.

x

x x

This physiological background should enable us to explore in a sensible way the hypothalamo-pituitary-gonadal axis.

As already stated hormonal abnormalities are found in only a minority of cases of infertility, but routine determination of plasma testosterone, LH and FSH and possibly prolactin seems warranted in the view of the important prognostic and/or therapeutic consequences of abnormal levels. Moreover in order to localize the origin or determine the nature of the defect, in selected cases additional hormonal explorations such as an HCG test, a GnRH test or an anti-estrogen test may be required . It is rare that decreased testosterone secretion is the direct cause of a deficient spermatogenesisbut a combined endo- and exocrine deficiency points towards other etiologies than an isolated oligozoospermia. Gonadotropin levels will indicate whether the lesion is primarily at the testicular or at the hypothalamo-pituitary level. Increased FSH levels in oligozoospermia point to an intact hypothalamo-pituitary function, but generally will only be observed when spermatogenesis is greatly impaired : indeed inhibin being produced by the Sertoli cells[5,8] increased FSH levels indicate impaired Sertoli cell function and almost certainly point to an irreversibly impaired spermatogenesis. On the other hand normal FSH levels can be found in aspermatogenesis, even when the cause is at the testicular level, as long as inhibin synthesis is intact. In the presence of low gonadotropin levels, a GnRH test will theoretically permit to destinguish whether the lesion is at the pituitary or at the hypothalamic level, whereas in the presence of a normal GnRH test, antiestrogens, competing for the estradiol receptor in the hypothalamus, should confirm a hypothalamic defect. Correct interpretation of all these tests requires however exact knowledge of all the possible interfering factors.

1. Testosterone

It is well known that testosterone secretion occurs episodically, in response to the episodic release of LH; the amplitudo of the resulting variation in plasma T levels is about 200% from nadir to zenith with a frequency of about 1 to 2 pulses in 6 hrs (9). Moreover testosterone levels show nycthemeral variations, levels in the late afternoon being ± 25% lower than in the morning[10], as well as seasonal variations, with highest levels in the fall[11]. ACTH[12], as well as corticoids[13] decrease plasma T levels, probably by a direct effect of cortisol on the Leydig cells. Stress factors as examplified by injection of a pyrogen, or physical exhaustion, as after a marathon run[14] cause an important fall of testosterone levels. Moreover chronic diseases may also decrease plasma androgen levels. Finally results should be interpreted in function of age of the patient a rapid decline of T levels being observed after the 6th decade of life[15].

2. HCG stimulation

This test will inform us about the secretory reserve of the Leydig cells and moreover permits to differentiate anorchism from bilateral cryptorchidism. In the young normal male a 5 days stimulation with 1000-3000 IU of HCG results in a doubling of T levels, but in normal elderly males the response is somewhat blunted[15]; moreover it should be realized that due to the absence of endogenous stimulation in hypogonadotropic hypogonadism or prepubertal boys, a longer stimulation may be required in these patients before obtaining plasma T levels comparable to those observed in normal males.

3. Gonadotropins

A differentiation of hypogonadropic hypogonadism from normal males is impossible by virtue of basal values alone. When T levels well within the normal range are found however, hypogonadotropism is practically excluded. Gonadotropins are released episodically[16,17], with an amplitudo ranging from 35 to 270% from nadir to peak and a frequency of 2-4 per 6 hrs for LH, whereas for FSH the amplitudo ranges from 1 1/2 to 2 fold. Only about 1 in 3 LH peaks however are followed within 1-2 hrs by a testosterone peak.

Hence borderline increased values should be checked by frequent sampling, and it is good practice to take 2 or preferably 3 blood samples with a 20 minutes interval and to have equivocal results repeated. It may be recalled that the MCR of hLH was calculated to be $\pm$ 25 ml/min/m^2 in normal men, and 20 ml in normal premenopausal women yielding a BPR of 81 IU/24 hrs in normal men, 40 in normal premenopausal women and 295 in postmenopausal women[18,19]. The plasma half life of hLH varies from 12 to 45 minutes, whereas the half life of FSH is $\pm$ 3 hrs.

Sex steroid hormone administration alters frequency and amplitudo of peaks, testosterone increasing amplitudo but decreasing frequency, whereas estradiol decreases pulse amplitudo without effect on frequency[17].

Before puberty gonadotropin secretion is low and prepuberty can be considered as a physiological hypogonadotropic state. The first sign of impending pubertal development is augmented LH secretion with sleep[20]. In elderly males on the other hand, basal LH and FSH levels are significantly increased in comparison to younger adults, probably a reflection of the aging proces affecting both the tubular and Leydig cell compartment;

this should be taken into account when interpreting results[15,21,22].

4. GnRH test

Several modalities have been advocated for this test : doses from 25 up to 500 ug of GnRH have been used and the polypeptide has been administered subcutaneously, intravenously or as a continuous infusion. Whereas continuous infusion undoubtedly gives additional information concerning the biphasic release of LH (which is not to evident for FSH)[23], generally GnRH is injected I.V. as a bolus, 100 ug of GnRH being the most frequently used dose.

A word concerning the analysis of the test : several ways of expression may be used : maximum level attained, maximum increase, maximum increase expressed as percentage of basal level, or cumulative response[24]. None of these types of analysis is completely satisfactory. The cumulative response might be the most satisfactory if all plasma samples are taken at equidistal time, so as to give equal weight to each point but, due to the fact that the rate of decline of hormone levels is influenced both by the disappearance rate and the continuing secretion[25] the interpretation may be ambiguous. Therefore we favor the absolute maximal increase. The most comprehensive study of the response to GnRH in adult males was published by Wollesen et al[25] who found that a dose response relationship existed for both the peak LH release and the total LH secretion over the range 1 to 3000 ug of GnRH, the minimal dose giving a significant response being 1.58 ug/subject. No dose response relationship existed for peak FSH release, but judged from total FSH secretion, the effects were dose related, the minimal effective dose being 20 ug.

The response varies in function of the age and sex of the subject studied. As far as prepubertal (stage P1) boys are concerned, it is generally accepted that LH release is minimal, whereas FSH release is similar in prepubertal, pubertal and adult males. Prepubertal and pubertal girls release more FSH than males at all stages of sexual maturation and the gonadotrophs of prepubertal girls are more sensitive to GnRF. As a consequence, in prepubertal boys the response to GnRF may be practically absent and differentiation from hypogonadotropic hypogonadism may be impossible[26].

The first event at puberty is probably the increased release of GnRH by the hypothalamus and as the degree of previous exposure to GnRH affects magnitude and quality of response, in peripubertal boys (and girls) there occurs a striking increase in the LH response, with a reversal of the FSH/LH ratio after GnRH between prepuberty and puberty[26,27]. In most cases the first sign of secondary sexual development occurs within one year after LH rises more than 2 ng/ml (LER 960) following 100 ug GnRH[26].

In adults the 95% confidence intervals for the peak response to an intravenous bolus injection of 100 ug were 400-800% of the individual mean base line LH concentration and 100-200% of the mean base line FSH concentration, with no significant change in serum T levels at any dose level[25]. Moreover there exists a positive correlation between peak LH response and basal LH level[21,25,28,29]. The LH peak is generally reached after 30 minutes (range 15-45) whereas the FSH peak is only reached after 60 minutes (range 30-90)[30].

In elderly males both basal gonadotropic levels and the absolute response to GnRH are higher than normal[15,31], but the relative response may be decreased[15,32].

5. Clomiphen test

After administration of Clomid[R], 100 à 150 mg/day for 10 days to adult males LH and FSH levels increase by 50-100%, with a parallel increase in T and E2 levels[33-36]. A slightly weaker increase was observed after treatment with tamoxifen 20 mg/day[36]; longer treatment (6 weeks) results in a slightly greater increase of LH, FSH, T and E2 levels. Whereas, due to the high sensitivity of the gonadostat before puberty, a response to clomiphen administration appears only at mid-puberty[37], tamoxifen, which has a much weaker estrogenic activity, is capable to activate the hypothalamo-pituitary gonadal axis in early puberty[36].

6. Prolactin

Prolactin levels do not change during development in boys but double in girls in late puberty; throughout life prolactin levels stay about 50% higher in women (5-20 ng/ml) than in man (4-12 ng/ml)[38]. Prolactin levels show important nycthemeral variations with maximum concentration between 5 and 7 a.m. and lowest between 10 a.m. and noon[39]. Its half life is very short (10 to 15 min.), which explains the effect of stress[40] increasing rapidly prolactin levels. Moreover, due to an increased TRF secretion, prolactin levels are high in hypothyroidism, whereas antidopaminergic drugs (phenothiazines, butyrophenones, metoclopramide etc.) cause hyperprolactinemia[41].

x

x x

Let's now consider the results of these investigations in our patients consulting either for primary or secondary in fertility, (defined as unprotected cohabitation for at least one year not resulting in pregnancy) and/or for impotence. The female partners of all the men in this study had been examined by a gynaecologist and were considered to be potentially fertile, although fertility in some of them might have been subnormal. Causes of infertility are manifold and classification is difficult, none being completely satisfactory. 615 cases have been analysed and results concerning basal hormonal levels are represented on table I.

From a group of 615 males consulting for infertility, hormonal abnormalities under basal conditions were observed in 30%. If we eliminate the patients with as a primary complaint impotence, either on an organic or psychiatric basis (n = 113), there remain 502 patients, in 183 of which (35%) an hormonal abnormality was observed. In 150 patients (30%) increased FSH levels were observed, and this of course was a secondary phenomenon to a primary spermatogenic failure. If we consider the findings according to sperm density, FSH levels were increased in 101/149 cases of azoospermia (68%), in 25/76 cases of oligozoospermia of less than 5 million (33%) in 9/35 (26%) cases of oligozoospermia between 5 and 10 million and in only 15 out of 242 (6%) of cases with more than 10 million spermatozoa per ml. In 62 cases (12%) LH levels were definitely increased, concerning essentially Klinefelter's syndrome (n = 26), testicular atrophy (n = 10) and anorchia (n = 4), whereas in 22 (5%) the increase was only marginal. Only in 3 cases increased LH levels were observed in the presence of normal FSH levels. Testosterone levels were decreased in 57 cases (11%), 14 of which in Klinefelter's S, 10 in testicular atrophy or anorchia, 13 in hypogonadotropic hypogonadism.

Increased LH levels with decreased T levels were observed in 35 cases, concerning mainly Klinefelter's syndrome (n = 14), male Turner (n = 2), anorchia and testicular atrophy (n = 10) and cryptorchidism (n = 6). Compensated hypoleydigism (increased LH and normal T) was observed in 31

TABLE I : INFERTILITY - FREQUENCY OF HORMONAL ABNORMALITIES

SPERM DENSITY:		AZOOSPERMIA				$0.1\text{-}5 \times 10^6$/ml				$5.1\text{-}10 \times 10^6$/ml				$>10 \times 10^6$/ml			
	TOTAL NUMBER	n	FSH↑	LH↑	T↓	n	FSH↑	LH↑	T↓	n	FSH↑	LH↑	T↓	n	FSH↑	LH↑	T↓
I. <u>DEFECTIVE SPERMATOGENESIS</u>																	
A. *TESTICULAR CAUSES*																	
1. MAINLY TUBULAR LESIONS																	
a. Chromos.abnorm.																	
- Klinef. S.	30	29	29	26	14	1	1	1	0	0	0	0	0	0	0	0	0
- Male Turner	2	2	2	2	2	0	0	0	0	0	0	0	0	0	0	0	0
b. Genetic abn.																	
- Steinert's D.	2	0	0	0	0	1	1	1	1	1	0	0	0	0	0	0	0
c. Cryptorchidism	67	26	21	3 (+6)	6	15	4	1	0	4	1	(1)	0	22	(8)	0	0
d. Testicul.atrophy (torsion, orchitis)	15	14	14	10	6	1	1	(1)	0								
e. Toxic.cytostatics	2	2	2	2	1	0	0	0	0.								
f. Idiopathic oligozoosp.	138	21	17	3 (+5)	0	25	6	1	(1)	8	(1)	0	0	84	0	0	0
2. COMBINED TUBULAR + LEYD.C.DEF.																	
- Primary : Anorch.	4	4	4	4	4	0	0	0	0	0	0	0	0	4	0	0	3
- Second : Hyperprolactin.	5	0	0	0	0	0	0	0	0	0	0	0	0	5	0	0	3
Hypogonadotr.hypog.	13	13	0	0	13	0	0	0	0	0	0	0	0	0	0	0	0

TABLE I continued

B. EXTRATESTICUL. CAUSES																	
VARICOCELE	170	14	8 (+1)	1 (+5)	1	33	9 (+2)	1 (+2)	1	22	7	(2)	0	101	6	0	0
C. GENERAL DISEASES																	
- Livercirrhosis																	
- Renal insuffic.	9	6	4	4	4	0	0	0	0	0	0	0	0	3	1	2	2
- Toxic.subst.																	
D. AUTOIMMUNE FACTORS																	
SPERM AGGLUTINATION	12	0	0	0	0	0	0	0	0	0	0	0	0	12	0	0	0
II. DEFECTIVE SPERM TRANSPORT																	
A. *ABSENCE EJACUL.DUCTS*	4	4	0	0	0	0	0	0	0	0	0	0	0	0	0	0	0
B. OBSTRUCTIVE LESIONS	14	14	0	0	0	0	0	0	0	0	0	0	0	0	0	0	0
C. PROSTATITIS	15	0	0	0	0	0	0	0	0	0	0	0	0	20	0	0	0
TOTAL	502	149	102	71	51	76	25	8	1	35	9	3	0	242	15	2	5

III. DEFECTIVE EJACULATION	n	FSH	LH	T
A. *ORGANIC LESION*				
1. PEYRONIE - HYPOSP. - FIMOSIS	2	0	0	0
2. DRUGS	3	0	0	0
3. PARAPLEGIA	6	3	0	4
4. HYPERPROLACT.	6	0	0	0
B. PSYCHIC IMPOTENCE - ANEJACUL.	96	1	(1)	1
TOTAL	113	4	(1)	5

( ) : Borderline increase

cases, whereas a decreased T level in the presence of normal LH was only observed 4 times.

Whereas it has been reported by Nankin et al[42,43] that in men with idiopathic oligozoospermia, mean testosterone concentration is lower than in normal men, this is not confirmed by our findings, as even in idiopathic azoospermia, all T levels were within the normal range, with a normal mean value.

As expected, the response to GnRH was increased whenever basal gonadotropin levels were high. It has been reported[43,44] that also in patients with oligozoospermia with normal basal gonadotropin levels, the response is excessive. The physiopathological significance of this observation is however unclear; it is nevertheless possible that an increased response indicates a more profound impairment of spermatogenesis and hence a poor prognosis.

In 13 cases out of 615 an isolated hypogonadotropic hypogonadism without loss of other endocrine functions was the cause of infertility; in two of these anosmia was observed (Kallmann's syndrome). Theoretically one would expect in these patients low gonadotropin and androgen levels, the latter showing a normal increase upon HCG stimulation; if the lesion is at the pituitary level one would expect an absent response to GnRH, whereas a lesion at the hypothalamic level would be expected to give a normal response to GnRH. However as far as HCG stimulation is concerned, one should realize that due to absent endogenous stimulation by LH, Leydig cells have not developed and that it may take a longer stimulation before a normal response of T levels is observed. As far as GnRH is concerned, this test evaluates the functional and not the anatomical state of the hypothalamo-pituitary unit[24]. Hence in patients with pituitary tumors but partially preserved gonadotropic function, the response to GnRH may be normal; on the other hand in hypothalamic disorders, due to the absence of previous endogenous priming, the response to GnRH may be deficient[24,30], the degree of previous exposure to GnRH affecting both magnitude and quality of response[26]. Moreover it has been suggested that in some cases, Kallmann's syndrome might involve both the hypothalamus and the pituitary[46]. It is not surprising therefore that several authors[47-49] reported that in hypothalamic disease, repeated stimulation with GnRH may finally lead to a response of the pituitary whereas others[46,50] did not observe any effect of prior priming the pituitary.

All our subjects with hypogonadotropic hypogonadism showed typical eunuchoidism and all of them had extremely low T levels, which responded to (prolonged) HCG stimulation.

In 3 of these patients the GnRH test gave a(n) (almost) normal response, suggesting a hypothalamic cause for the hypogonadotropism; this was confirmed by the absence of any response to either tamoxifen or clomiphen. In 6 patients no response was seen upon GnRH stimulation; in 2 of these prolonged GnRH stimulation with a depot preparation for 7 days, resulted in a normal response, suggesting again an intact pituitary; in 4 cases neither short nor long term GnRH stimulation resulted in an increase of gonadotropins : therefore a pituitary hypogonadotropic hypogonadism was diagnosed.

In 2 cases of Prader Willi syndrome (hypogonadism, hypomentia, muscular hypotonia and obesity) testosterone levels were extremely low with a moderate increase upon HCG stimulation; GnRH stimulation gave a normal response in both, but whereas Clomid 25 mg/day resulted in a normal response in one patient in the other a normal response was only observed after prolonged Clomid administration[50].

In obstructive oligozoospermia, hormonal levels were evidently normal.

In 113 subjects complaining only of impotence, hyperprolactinemia was observed in 6, 4 of which had marginally decreased testosterone levels, whereas of 6 subjects with posttraumatic paraplegia 3 had increased FSH and 4 a decreased T level.

CONCLUSIONS

Hormonal abnormalities were observed in 30% of the patients consulting for infertility or impotence. These occurred almost exclusively in patients with a sperm density below 5 million/ml, occasionally with a sperm density between 5 and 10 million and exceptionnally with a density over 10×10^6. This is in agreement with the conclusion of Smith & Steinberger[51] that it is of little value to evaluate hormone levels in men unless sperm counts are below 10×10^6/ml or total sperm count below 25×10^6.

In the majority of the cases the abnormality concerns increased FSH levels, a secondary phenomenon to impairment of Sertoli cell function. This finding has a high prognostic value as prognosis is uniformely bad whatever type of treatment is used. Moreover treatment with either anti-estrogens, GnRH or gonadotropins does not make sense when basal gonadotropin levels are increased. Increased LH levels occurred practically only when FSH levels were increased and almost exclusively in Klinefelter's S., testicular atrophy or anorchism, or operated cryptorchidism.

Decreased testosterone levels are most frequently found in testicular atrophy, Klinefelter's syndrome and in hypogonadotropic hypogonadism. The diagnosis of the latter requires more elaborate endocrine investigation, including GnRH and anti-estrogen tests.

From this survey it appears that whenever sperm counts are below 10 million/ml, FSH levels should be determined, as therapy and prognosis will be different whether normal or increased levels are found. In the presence of increased FSH levels, in operated cryptorchidism, and testicular a- or hypotrophy, complimentary investigations are required. Determination of prolactin levels on the other hand is only rewarding in patients complaining of (relative) impotence.

REFERENCES

1. Catt, K.J., Dufau, M.L. and Tsuruhara, T. (1972) J.Clin.Endocrinol. Metab., 34, 123.
2. French, F.S. and Ritzen, E.M. (1973) Endocrinology, 93, 88.
3. Catt, K.J. and Dufau, M.L. (1973) Nature New Biology, 244, 219.
4. Zanisi, M., Motta, M. and Martini, L. (1973) The endocrine function of the testes. Vol.I, Academic Press, pp.533.
5. Franchimont, P., Chari, S., Hazee-Hagelstein, M.T., De Brucke, M.L. and Duraisevani, S. (1977) The testes in normal and infertile men. Raven Press, New York, pp. 253.
6. Lugaro, G., Castellato, M.M., Mazzola, G., Faschini, G. and Carrea, G. (1974) Neuroendocrinol. 15, 62.
7. Bartke, A., Croft, B.T. and Dallerio, S. (1975) Endocrinology 75, 1601.
8. Steinberger, A. and Steinberger, E. (1977) The testis in normal and infertile men. Raven Press , New York, pp. 271.
9. Naftolin, E., Judd, J.H. and Yen, S.S.C. (1973) J.Clin.Endocrinol. Metab. 36, 185.
10. Dray, R., Reinberg, A. and Sebaoun, J. (1965) C.R.Acad.Sc.Paris, 261, 573.
11. Reinberg, A., Lagoguey, M., Chauffournier, M. and Cesselin, F. (1975) Ann.d'Endocrinol. 36, 44.
12. Rivarola, M.A., Saez, S.M., Meyer, W.J., Jenkins, M.E. and Migeon, C.J. (1966) J.Clin.Endocrinol.Metab., 26, 1203.
13. Doerr, P. and Pirke, R.M. (1976) J.Clin.Endocrinol.Metab., 43, 622.
14. Dessypris, A., Kuoppasalmi, K. and Adlercreutz, H. (1976) J.Ster. Biochem., 7, 33.

15. Rubens, R., Dhont, M. and Vermeulen, A. (1974) J.Clin.Endocrinol. Metab., 39, 40.

16. Nankin, H.R. and Troen, P. (1976) J.Clin.Endocrinol.Metab., 33, 558.

17. Santen, R. and Bardin, C.W. (1973) J.Clin.Invest., 52, 2617.

18. Pipperell, R.J., de Kretser, D.M. and Burger, H.G. (1975) J.Clin. Invest. 36, 118.

19. Kohler, P.O., Ross, G.T. and Odell, W.D.(1968) J.Clin.Invest. 47, 38.

20. Boyar, R., Finkelstein, J., Roffwarg, H., Kapen, S., Weizmann, D. and Hellman, L. (1972) N.Engl.J.Med. 287, 582.

21. Isurugi, K., Wakabayashi, K., Fukutani, K., Takayasu, H., Tamaoki, B. and Okada, M. (1973) J.Clin.Endocrinol.Metab. 37, 533.

22. Baker, H.W.G., Bremner, W.J., Burger, H.G., de Kretser, D.M., Dulmanis, A., Eddie L.W., Hudson, B., Keogh, E.J., Lee, V.W.R. and Rennie, G.C. (1976) Rec.Progr.Horm.Res. 32, 429.

23. Bremner, W.J. and Paulsen, C.A. (1974) J.Clin.Endocrinol.Metab. 39, 811.

24. Franchimont, P., Demoulin, A. and Bourguignon, J.P. (1975) Hormone Research 6, 177.

25. Wollesen, F., Swerdloff, R.S. and Odell, W.D. (1976) Metabolism 25, 845.

26. Grumbach, M.M., Roth, J.C., Kaplan, S.L. and Kelch, R.P. (1974) Control of the onset of puberty. John Wiley & Sons - New York, p. 115-166.

27. Garnier, P.E., Chaussain, J.L., Binet, L., Schumberger, A. and Job, J.C. (1974) Acta Endocrinol. 77, 422.

28. Von zür Mühlen, A., Köbberling, J. (1973) Horm.Metab. Res. 5, 266.

29. Wentz, A.C., Jones, F.G.S., Rocco, L. (1975) J.Obstetr. & Gynec. 45, 533.

30. Valcke, J.Cl., Mahoudeau, S.A., Thieblot, Ph., Pigue, L., Luton, J.P., Franchimont, P., Moreau, L. and Bricaire, H. (1974) Ann.Endocrinol. 35, 423.

31. Hashimoto, T., Miyai, K., Izumi, K. and Kumahara, Y. (1973) J.Clin.Endocrinol.Metab. 37, 910.

32. Snyder, P.J., Reitano, J.F. and Utiger, R.D. (1975) J.Clin. Endocrinol.Metab. 41, 938.

33. Bardin, C.W., Ross, G.T. and Lipsett, M.B. (1967) J.Clin.Endocrinol. Metab. 27, 1558.

34. Santen, R.J., Leonard, J.M., Sherins, R.J., Gandy, H.M. and Paulsen, C.A. (1971) J.Clin.Endocrinol.Metab. 33, 970.

35. Baker, H.W.G., Bremner, W.J., Burin, H.G., De Kretser, D.M., Dulmanis, A., Eddie, L.W., Hudson, B., Keoghs, E.J., Klee, V.W.R. and Rennie, G.C. (1976) Rec.Progr.Horm.Res. 32, 429.

36. Vermeulen, A. and Comhaire, F. (1978) Fertility & Sterility 29, 320.

37. Kulin, H.E., Grumbach, M.M. and Kaplan, S.M. (1969) Science, 166, 1022.

38. Yamagi, T., Shimamoto, K., Ishibashi, M., Kosaka, K. and Oremo, H., (1976) Acta Endocrinol. 83, 711.

39. Weitzman, E.D., Boyar, R.M., Kapen, S. and Hellman, L., (1975) Rec.Progr.Horm.Res. 31, 339.

40. Frantz, A.G., Kleinberg, D.L. and Noël, G.L. (1972) Rec.Progr. Horm.Res. 28, 527.

41. Lee, K.H., Amenomori, Y., Chen, C.L. and Meiter, J., (1976) Endocrinology 87, 667.

42. Nankin, H.R., Castaneda, E. and Troen, P. (1976) Idiopathic oligozoospermic men. Mosby Co. New York, pp. 370-374.

43. Nankin, H.R., Castaneda, E. and Troen, P. (1977) The testis in normal and infertile men. Raven Press, New York, pp. 529.

44. Snyder, P.J., Lipshulz, L.I., Greenberg, S.H.and Caminos Torres, R. (1977) The testis in normal and infertile men. Raven Press, New York, pp.539.

45. Winter, J.S.D., Tarasaka, J. and Faiman, J. (1972) J.Clin. Endocrinol.Metab. , 34, 348.

46. Zarate, A., Kastin, A.J., Soria, J., Canales, E.S. and Schally, A.W. (1973) J.Clin.Endocrinol.Metab. 36, 612.

47. Yoshimoto, Y., Moridera, K., Imura, A. (1975) N.Engl.J.Med. 292, 242.

48. Mortimer, C.H., McNeilly, A.S., Fischer, R.A., Murray, M.A.F. and Besser, G.M. (1974) Brit.Med.J. 4, 617.

49. Mortimer, C.H., Besser, G.M., McNeilly, A.S. (1974) J.Endocrinol. 61, LXI.

50. Tolis, G., Lewis, W., Verdy, M., Friesen, H.G., Salomon, S., Pagalis, G., Palatos, F., Fessasa, P.H., Rochefort, J.G. (1974) J.Clin. Endocrinol.Metab. 39, 1061.

51. Smith, K.D. and Steinberger, E. (1977) The testis in normal and infertile men. Raven Press, New York pp. 489.

Radioimmunology 1979, Ch. A. Bizollon, editor.

MODIFICATIONS OF 20 /17 HYDROXYPROGESTERONE RATIO AND ANDROGEN PLASMA LEVELS IN FEMALE HYPERPROLACTINEMIA AND HIRSUTISM.

GINO MAGRINI, FRANCOISE MEAN AND JEAN-PIERRE FELBER
Division de Biochimie Clinique, Département de Médecine, C.H.U.V., 1011 Lausanne, Switzerland

INTRODUCTION

Depending on the stage of the follicular phase, granulosa and/or theca cells may produce more or less estradiol, progesterone and androgens.

Progesterone (P) and 17αOH progesterone (17αOHP) were shown[1] to be major products of human granulosa cells from preovulatory Graafian follicles in control short-term cultures with endogenous and exogenous substrates. On the other hand, it is generally admitted that prolactin (PRL) influences steroidogenesis in women, and atypical PRL patterns have been implicated in abnormal ovarian functions. In cultured human granulosa cells, a biphasic action of PRL on P secretion has been reported[2].

Moreover, high activity of 20 hydroxysteroid dehydrogenase (20αOHSD), as observed in the secretory phase of the human menstrual cycle, leads to a decrease in intracellular P[3].

The metabolism of P into 20αOH progesterone (20αOHP) may thus be a local regulator of the molecular events initiated by P for the steroid to exert its action.

It was otherwise shown[4] that prostaglandin-induced luteolysis of rat ovary leads to an immediate decline in serum P, which probably triggers an increase in pituitary PRL which, in turn, stimulates 20 OH progesterone production. However, this hypothesis is in conflict with the inhibitory effect of PRL observed on 20αOHSD activity in vivo[5, 6] and in vitro[7].

In order to gather more data in this context, various groups of women presenting either hyperprolactinemia from different origins or hyperandrogenic hirsutism, were studied for their progestins and androgen levels.

MATERIALS AND METHODS

One group of women presenting hyperprolactinemia (H/PRL) from various origins (from moderately to highly elevated PRL levels) were studied before (8 women) and during (10 women) bromocriptine treatment (2 x 2.5 mg/day for 3 months). Plasma samples were obtained in middle-late follicular and/or luteal phases.

One group of 20 normally menstruating women was studied both in the middle-late follicular and in the luteal phase.

Two groups of hirsute women were studied, each patient presenting at least one elevated androgen level and normal PRL levels : 13 of the women had normal menstrual cycles and 19, irregular or no cycles.

Plasma samples were obtained in the morning (8 a.m.) in the middle-late follicular phase.

Plasma steroid levels (20αOHP, 17αOHP, testosterone (T), androstenedione (Δ_4), dehydroepiandrosterone sulfate (D-S), cortisol (F)) and PRL were measured by radioimmunoassay using specific antibodies[8].

RESULTS

In fig. 1, the mean 20α/17α ratio of plasma levels in the follicular phase decreased from 1.9 (controls) to 0.9 in the H/PRL group ($p = 0.025$), but returned to 1.8 during bromocriptine (H/PRL + CB) ($p < 0.025$). In the luteal phase, the 20α/17α ratio changed respectively from 2.1 to 1.5 and 2.5, but nonsignificantly.

The increase in mean absolute levels of 17 OHP from the control group to the H/PRL group was highly significant.

Figure 1

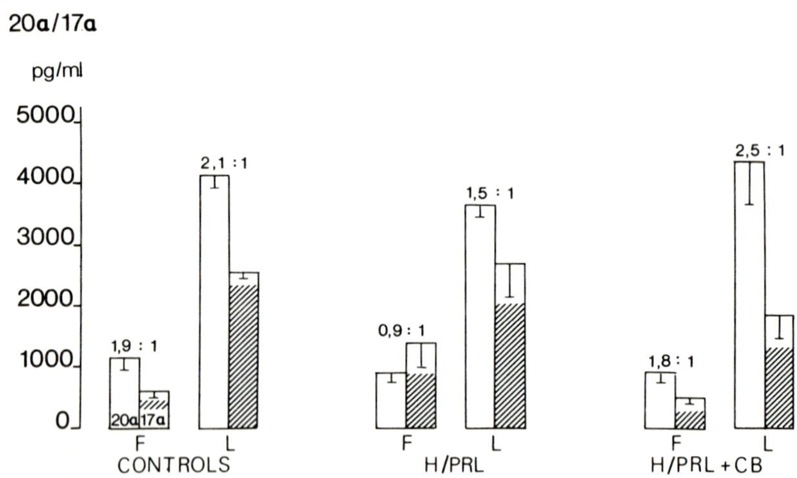

Hyperprolactinemic women before (H/PRL) and during bromocriptine (H/PRL +CB)
n=8 n=10

Figure 2

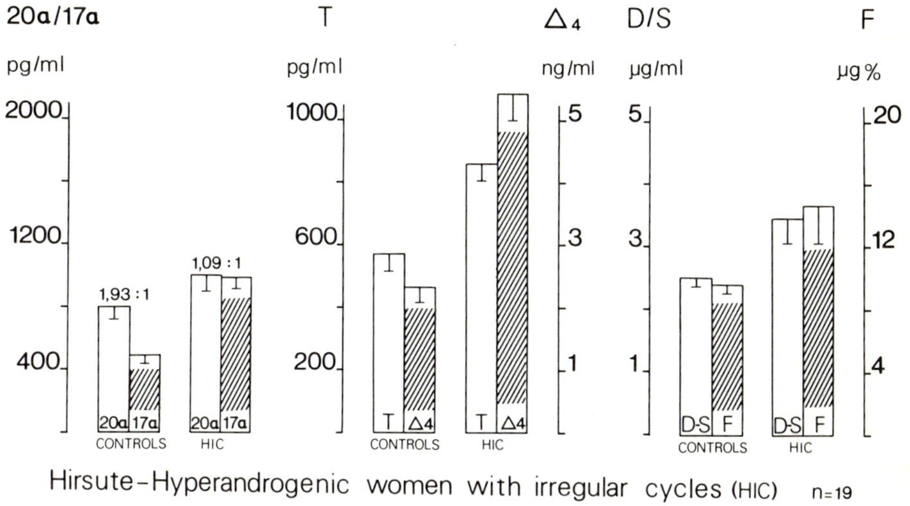

In the group of hirsute women with irregular cycles (Fig. 2), the 20α/17α ratio decreases significantly from 1.9 (controls to 1.09 ($p < 0.005$). Both mean testosterone and androstenedione levels were significantly increased, and mean D-S and cortisol, moderately increased. In the group of hirsute women with normal cycles (fig. 3), the 20α/17α ratio decreased, although nonsignificantly, from 1.9 (controls) to 1.47. Only mean Δ_4 levels were significantly elevated.

Figure 3

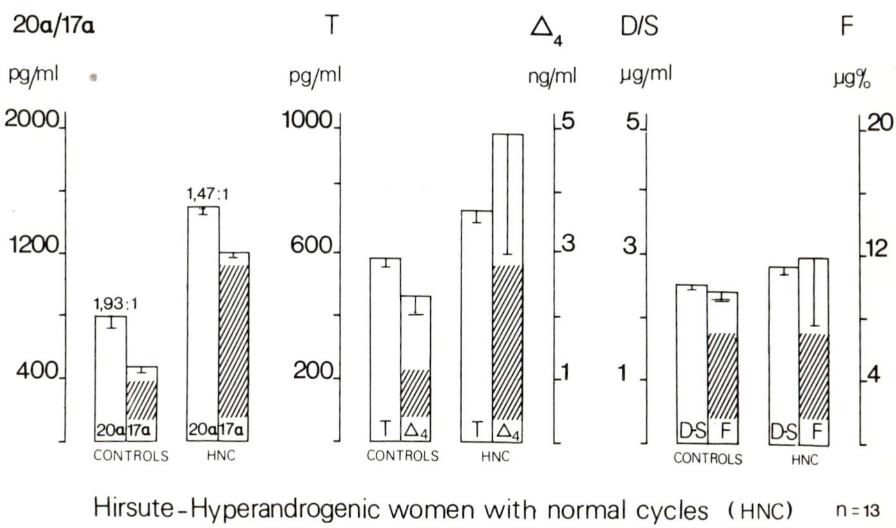

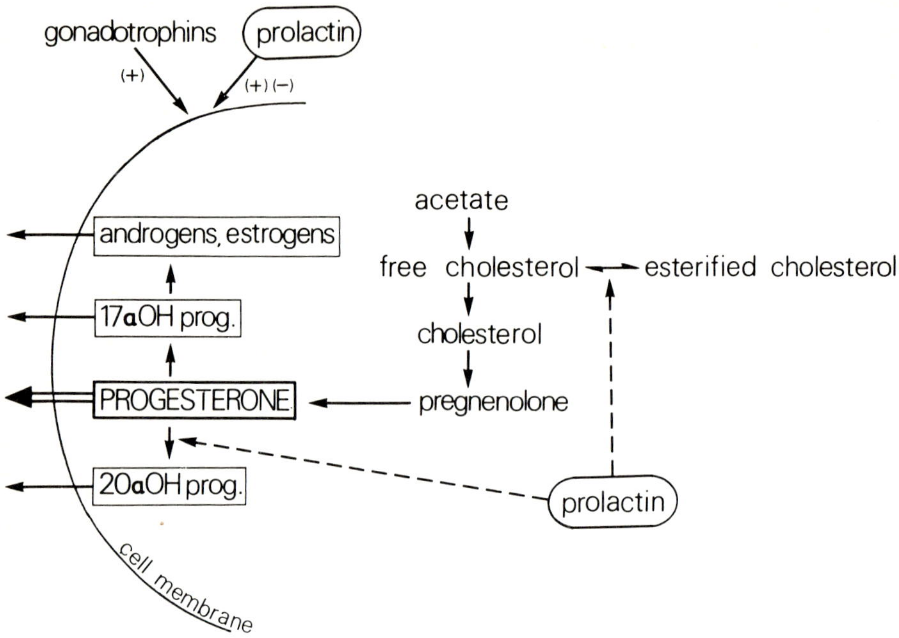

Fig. 4. Possible sites of action for PRL in the ovary.

DISCUSSION

In the group of 8 hyperprolactinemic women (fig. 1), the mean 20α/17α ratio of plasma levels in the follicular phase decreased significantly, compared with the control group of normal women in the same proliferative phase, but returned close to control values in the group of H/PRL + CB women during the bromocriptine treatment. In the patients in the luteal phase, the same trend of modifications in the mean 20α/17α ratio was observed. On the other hand, the decrease observed in the 20α/17α ratio was induced by an increase in mean absolute levels of 17αOHP (highly significant in the follicular phase), accompanied by a moderate mean decrease in 20αOHP ; reverse findings were observed during bromocriptine treatment.

These findings, suggesting possible modulating effects of hyperprolactinemia on the ratio between 20αOHP and 17αOHP plasma levels in favour of the 17αOHP formation, are in keeping with recent reports suggesting that PRL may play a role in regulating (and/or inhibiting) granulosa cells function and the activity of 20αOHSD[2, 4, 5]. Moreover, as 17αOHP is an androgenic precursor, increased levels may indicate a hyperandrogenic condition , sometimes reported in hyperprolactinemic women ; on the other hand, G.E. Abraham reported (which we also do in this study) elevated levels of 17αOHP in hirsutism. Our results, however, do not show a clear action of PRL on 20αOHP formation, but only a trend to inhibition, perhaps because of the limited number of patients studied. Other authors[5, 6] have suggested that PRL may have an inhibitory effect on 20αOHSD activity, in this step of modulation of the intracellular quantity of P, and others[4] reported a stimulatory role of PRL.

The significant decrease in the 20α/17α ratio also observed in the patients presenting strong hyperandrogenic hirsutism with cycle disturbances, suggests that both pathologies leading to hypersecretion of either PRL or androgens, might exert similar lowering effects on the 20α/17α balance of plasma levels ; this would indicate modifications of ovarian steroidogenesis in favour of this androgenic precursor, 17αOH progesterone.

ACKNOWLEDGEMENTS

The authors wisk to thank G. Chiodoni, P. Bianchi, A.M. Aeberhardt and D. Ganter for their excellent technical assistance, and F. Tapernoux for preparing the manuscript. Most plasma samples for this hormonal study were obtained from patients of Dr. P. Burckhardt and Dr. B. Ruedi, for which we are grateful.

REFERENCES

1 - Fowler, R.E., Fox, N.L., Edwards, R.G., Walters, D.E. and Steptoe, P.C.(1978) J. Endocr. 77, 171-183

2 - McNatty, K.P., Sawers, R.S., McNeilly, A.S. (1974) Nature 250, 653

3 - Pollow, K., Lübbert, H., Boquoi, E. and Pollow, B. (1975) J. Clin. Endocrinol. Metab., 41, 729-737

4 - Torjesen, P.A., Dahlin, R., Hug, E. and Aakvaag, A. (1978) Acta Endocrinologica, 87, 625-631

5 - Lamprecht, E.W. and Poyser, N.L. (1976). Physiol. Rev., 56, 595

6 - Strauss, J.R. and Stambaugh, R.L. (1974). Prostaglandins, 5, 73

7 - Lahav, M., Lamprecht, S.A., Amsterdam, A. and Lindner, H.R. (1977) Molec. Cell. Endocr., 6, 293

8 - Magrini, G., Ebiner, J.R. and Felber, J.P. (1979). Arch. Androl., 2, 141-156

© 1979 Elsevier/North-Holland Biomedical Press
Radioimmunology 1979, Ch. A. Bizollon, editor.

GONADOTROPINS AND THEIR MEMBRANE-BOUND RECEPTORS IN HUMAN TESTIS. STUDY IN PATHOLOGIC STATES.

R. ROULIER[1-2-3], A. MATTEI[2], P. FRANCHIMONT[4]

1 - Service d'Endocrinologie, Hôpital de la Conception, 13005 Marseille.
2 - Centre des Problèmes de la Reproduction Humaine, Marseille.
3 - Secteur des Hormones Protéiques, Service de Médecine Nucléaire, Institut Paoli et Calmettes, Marseille.
4 - Laboratoire de Radio-Immunologie, Université de Liège.

Testicular functions require secretion of pituitary gonadotropins. The first step of their action is binding to receptors in the testis. Interactions of gonadotropins with testicular receptors have been extensively studied in animal models. However, little information is available on the properties of the testicular receptors for gonadotropins in human testis. Accordingly, we felt that it was important to examine LH and FSH binding characteristics in human testis in order to study the variations of these characteristics in cases of male infertility.

Since investigative hormone studies in male infertility are presented in the report of A.Vermeulen, the discussion in this domain will be limited to our own conclusions based on the last years experience.

I MEASUREMENT OF GONADOTROPINS IN MALE INFERTILITY

Measurement of LH in such cases presents little practical interest as opposed to that of FSH whose relationship to spermatogenesis has been well established[1].

The diagnostic impact of FSH determinations should be studied in each of the three situations confronting the clinician after clinical evaluation and sperm examination :

A - Azoospermia and hypogonadism[2] :

In most of these cases secretory azoospermia resulting from primary testicular disorder is involved ; the latter is usually of constitutional origin (klinefelter syndrome, cryptorchidism...) or more rarely acquired (orchitis, radiochemotherapy), FSH levels are increased in agreement with results of testicular biopsy. The latter procedure is currently of no diagnostic utility.

Hypogonadotropic hypogonadism is much rarer and is generally functionnal in nature (Kalmann - Demorsier syndrome or idiopathic) and only exceptionnally tumor-related. In such cases diagnosis is achieved by clinical examination, whereas the low FSH and LH levels (basal and LHRH stimulated) furnish confirmative date.

B - Azoospermia with normal testicular volume[2] :

Differential diagnosis between secretory and obstructive azoospermia cannot usually be achieved on clinical grounds alone. Until recently, diagnosis was based on testicular biopsy showing either absent or arrested spermatogenesis (secretory azoospermia) or normal spermatogenesis (obstructive azoospermia). In the latter case, exploratory surgery in order to define the lesions and indicate possible corrective procedures was required.

Plasma FSH levels are increased in cases of secretory azoospermia and are normal in obstructive azoospermia. When confronted with borderline FSH values, LH-RH stimulation testing is useful : excessive response indicates FSH hypersecretion.

Measurement of baseline FSH levels and eventually LH-RH test lead to distinguishing between secretory and obstructive azoospermia, thus obviating testicular biopsy.

C - Oligospermia[2-3] :

Early aims of FSH and LH measurements centered on detection of partial deficiencies thus possibly justifying treatment with HMG-HCG whose effectiveness was well-known in cases of hypogonadotropic hypogonadism. In fact, no FSH deficiency can be evidenced, thus confirming the uselessness of treatment with HMG-HCG or clomifen citrate.

When sperm counts exceed 10 million/ml the FSH level is usually normal.

When sperm counts are less than 10 million/ml increased baseline FSH levels are encountered in 60% of cases, thus confirming the presence of primary testicular disorder. In such cases no therapy is currently available.

In cases of oligospermia increased FSH values confirm the severe prognosis.

II GONADOTROPIN RECEPTORS IN HUMAN TESTIS

Specific uptake of radioiodinated LH-HCG and FSH by testis has been reported in various animal species. Considerable information is now available on the characteristics of the membrane bound and solubilized gonadotrophin receptors[4-5-6-7-8] and their variations in different circumstances (sexual maturation[9-10-11-12-13], hypophysectomy[9], hormone[9-11-12], inter-actions[13]...) self regulation of Lh-HCG membrane receptors by their own hormone has also been demonstrated (see review of Tell et al[14]).

We first recall the methodology to evaluate gonadotropin binding in the normal human testis and then describe their modifications in pathologic states.

A - Gonadotropin receptors in normal human testis

. Methodology :

Preparation of (^{125}I) LH and FSH : unlabelled LH and FSH (a generous gift from Dr Schatz - Organon) were idoinated using the lacto-peroxydase method[15]. The specific activity determined by the trichloracetic precipitation varied from 50 to 70 uCI/ug for each hormone. The labelled gonadotropins were separated by gel filtration on a sephadex G 100 column (1 by 30 cm). Each of the eluted fractions was checked for binding to bovine testes cell membranes (FSH) or bovine corpus luteum kindly provided from F. Haour (LH). The fractions that exhibited the best binding were selected for use.

Preparation of testicular fraction for receptor studies : human testicular tissue was obtained from patients undergoing orchiectomy for prostatic cancer. None of the patients had received hormone therapy. Histological examination revealed normal spermatogenesis. Tissues were stored in liquid nitrogen until processed. Storage time varied from 24 hours to 30 days. Different durations of storage did not affect the degree of binding. The tissue was powdered in a thermovac apparatus. Homogenization was performed at 4°C in 10 mM tris-hydroxychloric acid buffer PH 7.8, containing 250 mM sucrose, 1mM $MgCl_2$, 1mM $CaCl_2$ by 10 up and down strokes in a glass teflon homogenizer. Homogenates were filtered through four layers of cheesecloth and centrifuged at 600 g for 20 min. Supernatant was further centrifuged at 20 000 g for 30 min. Protein content of the pellet was determined according to Zack and Cohen[16] modification of the method of Lowry et al[17]. This testicular preparation was used for the studies in this paper of testicular binding sites.

Determination of binding affinity and concentration of FSH and LH receptors: for binding sutdies, a fixed amount of testis homogenate (about 40 mg wet weight tissue) was incubated with increasing concentrations of unlabelled hormone, in the presence of a constant concentration of labelled hormone. The following reagents were added to 12 x 75 mm glass tubes : 100 ul hLH (1 - 200 ng/ml) or hFSH (1 - 200 ng/ml) in 25 mM tris-hydroxychloric acid buffer pH 7.2 containing 10 mM $MgCl_2$, 10 mM $CaCl_2$ and 0.2% B.A.S or 100 ul same buffer without unlabelled hormone ; 100 ul (^{125}I) hFSH or hLH (30 000 - 40 000 cpm) and 100 ul testis homogenate. Non specific binding was determined in the presence of 500 IU pregnyl or 7.5 IU pergonal per tube for the LH and FSH assays respectively. After vortex mixing and incubation at room temperature (22-25°C) for 8 h (LH) or 20 h (FSH), 2.0 ml ice-cold buffer were added to each tube. The tubes were vortexed and centrifuged at 3 500 rpm for 20 min. Supernatants were discarded and the pellets were washed and centrifuged one additional time to remove excess counts. The pellets were then counted in an intertechnique autogamma counter. Non specific binding was substracted from total binding to obtain specific binding. The binding inhibition curves obtained by this method were converted to scatchard plots[18] (bound to free hormone ratio VS bound hormone). The specific activities of the (^{125}I) hFSH and hLH preparations were adjusted for the addition of increasing amounts of unlabelled hormone. Linear scatchard plots were analyzed with the one site model. The apparent dissociation constants (kd) and the number of available receptor sites were calculated from the reciprocal of the slopes and x-axis intercepts, respectively.

RESULTS

A - Factors affecting binding :

Effects of time and temperature

As shown in Fig 1 the specific binging of (^{125}I) FSH and LH to human testicular receptor is dependent on both time and temperature - uptake of labelled FSH and LH was higher at 25° C than at 37° C - maximum binding was observed after 8 h for LH and 20 h for FSH. Continuing incubation resulted in a decreased binding which was greater at 37° C than at 25°C. This decrease, more marked for LH than for FSH, may be due to degradation of the receptors and/or the labelled hormone.

Effects of increasing concentration of protein : the extent of binding of (^{125}I) FSH and LH to human testicular membrane is proportional to the protein concentration reaching a maximum at 5 mg protein/ml for FSH and 8 mg/ml for LH.

Effect of PH : for both FSH and LH, binding capacity was maximum at pH 7.2 and decreased at higher and lower pH values.

Effects of enzymes : proteolytic enzymes such as trypsin and chymotrypsin abolished over 85% of the specific binding activity of LH and FSH receptor, while ribonuclease and deoxyribo nuclease treatment did not affect the receptor binding. At the high dose of 2,5 mIU used, phospholipase C resulted in virtually complete inhibition of receptor binding activity.

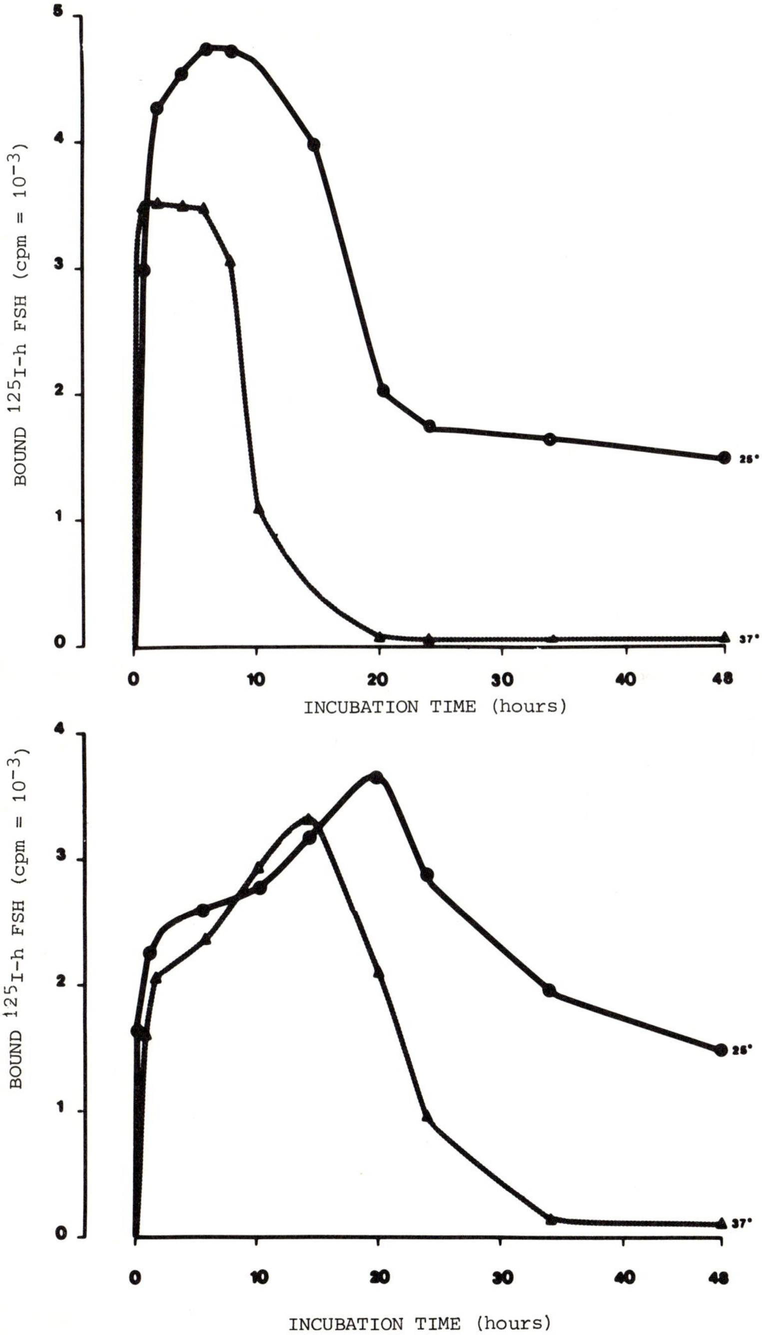

Fig. 1. Effects of time and temperature on iodo 125 FSH (upper part) and LH (lower part) binding to human testicular membrane receptor.

B - Characterization of binding of (^{125}I) FSH and LH to plasma membranes : binding of the hormone to the receptor was a saturable phenomenon (Fig 2)

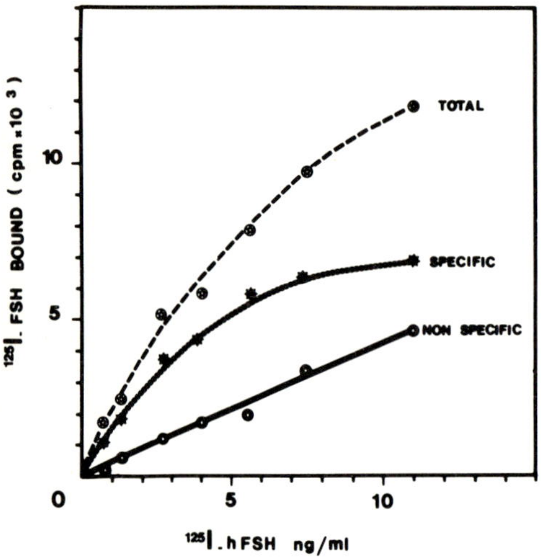

Fig. 2. ^{125}I FSH uptake by increasing labelled hormone doses.

Scatchard plots indicated a K_D of 1.10 x 10^{-10} M for FSH (Fig.3) and 2.6 x 10^{-10}M for LH (Fig.4) number of binding sites was on the order of 18.8 fMol/mg protein for FSH and 33.1 fMol/mg protein for LH

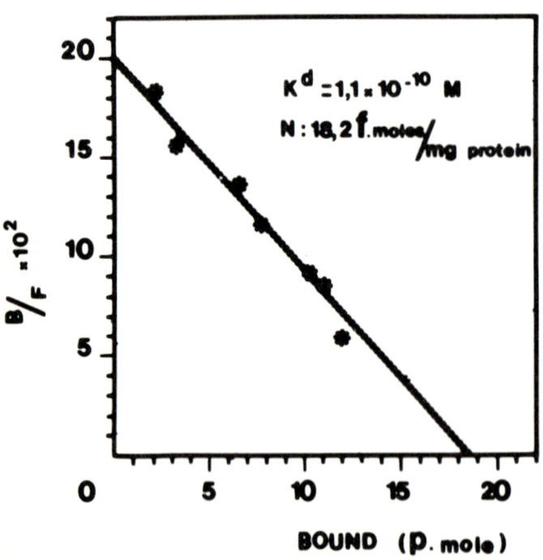

Fig. 3. Scatchard plot of hFSH binding on human testicular membranes.

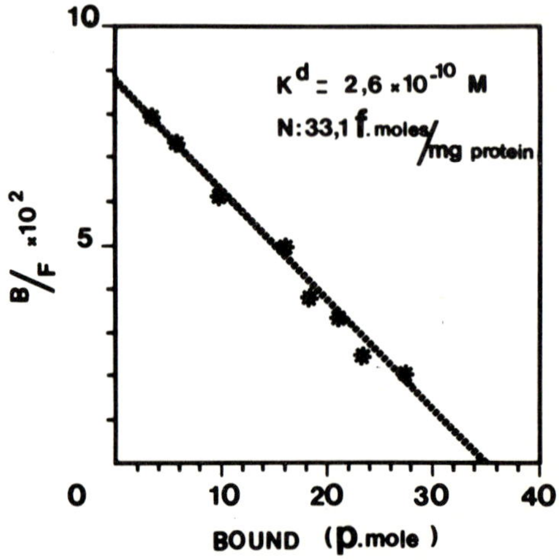

Fig. 4. Scatchard plot of hLH binding on human testicular membranes.

C - Gonadotropin binding specificity :

Gonadotropin binding is both tissue and hormone specific :

- tissue : very little hormone is bound specifically by other tissues in male genital tract (Fig. 5.), whereas up to 85% of the ^{125}I FSH bound by the testis can be competitively inhibited by an excess of unlabelled hormone.

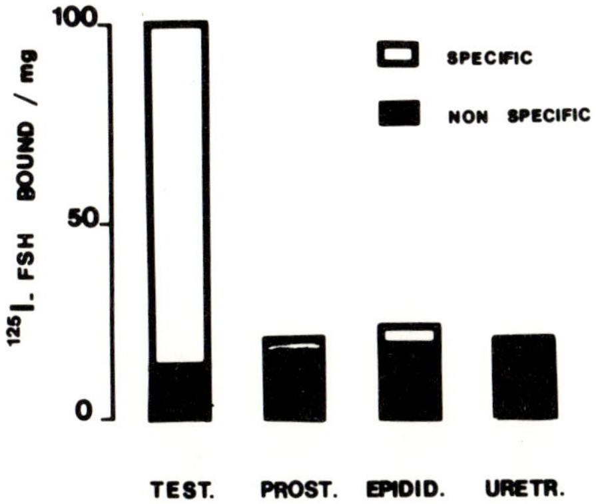

Fig. 5. ^{125}I hFSH binding on male genital tract.

- Hormone : displacement studies showed that both (^{125}I) FSH and LH were displaced specifically by homologous hormone (Fif. 6). Some of the displacement found with sub-units or other pituitary hormones may be due to contamination.

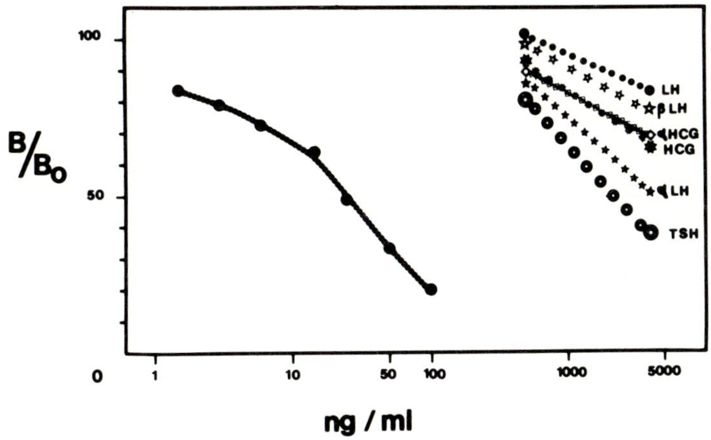

Fig. 6. ^{125}I hFSH binding specificity on human testicular membranes.

The general characteristics of the binding of ^{125}I hFSH and hLH on the plasma membranes of human testis are comparable to those reported in animal species for FSH and LH and in human for LH-HCG[19-20] : binding phenomenon is hormone and tissue specific and temperature, time and pH dependent. A single class of binding sites with a high affinity (10^{-10}M) and low capacity was evidenced. Additional studies are required however to eliminate low affinity, high capacity binding sites described in some species.

B - FSH membrane bound receptor in male infertility :

- Methodology :

. testicular biopsy : FSH binding was studied on testicular biopsy specimen obtained either during surgery (obstructive azoospermia, varicocele) or on the patient's request before accepting artificial insemination with donor sperm. At surgery, the specimen was devided in two parts in a 3/1 ratio for binding analysis and histological examination and immediately stored in liquid nitrogen wet weight ranged from 25 mg to 50 mg.

. Patients studied : 72 biopsies obtained from 42 patients (bilateral biopsy = 30 unilateral biopsy = 12). Patients were divided in three groups :

-first group (11 patients - 19 biopsies) underwent surgery for obstructive azoospermia. The histological examination revealed normal spermatogenesis and the FSH level was 3.1 $\pm$ 0.8 (S.D) mIU/ml) (N 8 mIU/ml) ;

-second group (16 patients - 28 biopsies) underwent surgery for varicocele sperm count ranged from 2 to 15 million spermatozoids/ml. Minimal lesions were found at biopsy. The mean FSH level was 5.4 $\pm$ 1.4 (S.D.) mIU/ml ;

- third group (15 patients - 25 biopsies) sperm count ranged from azoospermia to extreme oligospermia (< 1 M/ml). Marked lesions were found at biopsy. The mean FSH level was 19.3 $\pm$ 4.1 (S.D) mIU/ml.

. Preparation of plasma membrane fraction : the tissue was homogenized by a few strokes in a dounce hogenizer in 3 ml of buffer. The homogenate was centrifuged at 20 000 g for 30 min. The procedure was repeated one again and the final pellet was homogenized in tris-HCl buffer pH 7.2 containing 0.2% B.S.A in proportions corresponding to 30 mg of initial tissue in 1 ml of buffer ($\simeq$ 1 mg protein/ml).

. Gonadotropin binding was performed as previously described in methodology. Since only little testicular material could be obtained by biopsy binding was studied only in the absence of FSH and in the presence of an excess of cold hormone for determination of non specific binding. Results are expressed in fMOL/mg of initial tissue.

- Results :

In all three groups studied no signigicant difference was found between the left and the right testis (Fig. 7.)

In the three pathological groups :

results are summarized in Table I and shown in Fig. 8.

		Group I	Group II	Group III
n		19	28	25
Binding (fMol/mg/protein)	M	1.21	0.89*	0.39 **
	SEM	0.17	0.11	0.046

* N.S VS II

** p 0.0005 VS I

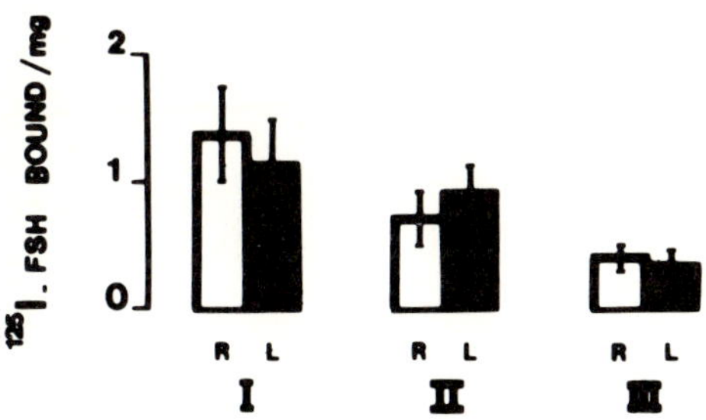

Fig. 7. ^{125}I hFSH human FSH binding in right and left testis for each group (for definition of the three groups, see text).

The evidence for decreased availability of FSH binding sites in cases where spermatogenesis is markedly depressed can only be discussed :

- decreased target cell number (sertoli cells and possibly spermatogia) ;
- increased occupancy of FSH binding sites (in this group FSH plasma levels are signigicantly higher than in the other groups. Fig. 9) ;

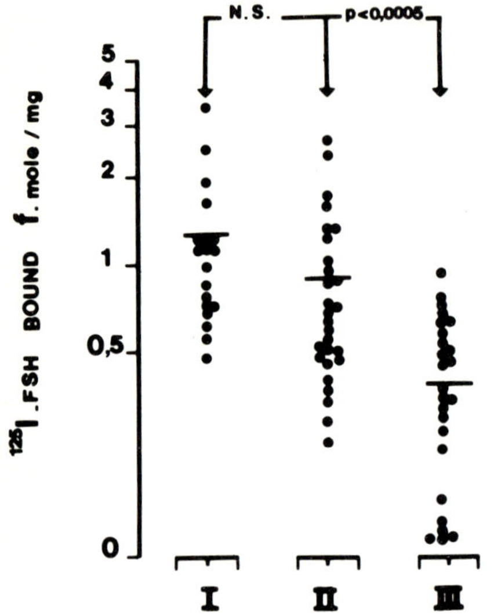

Fig. 8. ^{125}I hFSH binding in male infertility (for definition of the three groups, see text).

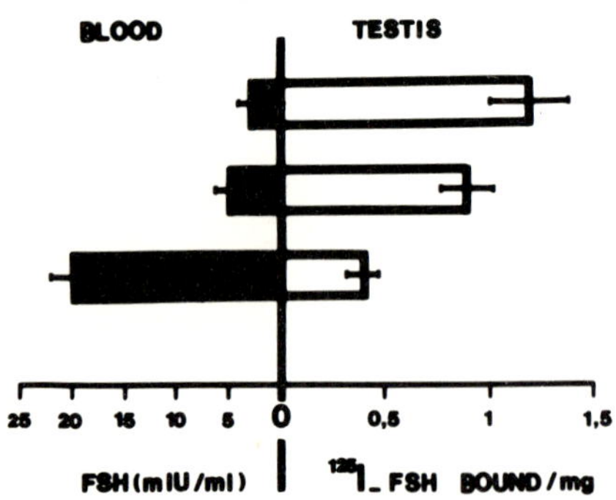

Fig. 9. ^{125}I hFSH binding and FSH plasma levels in male infertility (for definition of the three groups, see text).

- self regulation of membrane cell receptors by their own hormone inducing a loss of the receptors ;
- primary decrease of binding site number in some cases of male infertility.

Studies are currently in progress to evaluate these hypothetical mechanisms.

ACKNOWLEDGMENTS

To C. Andonian for her excellent technical assistance.

REFERENCIES

1. Franchimont, P., Millet, D., Vendrely, E., Legros, J.J. and Netter A. (1972) J. Clin. Endocrinol. Metab. 34 : 1003.
2. Roulier, R., Mattei, A. and Franchimont, P. (1976) Ann. Endocrinol. (Paris) 37, 407.
3. Roulier, R., Mattei, A., Duvivier, J. and Franchimont, P. (1978) Clinical Endocrinology, 9, 303.
4. Catt, K.J., Dufau, M.L. and Tsuruhara T. (1972) Biochim. Biophys. Acta, 279 : 194.
5. Charreau, E.H., Dufau, M.L. and Catt, K.J. (1974) J. Biol. Chem. 249 : 4189
6. Cheng, K.W. (1975) Biochem, J. 149 : 125.
7. Abou-Issa, H. and Reichert, L.E. Jr (1976) J. Biol. Chem. 251, 3326.
8. Abou-Issa, H. and Reichert, L.E. Jr (1977) J. Biol. Chem. 252, 4166.
9. Frowein, J. and Engel, W. (1975) J. Endocrinol. 64, 59.
10. Ketelslegers, J.M., Hetzel, W.D., Sherins, K.J., and Catt, K.J. (1978) Endocrinology, 103, 212.
11. Steinberger, A., Thanki, K.J. and Siegal, B. (1974) Hormone binding and targer cell activation in the testis (M.L. Dufau and R.R. Means Eds), 177, Plenum press, New-York.
12. Haugher, R.L., Chen, Y.D.I., Kelch, R.P. and Payne, A.H. (1977) J. Endocrinol., 74, 57.
13. Odell, W.D., and Swerdloff, R.S. (1975) Journal of steroid Bioch. 6, 853.
14. Tell, G.P., Haour, F. and Saez, J.M. (1978) Metabolism, 27, 1566.
15. Ketelslegers, J.M. and Catt, K.J. (1974) J. Clin. Endocrinol. Metab. 39, 1159.
16. Zack, B. and Cohen, J. (1961) Clin. Chim. Acta, 6 : 665
17. Lowry, O.H., Rosebrough, N.J., Farr, A.L. and Randall, R.J. (1951) J. Biol. Chem. 193, 265.
18. Scatchard, G. (1949) Ann. Ny. Acad. Sci. 51, 660.
19. Huhtaniemi, I.T., Korenbrat, C.C. and Jaffe, R.B. (1977) J. Clin. Endocrinol Metab. 44, 963?
20. Hsu, A.F., Stratico, D., Hosaka, M. and Troen P. (1978) J. Clin. Endocrinol. Metab. 47, 529.

Radioimmunology 1979, Ch. A. Bizollon, editor.

CLINICAL APPLICATION OF REFINED LH AND FSH ASSAYS TO HYPOSECRETORY STATES

W.M. HUNTER*, P. van LOOK[†] and D.T. BAIRD[†]
*MRC Immunoassay Team, 2, Forrest Road, Edinburgh, U.K.
[†]University Department of Obstetrics and Gynaecology, Edinburgh.

INTRODUCTION

The first measurements of the circulating levels of a given substance are usually concerned with hypersecretion. However, 'normal' levels generally represent a physiological median from which both upward and downward modulations are possible. Assays designed for measuring the former may not serve the latter purpose. For LH and FSH the major hypersecretory events such as the mid-menstrual cycle surge of LH secretion and the increases in FSH (and to a lesser extent in LH) which occur at the menopause are well described and are easily measured. Nevertheless the levels found in normal men, which might be considered as 'basal' with respect to these hypersecretory states are in fact markedly higher than the levels found in prepubertal children. The object of this paper is to show that assays designed to differentiate between prepubertal and adult LH (and to a lesser extent FSH) levels are useful not only for investigating problems of puberty but also for revealing important hyposecretory states, notably among patients reporting with secondary amenorrhoea.

ASSAY DEVELOPMENT

Seven laboratories were sent serum samples from six normal men and six small pools each of serum from prepubertal children. Although all laboratories were using the same standard and antiserum, the ratio of mean adult to mean children's levels varied from 1.5 to 4.3 and only two laboratories found a clear separation between the two groups. The levels recorded for the men's sera agreed fairly well, i.e. the variation was in the estimates on the prepubertal pools. This suggested that non-specific effects were intruding in most of the assays. Non-specific serum effects are well known to occur in certain RIA systems and assays for LH,

FSH[1,4] and TSH[2,3] are particularly susceptible. In the present LH and FSH systems which employ the highly sensitive and hormonally monospecific antisera supplied by Professor W.R. Butt, non-specific effects can be shown to be due to serum components of MW 200,000 and above. Sera from non-primates contain such material and with these sera responses are never found in the eluates in the 30,000 MW region (which is where the purified gonadotrophins appear). The activity present in human sera is a mixture of authentic gonadotrophin and high MW material which, by analogy with the non-human material, and because it fails to suppress in patients on gonadal steroids, is considered to be functionally unrelated to the glycoprotein hormones. We have been unable to eliminate these non-specific serum effects but we have investigated the assay conditions in some detail and found it possible to minimise the extent of their intrusion. The details are fully described elsewhere[4] and it will suffice if they are summarised:

1) Using tracer concentrations of 200 pg/ml incubate, equilibration was reached in 3-4 days at 4° or in 24 hrs at room temperature. There was no advantage in using 4°.

2) In delayed addition assays detection limit and non-specific effects were increased when antiserum concentrations exceeded an optimal level.

3) Both detection limit and the magnitude of non-specific effects were inversely proportional to the time employed for the first incubation up to a maximum of 16 hrs.

4) The time employed for the second incubation was without effect on the magnitude of the non-specific effects over the range 2-24 hrs, as was the concentration of tracer (range 0.2 - 2.5 ng/ml incubate). The position of the normalised standard curves (i.e. plots with B_o = 100% and NSB = 0%) were also unaffected through all such combinations.

5) The non-specific serum effects were minimised by including 100 µl of serum in an incubation volume of 200 µl. Dilution of serum increased these responses, without of course changing the specific responses found in normal male and post-menopausal serum samples, i.e. the non-specific effects and shallower response curves than the standards and consequently were relatively worsened by dilution.

6) Animal sera were entirely without effect when they were added immediately before addition of the second antibody.
7) Tracers were equally immuno-reactive (as judged by their subsequent reaction with dilutions of antibody normally used in the assays) after storage for 24 hr at room temperature in 50% animal serum and after storage in 2% animal serum.

We conclude that serum affects the assay system at the stage of the first incubation, i.e. it interferes with or inhibits the reaction of endogenous gonadotrophin with antibody.

By careful optimisation, as described above, we were able to develop routine procedures which required a total of 48 hr incubation (including 16 hrs at 4° for precipitation with second antibody). The table shows the complete separation of prepubertal from men's serum LH levels and the small overlap which is found between the FSH levels of the two groups.

TABLE 1
SERUM LH AND FSH LEVELS IN NORMAL MEN AND PREPUBERTAL CHILDREN

		LH iu/l		FSH iu/l	
	n	Mean	Range	Mean	Range
Normal men 20-50 years	100	5.7	2.7-14.0	3.2	1.4-8.4
Prepubertal children	71	0.85	<0.4-1.9	0.93	<0.3-3.0

ASSAY APPLICATION

We have used these assays for investigating patients presenting with both precocious and delayed puberty. The marked rise in LH which is seen at midnight (Fig. 1) which is the first measurable sign of the pubertal changes in the pituitary-gonadal system is easily measured and serves to reassure the paediatrician that changes are about to occur in a patient whose outward appearance is as yet prepubertal.

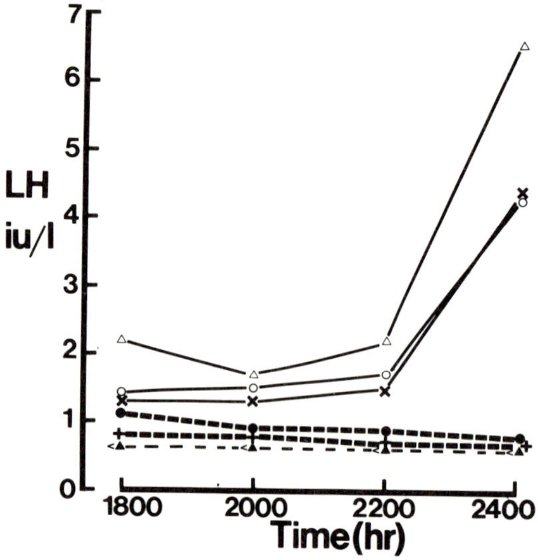

Fig. 1. Nocturnal serum LH levels in children being investigated for delayed puberty. The rise in LH levels provides reassurance that pubertal changes are imminent.

When these assays have been used to determine the hormonal status of patients with secondary amenorrhoea they have revealed a most interesting picture. Patients with a history of at least six months' amenorrhoea, those with high urinary gonadotrophins and those with evidence of cyclical activity as shown by urinary oestrogen determinations were excluded.

Fig. 2 shows the basal levels of LH and FSH in 50 cases of a series which eventually will consist of 140 consecutive patients. It will be seen that some 40% of patients had low basal gonadotrophin levels. The follow-up data on the first cases in this

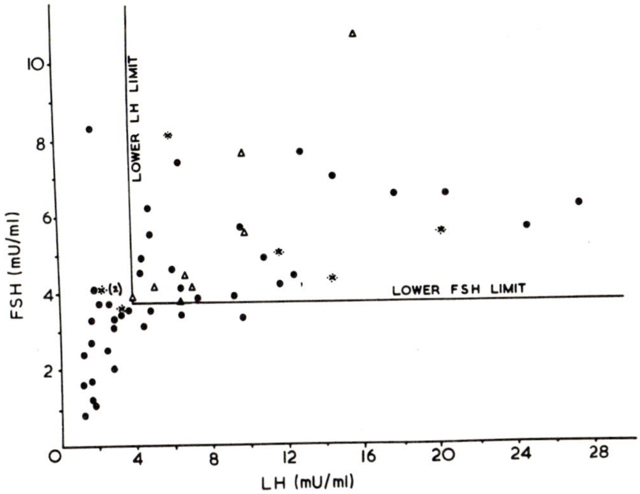

Fig. 2. Basal serum LH and FSH levels in normal women on days 3-5 of their cycles (△) and those found in 50 patients with secondary amenorrhoea. The latter were subdivided into patients with normal prolactin levels (●) and those with hyperprolactinoemia (✱).

series suggests that after removing patients with hyperprolactinoemia, patients with low basal gonadotrophin levels are (a) less likely to return spontaneously to episodes of vaginal bleeding than are those with normal levels and (b) very unlikely to show any ovarian response to Clomiphene. Those with low-normal levels may show follicular activity but are unlikely to ovulate, while patients with mid-high normal levels are likely to ovulate in response to Clomiphene therapy. Although the low-gonadotrophin group has a lower mean body weight than the remaining groups, this group is not confined to patients with a recognisable history of self-imposed weight loss.

The LH and FSH levels in response to LRF (50 μg) and to Clomiphene (on the fifth day of 100 mg/day) were measured in all cases. The information obtained did not add to the prognostic value which was already available from the basal determinations. This suggests that if the basal levels of LH and FSH are measured in assays which have been thoroughly optimised to operate in the region of hyposecretion, and ideally can go down one-tenth of the mean levels found in normal men, then it may be unnecessary to perform more elaborate stimulation tests in these patients.

REFERENCES

1. Hunter, W.M. and Bennie, J.G. (1973) Acta endocr. (Kbh.), Suppl. 177, p.97.
2. Hall, R. and Amos, J. (1971) Methods of assessing the sensitivity of h-TSH ntisera. In Radioimmunoassay Methods. Eds. K.E. Kirkham and W.M. Hunter. Churchill Livingstone, Edinburgh, pp. 143-147.
3. Spencer, C.A. and Challand, G.S. (1977) Clinical Chemistry 23, 584-588.
4. Hunter, W.M. and Bennie, J.G. (1979) J. Endocr. 80, 59-68.

QUALITY CONTROL IN RADIOIMMUNOASSAY

Radioimmunology 1979, Ch. A. Bizollon, editor.

ASSAY DESIGN AND QUALITY CONTROL

ROGER EKINS
Sub-Department of Molecular Biophysics, Department of Nuclear Medicine, The Middlesex Hospital Medical School, Mortimer Street, London, W1N 8AA.

INTRODUCTION

The objective of assay design (whether pursued at a theoretical or experimental level) is the development of assay systems which achieve maximal accuracy of measurement in minimal time of the concentrations of individual substances of interest - i.e. of specific analytes - within the constraints imposed by available reagents, technology and personnel. The term "maximal accuracy" is here used in the sense that measurements are made with minimal error, i.e. with minimal bias and with maximal precision (see 'Definitions'). 'Bias' and 'precision' are terms which respectively reflect the magnitude of systematic and random components of error deflecting assay results from the "true" or "correct" value: moreover the quantitative assessment of these parameters can only be made with the aid of statistical procedures which fall within the province of "quality control". It follows that, in "designing" an assay system in an experimental context - that is by making changes to the components of the system, or the concentrations at which individual components are used - the sole legitimate criterion by which any change can be judged is its effect on assay bias and precision as evaluated by the use of the statistical procedures of quality control.

Likewise, no theoretical analysis of radioimmunoassay (or of the 'saturation assay' technique in general) which purports to give guidance relating to the desirable characteristics of reagents (e.g. labelled antigen, antibody etc.) and the optimal concentrations at which these reagents should be used is valid unless it embraces a theoretical consideration of the errors that characterise such assay systems.

Though indisputable, these concepts have been widely ignored throughout the history of the development of these techniques, in relation both to the theoretical principles and the detailed experimental procedures which are commonly relied on in the field. As a result, the subject has been clouded by mythologies whose overall effect is to deflect attention from the critical factors which influence overall assay performance, as reflected in assay accuracy and in the overall time required to perform a measurement. The performance of current assay systems - though often tolerable - is thus of a lower standard than would be the case had the fundamental relationship between assay design and the assessment of assay performance been more widely recognised.

Misunderstanding of the fundamental principles of RIA design has also led, in practice, to the widespread adoption of assay procedures which - for example - demand repeated synthesis, at unnecessarily frequent intervals, of radiolabelled analyte (resulting in increased costs and radiation hazards); it has also led to a considerable misuse of radioisotope counting equipment, implying prolongation of assay turn-round times, and the unnecesary purchase of additional instrumentation. Finally, at a conceptual level, the frequent misrepresentation of the theoretical basis of RIA has had the consequence that newcomers to the field are generally presented with a set of dogmas which have little scientific validity, and which cannot be used as legitimate guidelines in the experimental development of efficient and "rugged" assay systems.

Such dogmas currently include items of scientific mythology typified by the following:

(a) maximal sensitivity in a RIA system is attained by using an antibody concentration which binds 33% (or 50%) of the labelled analyte at zero dose

(b) for maximal sensitivity the concentration of radioisotopically labelled analyte used should be "vanishingly small";

(c) a "pure" labelled analyte (i.e. labelled analyte which comprises 90% or more immunoreactive material) is essential for 'good' assay performance;

(d) samples originating in a RIA procedure should be counted for 10,000 counts

It has been the prime objective of instruction in my own laboratory for many years (and more recently in RIA Courses run under the auspices of the IAEA, WHO and British Council) to reveal the misconceptions underlying such mythologies and to establish a valid set of theoretical and practical guidelines enabling the experimenter to develop good assay protocols rapidly and with genuine understanding and insight. In particular, these courses have been intended to implant a number of principles relating to assay design which include the following:

(a) optimal assay design necessitates statistical assessment of the errors arising in a particular procedure.

(b) No evaluation of any change in assay protocol or reagents can be made without examination of the effect of the change on experimental errors in the procedure.

(c) The optimal amounts of antibody and labelled analyte used in an assay depend, inter alia, upon:

i. the relationship between the error in the response variable, and the magnitude of the response variable;

ii. whether 'bound, 'free', or 'free' and 'bound' radioactive fractions are counted and represent the response variable(s) for the system.

(d) Maximal assay sensitivity/precision/working range and minimal incubation time are attained using systems in which the misclassification of free and bound fractions approaches zero.

(e) In a well designed assay system in which misclassification of 'free' activity in the 'bound' fraction is minimised, and in which the 'bound' activity is 'counted', the optimal amount of antibody which yields maximal assay sensitivity approaches zero.

(f) The fraction of labelled analyte which is bound to antibody at zero dose in such a system will also approach zero (i.e. it will usually fall below 10% and may be as low as 1-2%).

(g) The concentration of labelled analyte which is required to attain maximal sensitivity/precision in the shortest incubation time may, in certain systems, be considerably greater than the concentration of analyte in the test sample (the theoretical optimum labelled analyte concentration may approach infinity).

(h) Reliable estimates may be made, in a well designed 'rugged' assay system, using labelled analyte containing large amounts (i.e. more than 50-80%) non-immunoreactive impurity.

(i) Acceptable precision (for example for clinical purposes) may be attained by counting samples for no more than 100 counts.

These and other precepts stem directly from an understanding of the very simple statistical concepts which underlie the correct design of RIA procedures. Nevertheless they appear heretical to many practitioners in the field, and it is frequently only with difficulty that widely accepted notions relating to the proper conduct of such assays can be overcome. It is the purpose of this presentation briefly to indicate both the fallacious nature of much of what passes as 'theory' in this field and the reasons why many of the mythologies referred to earlier have arisen. It is also intended to outline legitimate, scientifically valid, principles which should underlie the short-term and long-term development of RIA procedures in the laboratory. These principles will be illustrated by examples drawn from the experimental studies incorporated into the teaching courses given in my own laboratory and more recently those run under WHO/IAEA patronage.

DEFINITIONS

The fundamental source of much current misunderstanding concerning RIA design arises from confusion over the concepts of accuracy, bias, precision and sensitivity. Only if these concepts are clearly understood can the assayist embark upon a rational experimental strategy in setting up a particular assay procedure illuminated by a scientifically legitimate theoretical approach to assay design. These basic concepts will be discussed in turn:

Bias. The 'bias' of an assay result represents that component of its deviation from the 'true' or correct value which is due to systematic errors. Such errors can arise, for example, from the use of incorrectly diluted standards or of incorrectly calibrated pipettes. In a radioimmunoassay, 'bias' may typically be introduced into a measurement by the existence, in the sample under test, of a 'cross-reactant' which simulates the analyte in reaction with the specific antibody employed, leading to an incorrect estimate of the analyte concentration. 'Bias' is conventionally represented by the deviation of the mean of a large number of replicate determinations from the 'true' or 'correct' value for the measurement.

Precision. This term reflects the magnitude of the random components of error which deflect individual assay results from the true values. Such errors arise as a result of inconsistencies in the behaviour both of equipment (pipettes, etc.) and of assayist in the assay procedure: also (in radioanalytical methods) in consequence of the statistical nature of radioisotopic disintegration, and the consequent random errors of counting. The (im)precision of a measurement is usually represented by the standard deviation or coefficient of variation of a large number of replicate estimates.

Working Range. The 'working range' of an assay system is the range of concentrations over which errors of measurement (either consistent or random) fall within 'acceptable' limits. The definition of 'acceptable' error is a matter entirely within the discretion of the assayist, and the magnitude of 'acceptable' errors may be different at different analyte concentrations depending on the clinical (or other) purpose for which the assay result is intended.

Accuracy. This term is currently used in two senses:

(i) as indicative of absence of error in the measurement

(ii) as indicative of absence of systematic error (i.e. bias) in the measurement.

In sense (i), a measurement may be said to be 'accurate' because it is close to the 'true' result. This implies that the assay system displays minimal bias and is precise. In sense (ii), a measurement system may be said to be 'accurate' because the results it yields are unbiased. Individual measurements using such a system, may, however, be incorrect because of the occurrence of large random errors, i.e. because of assay imprecision.

Definition (ii) is that currently adopted by the International Federation of Clinical Chemists[1]; it is a definition which, however, leads to apparent absurdities such as the proposition that an assayist may be forced to adopt a less 'accurate' assay system in order to obtain results which are generally closer to the correct value (see Fig. 1).

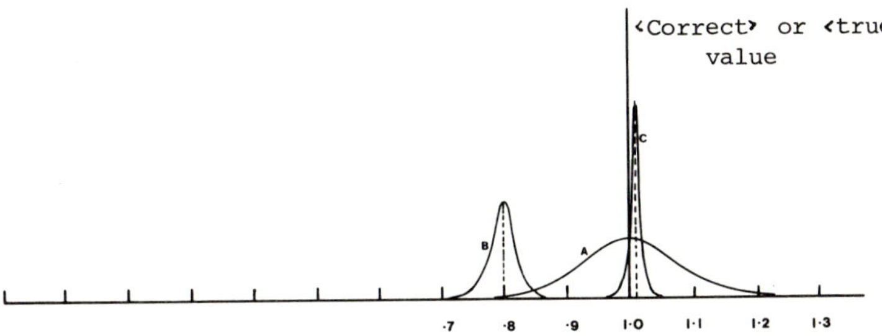

Fig. 1. Performance of three hypothetical assay systems. The 'true' or 'correct' assay result is represented by unity on the abscissa. Assay system B is strongly biased towards a lower value; C is slightly positively biased, but is extremely precise; A is unbiased but yields widely dispersed values. Of the three systems, C yields (singlicate) determinations which are generally closer to the 'true' value, albeit adoption of the IFCC definition of accuracy requires that system A is deemed the most 'accurate' system.

For this reason my personal preference is for definition (i) which implicitly embraces the concepts both of precision and bias. In so far as a numerical value can be assigned to this definition, it can be represented by:

$$\text{'Inaccuracy'} = \sqrt{(\text{Imprecision})^2 + (\text{Bias})^2}$$

where "Imprecision" is represented by the standard error of the mean of the replicates normally included in the assay protocol.

This value is a useful indicator of the overall reliability of the method in yielding results close to the true or correct values. Nevertheless because of the confusion that centres on the concept of 'accuracy' it is generally preferable to avoid the use of this term, and in further discussion in this paper, the specific terms 'bias' and 'precision' are used as indicators of assay performance.

Sensitivity. The sensitivity of an assay system is now generally accepted as being represented by the 'lower limit of detection', or 'minimal detectable dose', characterising tne system. The calculated value for the detection limit depends in practice upon the number of replicates employed in the measurement of samples, the level of confidence demanded, etc.; thus, for purposes of comparison of different methods it is generally preferable to define 'sensitivity' as the precision of measurement of zero dose, the magnitude of which, with appropriate numerical adjustment, essentially determines the minimal detectable dose. 'Sensitivity' thus defined represents in consequence merely a special case of the general concept of precision[2].

It is apparent that determination of each of the above parameters involves statistical analysis: thus, neither the precision of measurement of a defined analyte concentration, nor its bias, can be evaluated without the performance of replicate determinations (preferably large in number if reliable estimates are required).

MYTHOLOGIES

Much of the mythological content of RIA methodology arises from a misunderstanding of the above concepts. In particular, sensitivity has been (and continues to be) frequently equated with the slope of the dose response curve[3]; likewise precision has been defined as the slope of the response curve relating 'bound' radiolabelled analyte to the logarithm of the analyte concentration[3]. Such definitions, because they implicitly assume constancy of error (i.e. homoscedasticity) in the response variable, are untenable and lead to obvious absurdities; for example the shape and slope of dose response curves (and the variation in error along the curves) depend upon the coordinate frame in which they are plotted, so that a curve of steeper slope in one frame may be less steep in another. This can be illustrated, for example, by consideration of the effect in a RIA system, of changing the concentration of antibody in the system (Fig. 2). Thus, if results are plotted in terms of the fraction (or percentage) of label bound (b) v. H (analyte concentration), reduction in antibody results in progressive 'flattening' of the dose response curve and an apparent loss in 'sensitivity'. Conversely, if identical results are plotted in terms of 1/b v. H, reduction in antibody results in a progressive increase in slope of the dose response curve implying increase in 'sensitivity'. Clearly, the slope of the dose response curve per se constitutes an invalid basis on which logical conclusions can be reached with respect to the effect of change in antibody concentration on assay sensitivity.

Likewise the steepest portion of the B/F v. H dose response curve is at the point of zero dose; conversely the steepest portion of the F/B v. H response curve (theoretically) lies at infinite dose (assuming corrections for 'non-specific binding' and counter background are in each case applied to raw data). Thus the conclusion that maximal sensitivity for an assay system is obtained by employing vanishingly low concentration of labelled analyte[3] represents nothing more than an optical illusion stemming directly from a simplistic consideration of the B/F v. H response curve. A diametrically opposed conclusion could (equally illegitimately) be derived by consideration of the F/B v. H representation.

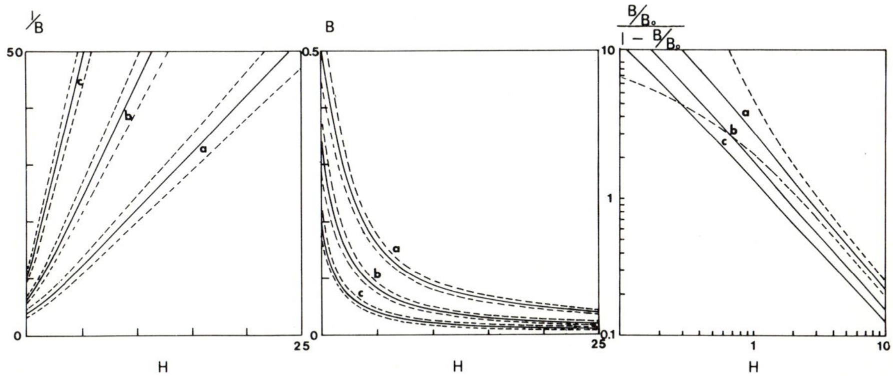

Fig. 2. Identical data plotted in terms of 1/B (reciprocal of fraction bound), B (fraction bound) and $\frac{B/Bo}{1-B/Bo}$ versus ligand concentration H on linear and log scales as indicated. Note typical non-uniformity of variance (heteroscedasticity) in each co-ordinate frame. Curves b and c represent 1:2 and 1:4 reductions in antibody with respect to curve a. Maximal slope at zero dose is observed with Ab concentration corresponding to c (1/B), to b (B): curves a, b, c display identical slopes in the log $\frac{B/Bo}{1-B/Bo}$ (logit B/Bo) representation, irrespective of antibody concentration.

Such conclusions typify the erroneous theoretical basis upon which much current RIA methodology is founded. A similar simplistic approach can frequently be observed to lie at the root of popular beliefs regarding, for example, the effects of degradation of labelled analyte ('reduction in percentage binding of label; reduced slope of dose response curve'); the effects of misclassification of free and bound activities ('non-specific binding'); the choice of optimal antibody concentration from antibody dilution curve data etc.

In each case, the fundamental logical flaw in the conclusion drawn from experimental observations is neglect of consideration of the error structure of the data.

OPTIMAL ASSAY DESIGN

Assay design is primarily concerned with the choice of reagents and protocol to maximise the precision of assay results and minimise their bias. The minimisation of bias represents a philosophical conundrum since, in the great majority of situations in which RIA methods are used, the 'true' value of the measurement is unknown; indeed it is often (currently) unknowable since no 'reference' technique usually exists which enables a methodologically independant estimate to be made. Nevertheless experienced assayists are widely familiar with the general strategies which must be adopted to reduce bias. These include the selection of highly specific antibody, the choice of a closely similar incubation milieu for standards and unknowns, the rigorous standardisation of physical parameters governing the assay procedure (e.g. temperature, times of incubation, instrument performance) etc. The adoption of these measures does not, however, guarantee that an indivdual result will be unbiased.

It is not, however, the purpose of this paper to dwell extensively on the question of assay bias, and it is assumed henceforth that all necessary conventional measures have been adopted to minimise this type of error. The problem of precision nevertheless remains, and, in particular, the question of the optimal choice of reagents which maximise the 'precision of measurement of the target concentration' - or 'target range of concentrations' - which represents the prime objective of the measurement.

The choice of optimal concentrations of reagents based upon theoretical analysis or upon computer optimisation techniques has been discussed at intervals either by myself or my collaborators[4,5] (and more recently by Rodbard[6]) since the earliest inception, in 1954, of the saturation assay principle in my own laboratory. Central to these theoretical analyses has been a consideration of the influence of the 'error structure' of an assay system on its optimum design. For many years such analyses have pointed to the sub-optimal nature of conventional assay methodology based upon the simplistic concepts discussed earlier in this presentation. However, perhaps because of their mathematical complexity, the conclusions emerging from these studies have failed to be assimilated and acted upon by the majority of workers in the field. More recently, therefore, the principal aim of our (including WHO and IAEA Courses) teaching in the field has been to present these fundamental design concepts in a more digestible form, whereby they can be understood and acted upon by those who cannot readily comprehend mathematical reasoning.

THE RESPONSE ERROR RELATIONSHIP (RER)

This, quite simply, represents the relationship between the random error (standard deviation or variance) in the response metameter and the magnitude of the response (see Fig. 3).

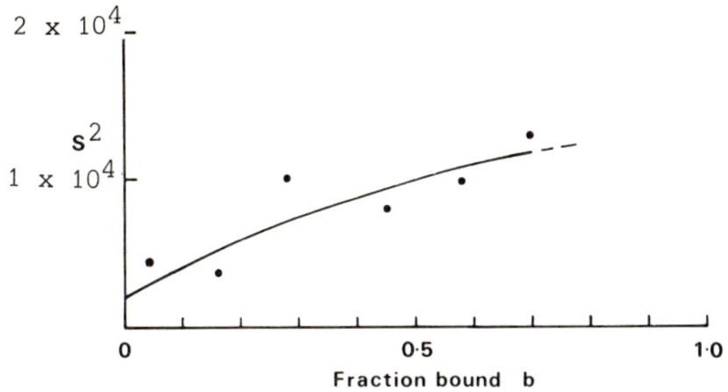

Fig. 3. Response error relationship (RER). Plot of error in response variable as a function of response. In this illustration 'error' is represented by the variance (standard deviation^2) in the response; it is equally acceptable to plot the standard deviation per se.

In essence, it represents the shape of the error envelope which surrounds the dose response curve as illustrated in Fig. 2 (a similar envelope surrounds, for example, antibody dilution curves). The characterisation of this relationship for any particular assay system ideally requires the acquistion of a considerable amount of data, which can be derived in two different ways. In the first approach, a large number (e.g. ten or more) replicate measurements may be made at each of (for example) ten representative points along the dose response curve, and the calculated standard deviation in the response metameters at each point plotted against the corresponding response. The setting up of assays specifically to evaluate the form of the RER in this manner has comprised a standard procedure in assay development in my own laboratory for a number of years[7]. Alternatively by plotting the standard deviation in the response calculated from replicates (e.g. duplicates or triplicates) against the mean of each set of replicates (using both standards and unknowns) and subsequently 'binning' the resulting data points, the shape and position of the RER can be readily perceived. Clearly the greater the number of sample tubes included within an assay (whichever of the above procedures is adopted) the less statistical uncertainty will attach to the form of the RER.

The determination of the RER is also an essential pre-requisite to the 'weighting' of 'standard' data points for the computer fitting of dose response curves. More detailed descriptions of the calculations involved - particularly in the context of computer data processing - have been published by Rodbard and his colleagues (e.g. 8); nevertheless the calculations involved, albeit somewhat laborious, are exceedingly simple and readily performed 'manually'

The shape of the RER plot clearly depends, inter alia, upon the particular response variable that is chosen for the plotting of dose response curves. For example, the curve relating S_b v. b (standard deviation in 'fraction bound' v. 'fraction bound') is of a different form from that relating $S_{\text{logit b/bo}}$ v. logit b/bo (where bo is the fraction bound at zero dose), and logit b/bo is the response metameter. In certain circumstances, the RER may be represented approximately by a simple mathematical expression such as $S_b = \alpha + \beta b$

For the purposes of illustration both in this presentation and in evaluating experimental data generated during RIA training courses, a simple linear relationship between the standard deviation in fraction or percentage of labelled analyte 'bound' to antibody (S_b) and the magnitude of the bound fraction (b) has been generally assumed.

THE PRECISION PROFILE

The precision profile[9] of an assay system (see Fig. 4) comprises a plot of the precision of measurement of the analyte concentration against the corresponding analyte concentration.

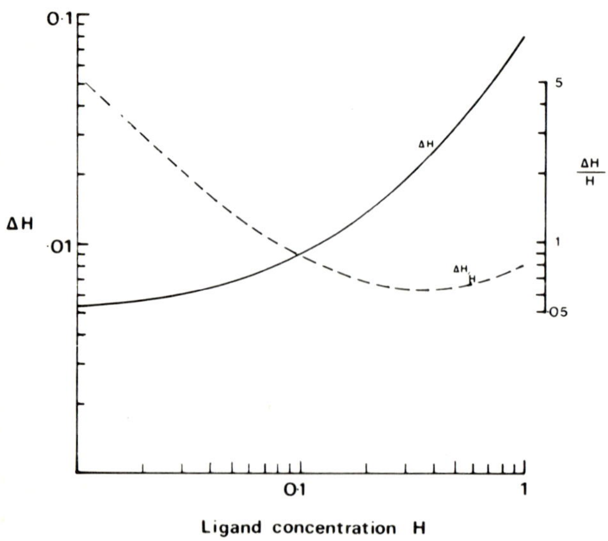

Fig. 4. Precision Profile. Plot of error (ΔH) or relative error ($\frac{\Delta H}{H}$) in dose as a function of dose (H).

It may be portrayed in terms of the absolute or relative error in the measurement (i.e. standard deviation of coefficient of variation) and either (or both) of these variables may be plotted on arithmetic or logarithmic scales, whichever is the more convenient. Evaluation of the precision profile can be accomplished in several ways; nevertheless for a variety of reasons it is useful to establish the profile by calculating, at a series of arbitrarily selected analyte concentrations:

(a) the slope of the dose response curve (dR/dH)

(b) the standard deviation (S_R) of the response metameter at the corresponding point of the curve.

Division of S_R by the slope yields the standard deviation of the analyte measurement (S_H) for each selected analyte concentration thus enabling the precision profile to be plotted.

Performance of these calculations clearly necessitates information regarding the form of the error envelope which surrounds the dose response curve i.e. of the RER. It should be emphasised that acceptably reliable estimates of the random error arising at any point of the dose response curve can only be derived from the RER; not from individual estimates based on a small number of replicates at a particular point.

The fundamental importance of the precision profile is that the effect of any change in assay procedure, reagent concentrations, quality of reagents etc. can only be evaluated by examination of the resulting change in the profile. For example, a change in antibody concentration may have the effect of altering the profile from curve a to curve b (Fig. 5). The implication of such a change is a loss of sensitivity in assay b ($(S_{H=o})_a < (S_{H=o})_b$) but an increase in precision in values greater than 15 ng/100 ml.

Likewise changes in purity of label, amount of label used, separation procedure, or the effect of misclassification of free and bound activities can only be judged by their effect on the profile.

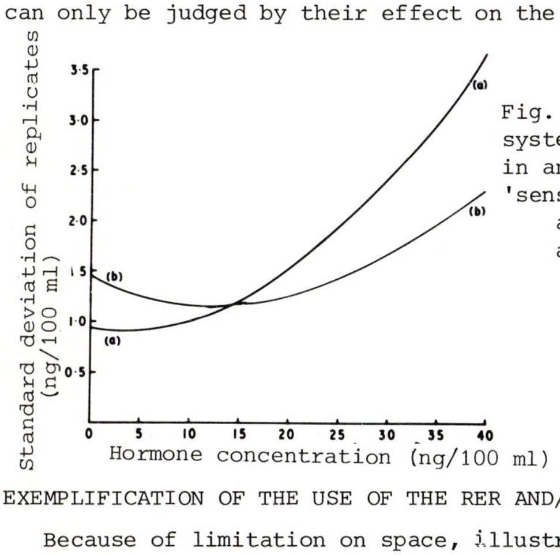

Fig. 5. Precision profiles in two assay systems reflecting (for example) changes in antibody concentration. Note 'sensitivity' of:
assay a = 0.95 ng/100 ml
assay b = 1.45 ng/100 ml

EXEMPLIFICATION OF THE USE OF THE RER AND/OR PRECISION PROFILE

Because of limitation on space, illustration of the application of these concepts must be restricted to two examples taken from practical experiments included in RIA teaching courses conducted in my own laboratory, and subsequently in WHO and IAEA courses.

Exp. 1. Choice of antibody concentration. This study is designed to demonstrate the statistical analysis that is obligatory in a rational choice (Fig. 6) of antibody concentration for use in an RIA. (Two irrational methods of selection are illustrated in Fig. 7).

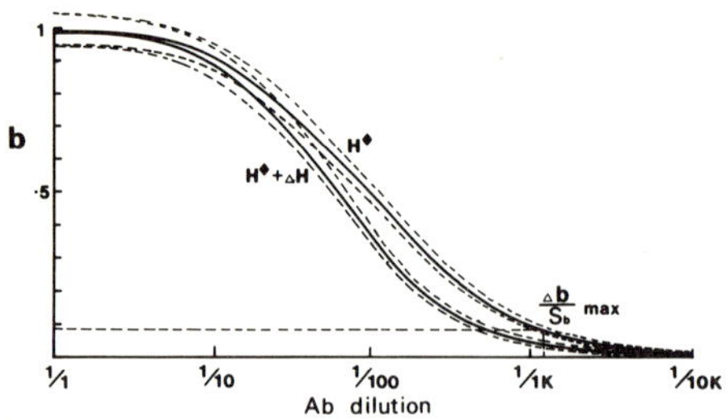

Fig. 6. Rational choice of optimal Ab dilution yielding maximal assay sensitivity. H♦ represents the Ab dilution curve obtained with labelled analyte only, H♦ + ΔH the dilution curve in the presence of an incremental concentration ΔH. Optimal Ab is that at which Δb (change in 'fraction' of label bound) divided by error in measurement of fraction bound (estimated standard deviation S_b) is maximal. To achieve maximal precision of any target analyte concentration, the 'base' dilutions (H♦) must be incubated with an amount of inactive analyte equal to the target concentration.

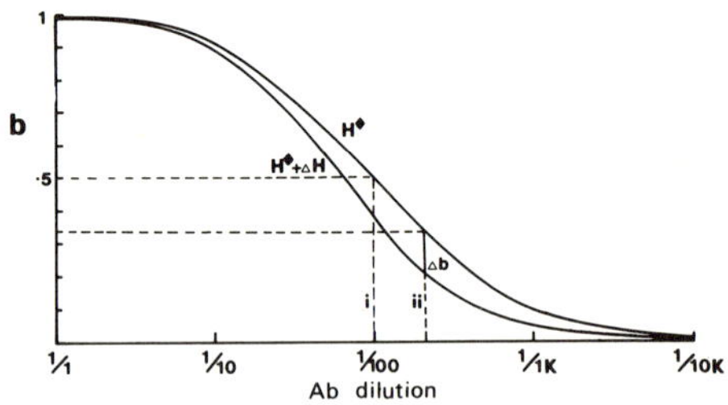

Fig. 7. Two conventional modes of choice of working antibody dilutions, neither of which is based on optimisation of assay performance parameters.
i) dilution which binds 50% of a low concentration of labelled analyte
ii) dilution which displays maximal change in 'bound' label in response to a small increment (ΔH) in analyte concentration (i.e. $\frac{db}{dH}$ maximal). This dilution binds 33% of low concentration of labelled analyte.

In the particular study illustrated in Figs. 8, 9, 10, the immediate objective was the choice of antibody concentration maximising the sensitivity of a T4 assay relying on cellulose-coupled Ab; analogous experiments may be devised to yield the optimal Ab concentration to yield maximal precision of measurement of any target analyte concentration. The optimal Ab concentration is that at which the change in the response variable (Δb, assuming 'bound' radioactivity is estimated) following addition of a small concentration (ΔH) of inactive analyte to incubation tubes, divided by the error (S_b) in b_o is maximal (or $\frac{Sb_o}{\Delta b}$ is minimal).

In practice, two Ab dilution curves are plotted (Fig. 8) representing determinations of labelled analyte binding in the absence and presence of a low concentration of inactive analyte. The error envelope surrounding each dilution curve is also evaluated by examination of the RER (see Fig. 9). A plot of $\frac{Sb_o}{\Delta b}$ is shown in Fig. 10, illustrating the conclusion that the optimal concentration of Ab to maximise assay sensitivity in the system is of the order of 1/2000,000 yielding 'zero dose binding' (bo) of the order of 5%.

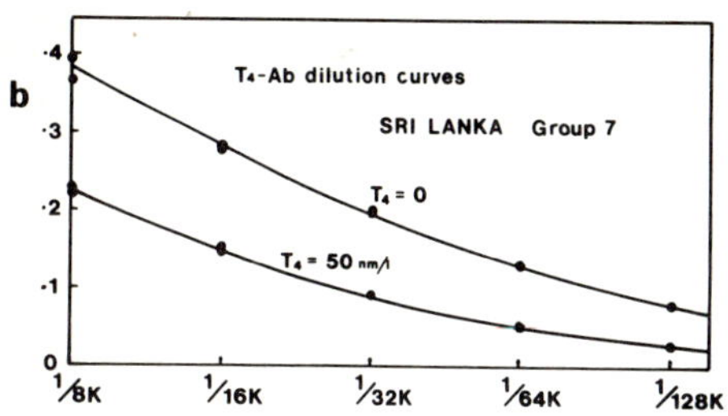

Fig. 8. Typical T4-antibody dilution curves obtained by students in a RIA teaching course (Sri Lanka, 1979). T4-antibody was coupled to microcrystalline cellulose; antibody precipitates were subjected to a single buffer wash. No correction for counter background or 'non-specific' binding was applied to the raw data plotted in this diagram. Heteroscedasiticy is perceptible, but differences between duplicates are obscured largely by the scale of this representation.

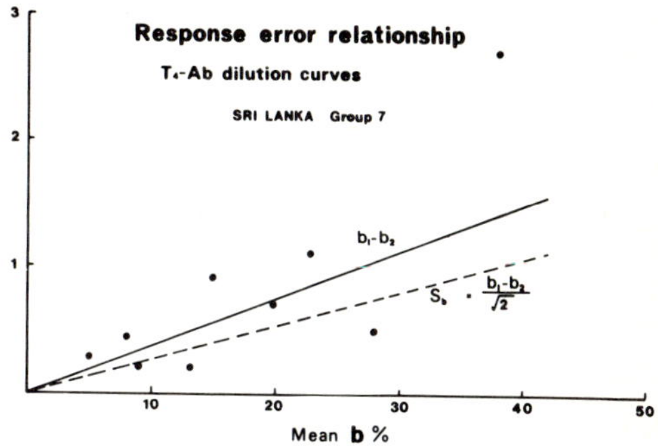

Fig. 9. Differences between duplicates (b_1-b_2) in the Ab dilution experiment portrayed in Fig. 8 plotted against mean % bound. An estimate of the standard deviation in '% bound' (S_b) is derived by dividing differences between duplicates by $\sqrt{2}$. Note that, because no corrections for non-specific binding and counter background have been applied, the standard deviation of ('% bound') at zero must also be zero. These data are commensurate with a constant coefficient of variation in measurement of label in the bound fraction.

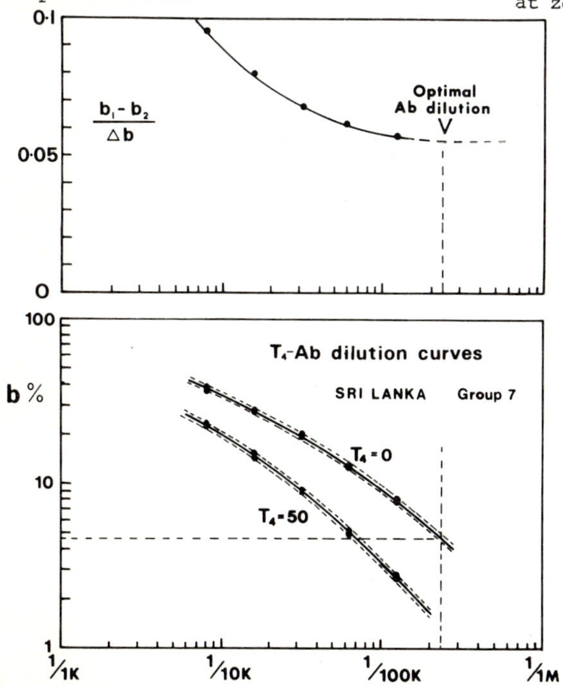

Fig. 10. T4-antibody dilution curves plotted in terms of log (% bound). In this presentation, the curve display homoscedasticity (reflecting constancy of the coefficient of variation in measurement of % bound). Minimal $\frac{b1-b2}{\Delta b}$ (or $\frac{Sb}{\Delta b}$) is observed at an antibody dilution in the order of 1/220,000: the antibody dilution curves are approximately parallel at this dilution. Note that maximal sensitivity is obtained with a antibody dilution such that less than 5% of the label is bound at 'zero dose'.

Exp. 2. Choice of Assay System. This experimental study is designed to select the best combination of reagents/assay protocol from amongst eight possible alternatives. The alternative protocols are generated by taking combinations of high or low antibody, pure and (50%) impure label, 'good' (2% non-specific binding) and 'bad' (8% n.s.b.) separation systems. Each student is thus provided with one of the eight possible combinations (e.g. high antibody, impure label, bad separation system) and with sufficient reagents to assay approx. 50 'unknown' samples (in duplicate) and 7 standards. The objective of the study is to evaluate which particular reagent combination is (a) most sensitive (b) yields an estimate of highest precision for a specified analyte concentration, (c) possesses the widest working range. A group of 32 students is ideal in such a study: each individual reagent combination can thus be evaluated by each of 4 individual students, thereby tending to reduce the effects of individual variations in expertise.

Having performed the experiment, each student is required to plot dose response curves in a variety of co-ordinate frams (e.g. %b v. analyte; 1/%b v. analyte; logit b/bo v. log analyte; log $(\frac{1}{b} - \frac{1}{bo})$ v. log analyte) and the effects of the changes in reagent composition on the dose response curves in each frame compared. Subsequently the statistical manipulations required to calculate the RER for each reagent combination, and the corresponding precision profile, are performed. Fig. 11 illustrates the results obtained with a group of 16 student pairs in such a study carried out in Costa Rica in 1977.

DISCUSSION

These two examples illustrate the statistical calculations that must underlie any logically defensible approach to assay design. In the limited space available it is impossible to discuss in detail the range of statistical information which is derivable from the second of the two studies, which includes evaluation of intra-assay, inter-assay and inter-method variation, the recognition of outliers etc. The principle concept that this particular exercise is intended to convey is that decisions relating to choice of reagent concentrations, and conclusions regarding the effects on assay performance of changes in (for example) tracer purity, separation procedure etc. can only be made as a result of a formal determination of the effect on the precision profile of the system. A second particular objective of this study is the demonstration that as 'non-specific' binding (i.e. misclassification of 'free' activity as 'bound') is reduced, the optimal amount of antibody required to yield highest sensitivity falls and the vulnerability of the assay system to the effects of tracer impurity is minimised.

Unfortunately a wide variability in experimental expertise amongst the students engaged in the study from which the results presented in Fig. 11 were drawn coupled with the logistic problems arising in setting up an exercise of this type in a distant laboratory possessing limited facilities have tended to obscure the particular conclusions that can be drawn from a study of this kind. (Similar difficulty has arisen in the detailed interpretation of similar studies set up as part of other teaching courses, albeit the fundamental principles relating to the analysis of assay design changes have always been successfully conveyed). Nevertheless, examination of the curves shown in Fig. 11, indicates that the best overall assay performance was

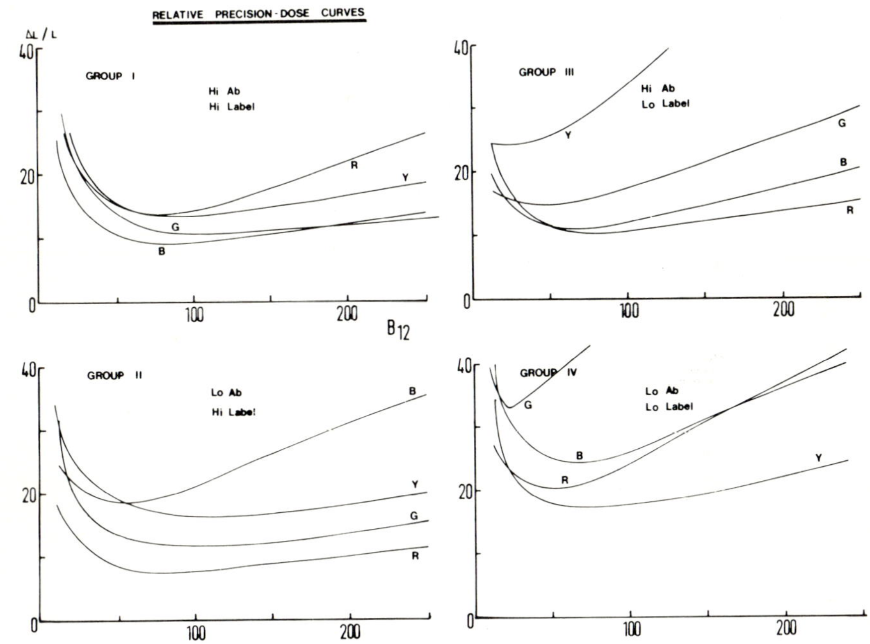

Fig. 11. Precision (coefficient of variation) profiles obtained by 16 student (pairs). 'Hi Ab' indicates assays in which twice the concentration of antibody as compared with 'Lo Ab' was employed. 'Lo label' refers to assays in which the label was approximately 50% degraded and non-immunoreactive. In each group assayists R and B employed a 'good' separation system (2-3. n.s.b.); G and Y a 'poor' separation system (8-10% N.S.B.)

obtained using a combination of high purity label, a low concentration of antibody and a 'good' separation system (Group IIR), although another student (pair) (Group IIB) obtained a much poorer precision profile using an identical assay system. However, it can also be observed that closely comparable precision profiles were obtained by students using degraded label of which only 50% bound to the binding reagent when a 'good' (2-3% non-specific binding) separation system was employed (Group III R and B). The most imprecise systems were generally obtained by students using impure label and a poor (10% non- specific binding) separation system and a 'low' binding protein concentration (Group IV).

Perhaps the most important general conclusion that can be drawn from the results of this particular study is that the experimental skill of the individual assayists was a more important determinant of assay performance than choice of antibody concentrations, separation procedure or purity of label. However, it must be recorded that, although the participants were, to a greater or lesser degree experienced in performing radioimmunoassays, they had never employed the particular procedure nor, in many cases, the type of semi-automatic pipettes with which they were furnished. Ideally such a comparitive trial would be performed by a more homogenous group having had reasonable practical experience of the particular procedure under examination.

The first study illustrated in Fig.10 was performed by an equally heterogenous group of students, some of whom had never previously performed an immunoassay. Nevertheless the results of all participating students were virtually identical to those represented here, illustrating the 'ruggedness' of solid-supported antibody techniques in the face of operator inexperience. Because of the low 'non-specific' binding characteristic of 'solid-phase' systems, the coefficient of variation in the observed response variable (% bound) is virtually constant; under these circumstances it can be demonstrated theoretically that maximal sensitivity is attained using an antibody concentration tending towards zero[6] with a comcommitant approach towards zero of the 'zero dose binding'. It should be noted that approximately twenty-five times less antibody is optimal under the conditions of this study as compared with that demanded in 'conventional' assay designs.

Aside from the improvement in sensitivity and reduction in antibody usage stemming from the use of solid-linked antibody, low 'non-specific binding' RIA systems, it may be demonstrated that assay working range is improved, susceptibility to degradation of label is reduced, incubation time is shortened, and the overall ruggedness of assays (as revealed by inter-assay precision profiles) is improved.

It is, however, impossible to examine each of these claims in detail in this short presentation. The fundamental point that I have endeavoured to illustrate is that the detailed formal evaluation of RIA performance using the statistical procedures embodied in quality control forms the only scientifically legitimate basis for RIA design, both in terms of choice of reagents and the concentration at which they should be used, and in the more general strategic development of simple rugged, reliable RIA procedures. The conventional approach to assay design, based upon a simplistic consideration of dose response curves is based upon nothing more than scientific mythology; adherence to this mythology has had the effect, inter alia, of diverting attention from critical factors (e.g. non-specific binding effects) which critically affect assay performance and of significantly reducing the reliability, clinical usefulness and practicability of these procedures.

REFERENCES

1. Buttner, J. "et al". (1978) Clin. Chem., 24, 1213.
2. Ekins, R.P. "et al". (1970) Statistics in Endocrinology, M.I.T. Press, Cambridge, Mass., p. 345.
3. Yalow, R.S. and Berson, S.A. (1970) Statistics in Endocrinology, M.I.T. Press, Cambridge Mass., p. 327.
4. Ekins, R.P. (1963) Ph.D. Thesis, University of London.
5. Ekins, R.P. and Newman, G.B. (1970) Acta Endocrinol., 64, 11.
6. Yanagishita M. and Rodbard, D. (1979) Analytical Biochem. (in press).
7. Albano, J.D.M. "et al". (1972) Acta Endocrinol. 70, 487.
8. Rodbard, D. (1978) Radioimmunoassay and Related Procedures in Medicine, Vol. II. International Atomic Energy Agency, Vienna, pp. 21-38.
9. Ekins, R.P. (1976) Hormone Assays and Their Clinical Application, IV Edition, Churchill Livingstone, pp. 1-72.

Radioimmunology 1979, Ch. A. Bizollon, editor.

RESULTS FROM SOME EXTERNAL QUALITY CONTROL SCHEMES

P. GORDON MALAN
Sub-Department of Molecular Biophysics, Department of Nuclear Medicine, The Middlesex Hospital Medical School, Mortimer Street, London, W1N 8AA, U.K.

INTRODUCTION

Immunoassay techniques have only relatively recently moved from the research laboratory into the routine hospital or diagnostic laboratory. The need to establish stable, reliable results from these techniques has lead to introduction of methods by which assay performance may be assessed: this is possible by use of suitable quality control procedures. Quality control of immunoassay is not a very different problem from similar assessment techniques used in industry and laboratories around the world to establish acceptable limits for performance, or for the 'quality' of products or results. Since any laboratory technique is subject to errors arising from variations or inaccuracies in the equipment, reagents and personnel, it is essential to adopt statistical procedures to assess the limits within which results may be considered to be acceptable. It is statistically convenient, and also of practical benefit, to separate the assay errors into random error and bias error components. Bias errors are those which arise from systematic variations such as incorrectly calibrated pipettes, etc., and these errors may usually be corrected when their source is ascertained. Random errors on the other hand arise from statistical fluctuations or variations over which the experimenter has little control, except to minimise errors from this source e.g. by using better quality pipettes. In this presentation, the terms precision or imprecision are used to refer to errors arising from the random component, while bias is the deviation measured from some accepted reference point such as the 'true', 'correct' or concensus mean value for analyte concentration. Accuracy is not used here as it is an ambiguous term, and we prefer to reserve this word to refer to a combination of precision and bias errors.

A laboratory can only claim to produce reliable results if it performs suitable techniques of assay assessment in the form of internal quality control (QC) with each assay run. In an attempt to assess inter-laboratory performance, external QC schemes have been introduced for many immunoassays on a National basis in the United Kingdom. Some of the results from those schemes in which our laboratory is involved will be used to illustrate the status of certain assays, and also deficiencies in existing external QC schemes for thyroxine (T4), triiodothyronine (T3), digoxin, parathyroid hormone (PTH) and human placental lactogen (hPL) assays. In contrast to results from these external QC schemes in the UK, a limited trial has been performed in collaboration with certain laboratories around the world who perform luteinising hormone (LH) and estradiol (E2) assays using matched reagents and standard assay protocols, as part of the WHO Reproductive Hormone Programme. The results obtained in these different schemes will be compared to illustrate the need to establish and define the characteristics of assay performance before it is possible to obtain more reliable and uniform results in an external QC scheme.

ORGANISATION OF QC SCHEMES

U.K. National QC Scheme. The Department of Health is advised by professional committees in matters relating to laboratory tests and other services offered as part of the National Health Service. A small Advisory Panel comprising representatives of the relevant Professional Organisations in the UK is responsible for monitoring the performance of laboratories through external QC schemes. Organisation, daily administration and reporting of results to the Advisory Panel has been placed in the hands of individual experienced laboratories for the external quality control of most immunoassays. Our laboratory is responsible for organising the thyroxine (T4) and triiodothyronine (T3) QC schemes, and we also provide data-processing facilities for other schemes which are organised and administered by the following centres: Digoxin - St. Luke's Hospital, Guildford Surrey (Dr. G. Mould): PTH - Royal Postgraduate Medical School, London (Drs. K. Mashiter and C. Hillyard): hPL - St. Bartholomew's Hospital, London (Dr. I. Pull).

In general, three or four liquid human serum QC pools are distributed to participants at monthly intervals. It is the intention of these schemes that QC pools should be treated identically to other patient samples within the receiving laboratory. The organising laboratory ensures that a variety of QC pools are available for distribution in some pre-arranged pattern so that an estimate of both within- and between-assay performance may be made, although participants are not informed of the expected results before the pools have been assayed. Most of these schemes have been in operation for two or three years, and it appears to take about six months before a scheme has settled down to a state where a reasonable assessment of performance may be made. The organising laboratory acts in an advisory capacity to monitor and assist participants where possible.

World Health Organisation (WHO) Trial. As part of the WHO Reproductive Hormone Programme, attempts are being made to examine results and improve on the performance of various assays used by participating laboratories in projects coordinated by Mr. Peter Hall. To this end, organisation of matched assay reagents and standard assay protocols have been developed and distributed by Dr. S.L. Jeffcoate and Mr. S.B. Sufi (Chelsea Hospital for Women, London). In addition to participating in conventional external QC schemes (which will not feature in this discussion), a limited trial involving ten laboratories around the world was conducted for luteinising hormone (LH) and estradiol (E2) assays. Laboratories were provided with matched reagents, assay protocols, etc., and were asked to perform assays comprising a maximum of 50 samples in duplicate. In addition to the standard curve and non-specific binding tubes, three groups of 3 different QC pools were to be included with each assay to enable a check for 'drift' to be made. The laboratories returned their raw data as counts recorded for each assay tube, and this was processed on our immunoassay data-processing program using a multiple binding-site curve-fit based on the Law of Mass Action[1]. The computer program also produces an extensive within-assay error analysis, and both within- and between-assay analyses of the QC pools are also performed.

The objects of this trial were to (i) assess the performance of the LH and E2 assay methods, (ii) derive information about the performance characteristics of different laboratories, (iii) identify those procedures within assays where individual laboratories were encountering difficulties, and (iv) define practically attainable goals for assay and laboratory performance.

METHODS OF DATA ANALYSIS

The techniques used to analyse returns from the QC schemes are those summarised by Youden and Steiner[2], and include parametric and non-parametric tests and analysis of variance procedures. Youden's X-Y analysis was used to derive estimates of the precision and bias characteristics of each laboratory's performance when the same QC pool was distributed on only two occasions, for example when an estimate of the within-assay errors was required. Tests for outliers were performed using Youden's criterion (the difference between two results exceeding 2.5-times the average difference for all laboratories), and Dixon's Test[2]. All of the tests and analyses performed have been programed in FORTRAN, and the results for each laboratory are expressed as a precision and a bias component of error. Unless otherwise stated, bias was assessed relative to the concensus mean of all results, while precision was estimated from the scatter of repeated determinations on the same QC pool. In the case of Youden X-Y analyses, the distance of a result from the concensus mean along the 45° diagonal is considered to be an estimate of the bias for that laboratory, while the perpendicular distance of the result from this line is the precision component of error. (The direct distance of any result from the overall mean may be considered to be the accuracy, by our definition of this term).

RESULTS

External QC Schemes

A record of the time taken to return results to the organiser is made, and for most assays and laboratories an average turnaround time of about 14 days is achieved: however, this ranges from a few days up to several months. Particularly long delays are experienced from some PTH participants. It is noteworthy that postal delays usually account for only one or two days in each direction, with surprisingly few lapses of three or more days in the mail.

Estimation of Bias. There are several reasons for using the concensus mean as a reference point for assessing bias in these schemes. First, different antisera do not have the same affinities for a particular antigen, and so different reagents and methods would be expected to yield slightly different results. Second, a single species of substance comprising the analyte is seldom present alone in serum, as it is often accompanied by various metabolites which can cross-react with the antiserum used. Third, standards are often prepared from non-serum sources, and so they can differ significantly from circulating forms of the analyte. For these and other reasons, the concensus mean of the results from all participants is a suitable reference point against which to assess bias. However, once a suitable reference method is established and accepted, it is probably better to assess bias relative to the reference method.

Method Differences. Many laboratories use a variety of different methods, and even when using the same method they often alter the conditions of assay, so it is often difficult to identify a 'reference group' of laboratories unless they are using a commercial kit. The results shown in Fig. 1 illustrate this point with reference to the digoxin QC scheme. These Youden plots show the results obtained by each laboratory on two different occasions for each of two QC pools, and the results in Fig. 1b were obtained after a report summarising the differences between the two digoxin kits was circulated. The cross-wires at the centre of the diagrams show the concensus mean (± 1 standard deviation), after excluding the results in parentheses which were flagged on Youden's criterion as being excessively imprecise (P< 4.6%). The dashed circles show the one standard deviation limits obtained by the pooled results from those laboratories using each of the two commercial kits for digoxin, labelled R and Y respectively. It can be seen that kit R produced a slight negative bias, while kit Y yielded a slight positive bias (Fig. 1a) which has been virtually eliminated over the course of a year (Fig. 1b). These digoxin results, of which those shown in Fig. 1 are merely representative examples, were obtained at all concentrations of digoxin over the range of these assays.

Distribution of QC pools spiked with digitoxin showed that the commercial antisera, and only <u>some</u> of the other antisera used, did not cross-react significantly. One antiserum in particular yielded values of about 6 nmol/l for digitoxin-spiked serum, while most other assays registered less than 1 nmol/l.

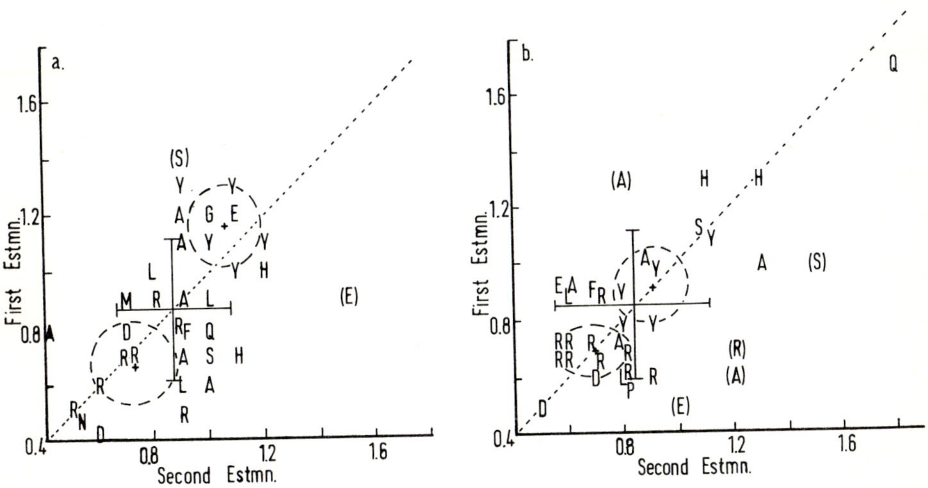

Fig. 1. Youden X-Y plots of results from the UK National Digoxin QC Scheme. Each QC pool was distributed on two occasions represented by results plotted on the Y- and X-axes respectively (nmol/l). (a) Pool 22; (b) Pool 25. Letters indicate different methods used by participants.

Within-Assay Errors. The frequency of sampling laboratory performance is relatively low in these external QC schemes with only one distribution of QC pools per month. However, a particular group of QC samples would be expected to be inserted into the same assay as soon as practicable after they are received by the participating laboratory. Thus, if two samples of the same QC pool are sent out on one occasion under different identity codes, these results can be used to assess the within-assay precision using Youden's analysis. Results from the PTH and iodothyronine QC schemes show that a large proportion of the laboratories do not employ sufficiently rigorous internal QC checks on assay performance, as the imprecision is often very much greater than 20% and several laboratories are also flagged on successive occasions: some laboratories admit to performing no internal quality control checks whatsoever. We have now circulated recommendations for internal QC to all participants in the iodothyronine schemes.

Comparison of Performance. It is fairly obvious that before it is possible to assess the significance of bias of assay results, it is first necessary that the estimates are obtained with a reasonable precision. This was possible with the two digoxin kits shown in Fig. 1, but not with the other methods used as the latter results were not estimated with sufficient precision. Note that imprecision or precision is usually expressed numerically as a coefficient of variation (percentage relative standard deviation) of several estimations.

In comparing laboratory performance, it is first important to consider the use to be made of the assay. This is illustrated for the hPL assays, which are used by most laboratories for mid-pregnancy testing where placental lactogen levels are moderately high: however, since one centre employs a more sensitive assay, predominantly as a tumour-tissue marker, it dilutes all serum samples and therefore has a consistently greater imprecision double that of the other laboratories (usually about 6%).

A second example where comparisons are inappropriate occurs in the PTH QC scheme. One participant, without warning or explanation, started using an N-terminal antiserum and began to report results in units which differed by a factor of 100 from the C-terminal antiserum used by all other laboratories. Only two of the 14 PTH participants achieved an overall precision of $<30\%$, and half of the laboratories were unable to distinguish between serum spiked with 0.5 and 1.0 ug PTH/l, including the laboratory which had switched methods. To attempt to introduce such a major alteration while the agreement between PTH assay results was already poor, without also ensuring that the C-terminal assay is maintained in parallel with the new N-terminal assay, makes comparisons impossible.

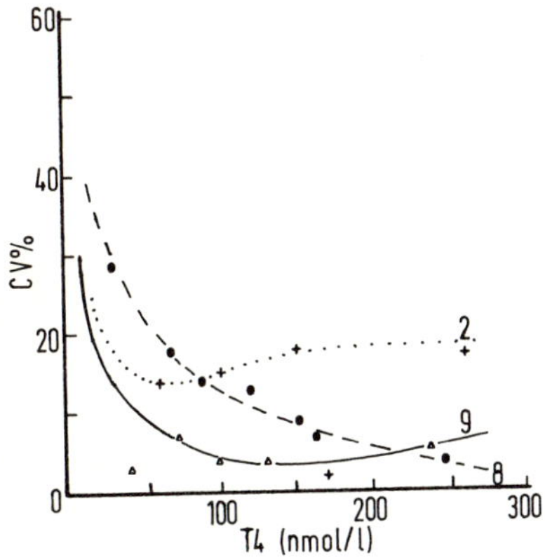

Fig. 2. T4 precision-dose profiles.

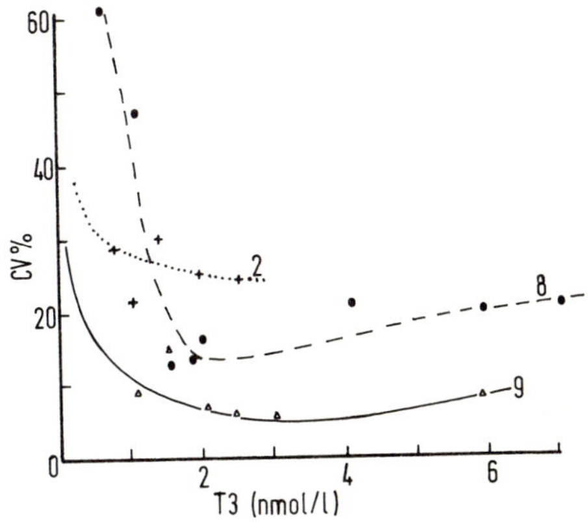

Fig. 3. T3 precision-dose profiles.

Results from three laboratories in the UK National QC Schemes for T4 and T3, with coefficients of variation plotted against hormone concentration. The results were grouped into narrow ranges of hormone concentration and the median results are plotted to minimise the influence of outlier estimates.

Some typical results from the T4 and T3 QC schemes are shown in Figs. 2 and 3. The normal range for T4 extends from about 50 to 150 nmol/l, while that for T3 covers the range from about 1 to 3 nmol/l. Some laboratories employ a strategy for assessing thyroid function, and assay for T4 first to determine whether it is then necessary to assay for T3 or TSH. The latter assays are used to discriminate borderline-high or -low T4 results so that a greater certainty in diagnosis of hyper- or hypo-thyroidism, respectively, may be made. Thus, maximum precision is required for T4 in the region of 50 and 150 nmol/l, while that for T3 occurs in the region between 2 and 4 nmol/l. Numbers next to the curves in Figs. 2 and 3 are the laboratory identity codes, as these schemes are anonymous and confidential to the participants. Laboratory 9 has a good precision of <10% and it is nearer to 5% over the range of interest for both assays. For T4, laboratory 8 has an unacceptably high imprecision of about 20% at the low range and a moderate precision in the high range, while laboratory 2 has an unacceptable imprecision over the entire assay range. Both laboratories 2 and 8 had very poor precision in the T3 assay and Lab. 2 made no returns for the high QC pools, which is why this curve does not cover the same range as those for the other laboratories.

With T4 assays, it is essential to obtain good precision at both ends of the normal range, while with T3 it is usually only important to estimate results precisely at the high-normal end of the range. Consideration of what constitutes satisfactory performance depends to some extent on the eventual use of the assay, and also upon the costs in terms of development effort and the resources available to perform the service assay. Thus, a precision of about 5% in the discriminating ranges may be considered satisfactory to enable decisions to be made relating to thyroid function, whereas estimates with associated errors of 20% may be permissible outside these critical ranges. As Figs. 2 and 3 show, the precision-dose profiles are not constant over the ranges of analyte concentration. This is the principal reason why we have not expressed the results as a cumulative coefficient of variation, or as a variance index score which Whitehead[3] has introduced for each laboratory in his clinical chemistry external QC schemes.

The present status of immunoassays is such that summary results from external QC schemes are so condensed that participants gain very little information of use to them in improving their performance. In addition to misunderstanding the role of external QC and its relationship with internal QC procedures, there is often disbelief that external QC usually reflects the general performance of the assay or laboratory. Differences in assay methodology are often offered as explanations to excuse poor performance, and in some cases "recommended assay methods" and reagents are provided by scheme organisers to assist participating laboratories. Before this is done, however, it is essential that the recommended procedure is thoroughly validated, and the assay must also be extremely 'rugged' to environmental and operator perturbations, as well as having an acceptable precision-dose profile.

WHO LABORATORY TRIAL

Matched reagents and standard assay protocols were used by selected participants in the WHO Reproductive Hormone Programme for LH and E2 assays. Organisation of this scheme and the techniques used in the analysis were described in the results section. A sample of the results obtained will be used to illustrate two points. First, the value of rigorous internal assessment of assay performance will be described. Second, the benefit of employing standard assay reagents and protocols in assessing laboratory performance and in providing defined characteristics of acceptable performance will be outlined.

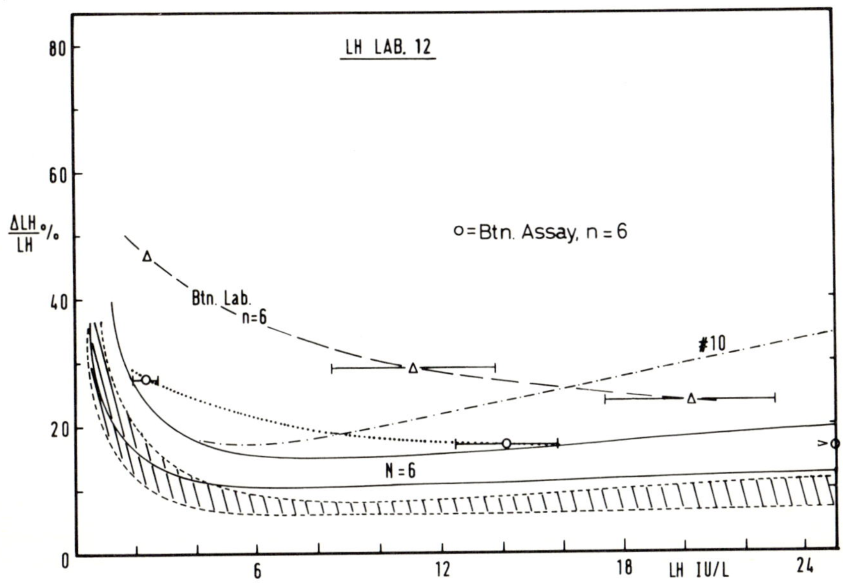

Fig. 4. Precision-dose profiles for an LH assay using WHO matched reagents and a standard assay protocol. Note: results are for singleton estimations, and the precision should be divided by $\sqrt{2}$ to correct the results for determinations in duplicate.

One of the set of results obtained in the WHO trial is shown in Fig. 4. The lower hatched envelope shows the within-assay relative precision-dose profile (RPDP) obtained by the 'best' laboratory (number 40). Laboratory 12 produced a slightly higher within-assay RPDP envelope, shown as the two continuous lines on either side of N=6, which is the number of assays performed. This upward shift in the RPDP envelope, and an examination of the raw data, suggested that Lab. 12 has a problem in the separation stage of their assay. The RPDP for one assay (# 10) is seen to be quite different from RPDP's of the other assays, and this fact, along with statistical flagging of the quality control results enabled us to reject this particular assay from subsequent analyses. Between-assay and between-laboratory RPDP's are also shown on Fig. 4, and attest to the overall relatively poor performance of this assay. In fact, of the six laboratory results examined, only the results from laboratory 40 showed reasonable within- and between- assay precision of $<20\%$ at 2 IU LH/l, which decreased to $<10\%$ at higher LH concentrations (after dividing by $\sqrt{2}$ to correct for determinations in duplicate). Examination of the LH QC data showed that only laboratory 40 was capable of determining LH concentrations with an acceptable precision, which suggests that the assay method is not sufficiently 'rugged' to be used as a generally recommended procedure in its current form.

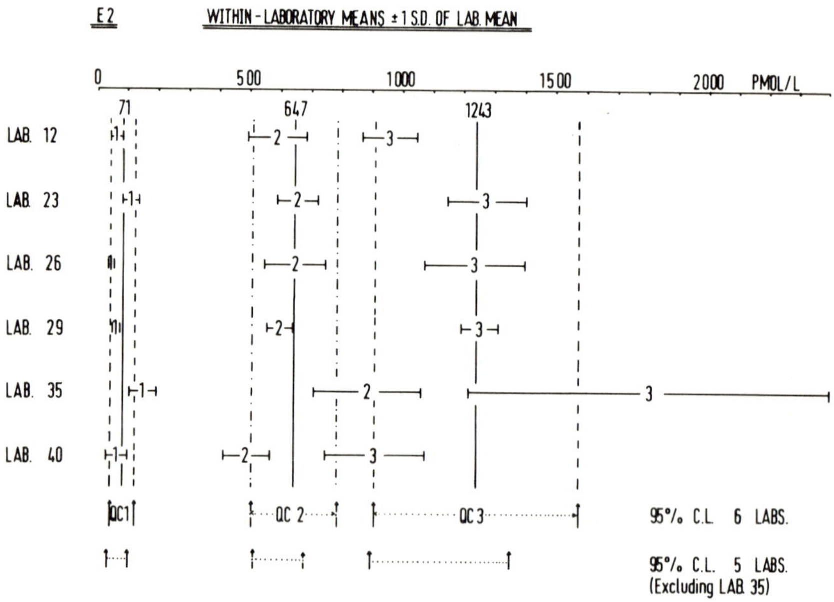

Fig. 5. Bias plots for three QC pools assayed by six laboratories in the WHO E2 trial.

A bias plot for E2 QC results is shown in Fig. 5. For this assay laboratory 29 produced the 'best' within-laboratory RPDP's, and laboratory 35 yielded unacceptable results. Laboratories 12 and 40 appear to have problems in recovery during the extraction stage of the assay procedure, as they have a consistent negative bias: except for the latter point, the E2 assay procedure appears to be moderately 'rugged'.

SUMMARY

External Quality Control Schemes can only give a guide to the average performance of a particular laboratory over a period of time. It is the duty of the organiser to ensure that the appropriate assessments and comparisons of performance are made in external QC schemes, but it is also necessary to assist participating laboratories who are experiencing difficulties. Unless participating laboratories apply strict statistical criteria of acceptability of assay performance within their laboratories, they will always perform relatively poorly in external QC schemes. Provision of matched assay reagents or recommended procedures is helpful to participants, but these assay methods must be thoroughly validated and also 'rugged' if they are to be of use. The value of external QC schemes lies in providing an approximate, overall comparison of assay and laboratory performance, and also in fostering contacts and exchanges of information between participants. This process should speed the development of simple, rugged immunoassay systems, and lead to a more rapid unification of results obtained from different centres.

ACKNOWLEDGEMENTS

I am grateful to participants and organisers of the various schemes quoted here for permission to use their results, and particularly to the WHO for financial support for part of this work. I am indebted to Professor R.P. Ekins for many fruitful discussions and encouragement, and to Martin Neill and Christine Redford for their hard work on the WHO and iodothyronine results, respectively.

REFERENCES

1. Malan, P.G., Cox, M.G. and Long, E.M.R. (1978) Radioimmunoassay and Related Procedures in Medicine, Intnl. Atomic Energy Agency, Vienna, pp. 425-436.

2. Youden, W.J. and Steiner, E.H. (1975) A Statistical Manual of the A.O.A.C., The Association of Official Analytical Chemists, P.O. Box 540, Benjamin Franklin Station, Washington, D.C. 20044 (price $5.00).

3. Whitehead, T.P. (1977) Quality Control in Clinical Chemistry. J. Wiley & Sons, New York.

Radioimmunology 1979, Ch. A. Bizollon, editor.

A NATIONAL QUALITY CONTROL SCHEME FOR SERUM HGH ASSAYS

W.M. HUNTER and I. McKENZIE
MRC Immunoassay Team, Edinburgh, U.K.

INTRODUCTION

The Department of Health established the Supraregional Assay Service (SAS) in January 1974. The objects were: (a) To provide a nationwide analytical service using centres which would receive samples sent by post. The Scheme was to function as a 'consultant service', i.e. the 'customer' had a right to the analysis but was expected to authenticate his request if asked. (b) The SAS centres were also expected to bring the existence and clinical value of the Service to the attention of clinicians and referring laboratories and were also expected to advise on the clinical interpretation of the analytical results. A booklet was produced describing the Service and containing an outline of the clinical situations in which each assay was known to be useful, together with details of the samples required including descriptions of any necessary dynamic tests. (c) The SAS laboratories were to assist in training staff from other laboratories as and when the assays were 'devolved' to Regional or District level. It soon became apparent that some attempt to co-ordinate the quality of the analyses was necessary, not least because samples from a given centre might on different occasions go to different SAS centres. In the Autumn of 1975 the SAS established a Quality Control Sub-Committee and the intra-laboratory QC Scheme for Growth Hormone (HGH) assays which is described here has served, in many respects, as a pilot scheme for protein RIA.

Objects of the Quality Control Scheme

The Scheme was designed both to assess and where necessary assist participants to improve both their analytical and interpretative performance. Thus, unlike the manufacturer whose QC is concerned with ascertaining that replicates of his product are within his design specification, we suspected (correctly) that performance might in some instances be inadequate because of poor assay design. We were anxious to separate these problems from inadequacies in laboratory management. In order to allow this separation we required completion of a detailed method questionnaire before participation began so that imperfections of performance could be related to assay design.

Participation

Participation is open to all U.K. laboratories whether 'research' or 'service' and in both the private and public sectors.

Use of common standard

The only technical pre-condition for entry to the Scheme was preparedness to report results in terms of the International Reference Preparation (IRP) 66/217 available from the National Institute for Biological Standards and Control, Holly Hill, London, N.W.3. Initially it was recommended that this material be used as the laboratory standard or a laboratory standard (e.g. in a Kit) could be calibrated against it. Later (see below) important advances were brought about by introducing a working standard.

Clinical uses of HGH assays

We indicated from the outset that the Scheme would assess and monitor performance for the main clinical uses which were described as: (1) To assess a patient's ability to secrete appropriate amounts of HGH in well-defined stimulation tests: median normal peak responses, e.g. to intravenous insulin 0.1 U/kg, are in the region of 30 mIU/l. The dividing line between normal and partial deficiency is variously quoted as 10-20 mIU/l. These purposes call for (a) detection limit of about 1 mIU/l, and (b) good precision over the range 1-30 mIU/l. (2) To confirm or deny the presence of an acromegalic picture: this disease is characterised by continuously elevated plasma HGH levels, which may rise in response to positive stimuli but typically show impaired or absent suppression during hyperglycaemia. Normal subjects suppress to <1 mIU/l, although the levels may rise again immediately. Clinically apparent acromegaly has been seen in untreated patients in association with HGH values which are maintained at levels at any point within the range 3-1000 mIU/l. Individual patients generally maintain rather constant HGH levels both within and between days. An assay designed to serve these patients needs to show good specificity down to 1 mIU/l in order to distinguish patients in the lowest range from normals. It also needs good precision throughout the acromegalic range (3-1000 mIU/l). This is because there is no simple treatment of certain efficacy for acromegaly and clinicians may find the changes in patients' post-treatment HGH levels a valuable index for monitoring therapy.

Material for distribution

The distributed material consisted of excess plasma and serum which remained after sample analysis and also, and latterly exclusively, of serum samples from donors.

Recommended assay procedure

Early in 1976 the SAS Quality Control Sub-Committee decided that the best means of minimising between-laboratory differences in numerical values lay in unifying assay reagents and procedures rather than in step-by-step dissection and correction of the causes of the differences. Accordingly, this laboratory identified a suitable antiserum to HGH and obtained a large pool of donkey anti-rabbit IgG. A 'recommended procedure' was developed: detailed protocols together with supplies of first and second antibody were made available to U.K. service and research laboratories in June 1976. By April 1979 15 participating laboratories indicated that they were using the recommended procedure.

OPERATION OF THE SCHEME

Three samples were sent out every 2 weeks. Laboratories were asked to treat them just as they would treat regular samples and to report their numerical results and also to indicate what interpretation would accompany their report for each sample if the result had been obtained in a sample taken 90 min. after a 50 g oral glucose load and similar values were found in 30 and 60 min. samples in a patient who was being considered as possibly acromegalic.

A computer printout displaying the results was sent out four weeks after sample despatch. The laboratories were given single or double letter codes. The code letters were used as the symbols on all scattergrams and statistical listings. The following is a typical (shortened) example of the printout for a single sample (a normal report would contain this information on each of three samples).

Materials: Sample 232 = Recovery Pool B4: 3rd Distribution.

Sample	Reference Group Mean Value mIU/l	Recommended Procedure Mean Value mIU/l	Recommended Interpretation If from GTT for ? acromegaly
232	25.1	24.4	Abnormal: consistent with acromegaly. If untreated, patient is at 25th centile for this disease.
Recovery pool	Correct value 25.0 mIU/l		
Mean recovery	100.4%	97.6%	

```
 --+--+--+--+--+--+--+--+--+--+--+--
           REC. PROCEDURE LABS.


               AE    M
         R AG AH X     F AR AD
 --+--+--+--+--+--+--+--+--+--+--+--
              OTHER LABS.


               AP
               AD
               AE AA
    SA         X  Z  Y AR
    N  U AG AH P  L  M PL AD PI
 --+--+--+--+--+--+--+--+--+--+--+--
             REFERENCE LABS.

                     J
                     F
       R        D  K A  E
 --+--+--+--+--+--+--+--+--+--+--+--
 15.0  17.8  21.1  24.9  29.5  35.0
           Serum HGH mIU/l
```

```
REFERENCE LABS
 MEAN    25.1   SD 3.7  CV 14.6%  MEDIAN 26.1  RANGE 18.0 TO 28.7
OTHER LABS
 MEAN    24.4   SD 4.9  CV 20.3%  MEDIAN 23.7  RANGE 16.0 TO 34.6
REC. PROCEDURE LABS
 MEAN    24.4   SD 4.6  CV 19.0%  MEDIAN 23.5  RANGE 18.0 TO 32.0
OVERALL
 MEAN    24.6   SD 4.6  CV 18.6%  MEDIAN 24.5  RANGE 16.0 TO 34.6
```

CLINICAL INTERPRETATION SCORE

```
              REFERENCE LABS                   OTHER LABS
                                                            AA
                                                            AR
                                                            AP
                                                            AO
                                                            AH
                                                            AG
                                                            AE
                                                            AD
                                                            Y
                           R                                X
                           F                                U
                           E                                P
                           D                             Z  M
                        K  A                             N  L
+--+--+--+--+--+--+--+--+--+--+--+--+--+--+--+--+--+--+--+--+--+--
               1  2  3  4  5                    1  2  3  4  5
```

SCORE 5 = ACCURATE & PROVIDING ALL NECESSARY INFORMATION
SCORE 4 = ACCURATE BUT LACKING SOME VALUABLE INFORMATION
SCORE 3 = IMPRECISE AND LACKING SOME VALUABLE INFORMATION
SCORE 2 = INADEQUATE
SCORE 1 = MISLEADING

RANKED LISTING OF CUMULATIVE PRECISION (CV)

Data for 3 labs each at top, middle and bottom of the table

6 MONTH CUMULATIVE CV, LAB F: 6.82% ON 5/5 POOLS AND 19/19 RESULTS

6 MONTH CUMULATIVE CV, LAB K: 7.77% ON 4/5 POOLS AND 16/19 RESULTS

6 MONTH CUMULATIVE CV, LAB E: 8.02% ON 4/5 POOLS AND 15/19 RESULTS

....

6 MONTH CUMULATIVE CV, LAB PL:13.04% ON 5/5 POOLS AND 19/19 RESULTS

6 MONTH CUMULATIVE CV, LAB B: 14.77% ON 3/5 POOLS AND 13/19 RESULTS

6 MONTH CUMULATIVE CV, LAB L: 15.28% ON 5/5 POOLS AND 19/19 RESULTS

....

6 MONTH CUMULATIVE CV, LAB C: 41.61% ON 4/5 POOLS AND 15/19 RESULTS

6 MONTH CUMULATIVE CV, LAB Z: 45.36% ON 4/5 POOLS AND 15/19 RESULTS

6 MONTH CUMULATIVE CV, LAB W: 61.24% ON 3/5 POOLS AND 12/19 RESULTS

RANKED LISTING OF CUMULATIVE BIAS (%)

Data for 3 labs each at top, middle and bottom of the table

6 MONTH CUM RELATION TO REF MEAN: LAB U, (30 RETURNS) -34.0±20.3%
6 MONTH CUM RELATION TO REF MEAN: LAB N, (26 RETURNS) -30.8±16.3%
6 MONTH CUM RELATION TO REF MEAN: LAB AO, (22 RETURNS) -25.2±22.4%
....
6 MONTH CUM RELATION TO REF MEAN: LAB PJ, (24 RETURNS) -1.4±16.4%
6 MONTH CUM RELATION TO REF MEAN: LAB D, (29 RETURNS) 0.0±19.6%
6 MONTH CUM RELATION TO REF MEAN: LAB I, (26 RETURNS) 1.9±34.2 %
....
6 MONTH CUM RELATION TO REF MEAN: LAB AD, (29 RETURNS) 14.5±26.0%
6 MONTH CUM RELATION TO REF MEAN: LAB L, (28 RETURNS) 19.0±18.2%
6 MONTH CUM RELATION TO REF MEAN: LAB PI, (29 RETURNS) 19.7±29.9%

RESULTS

The first distribution

Three samples were sent out in June 1975. 17/20 laboratories returned results. Soon after our report was sent out two laboratories indicated that they were using incorrect standards, one requesting a correction of x 1.25 and the other of x 2. The results obtained are shown in Table 1 after correction of these errors.

TABLE 1

HGH LEVELS (mIU/l) RETURNED ON FIRST GROUP OF SAMPLES

Sample	All laboratories (n = 17)			SAS laboratories (n = 9)		
	Mean	CV	Range	Mean	CV	Range
1	21.6	27		19.2	9.4	
2	5.0	61	<1-9.8	2.4	69	<1-5.5
3	10.9	33		9.0	14	

Sample 2 was pooled from samples assaying at <1 mIU/l in our own laboratory: 3 laboratories found values of <1 and a further 5 found 2 mIU/l or less. It was suggested that the true value was indeed <1 mIU/l and that results above this were non-specific. Much more evidence on base-line performance was accumulated during the first 6 months. The overall agreement and the incidence of considerable positive bias as indicated by the results on low pools argued against accepting the overall mean as a 'target' value at which participants might be encouraged to aim. The 9 (eventually 11) SAS laboratories did show good agreement and their base-line performance was better. The SAS laboratories therefore provided a 'reference group' whose mean values could so serve. Although these laboratories were identified before the Scheme started, they served as a reference group only because their performance could be seen, by clearly defined criteria, to merit such use.

Baseline performance: results on HGH-free pools

Samples containing <1 mIU/l HGH are frequently distributed and in the first months of the Scheme these included samples from normal subjects 90 min. after glucose because responses found for these could more easily be arraigned as non-specific. The completed method questionnaires made it possible to examine the mechanism giving rise to these non-specific responses.

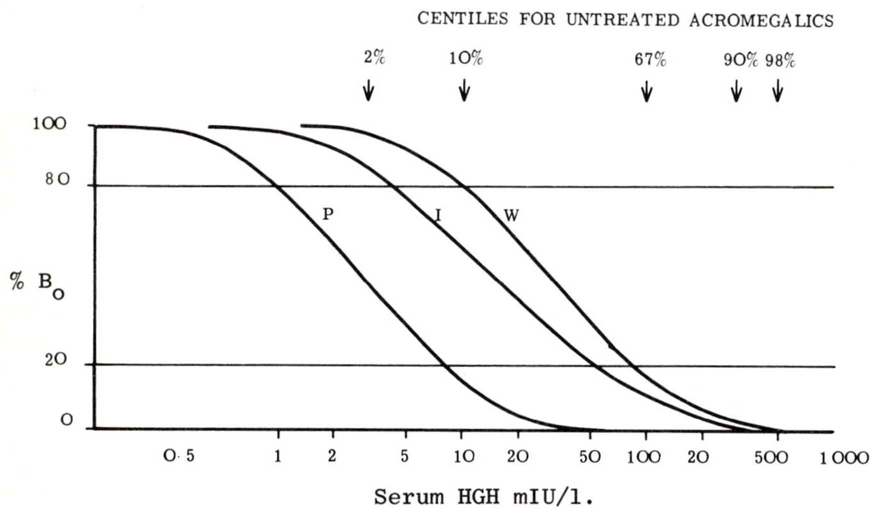

Fig. 1. Variation in concentration range of standard curves. Curves from laboratories P, I and W are shown.

Fig. 2 shows that the level of non-specific effects found by different laboratories on pools which actually contained no HGH (<1 mIU/l) was related to the range covered by their respective standard curves, i.e. to the position (left to right) of the curves in Fig. 1.

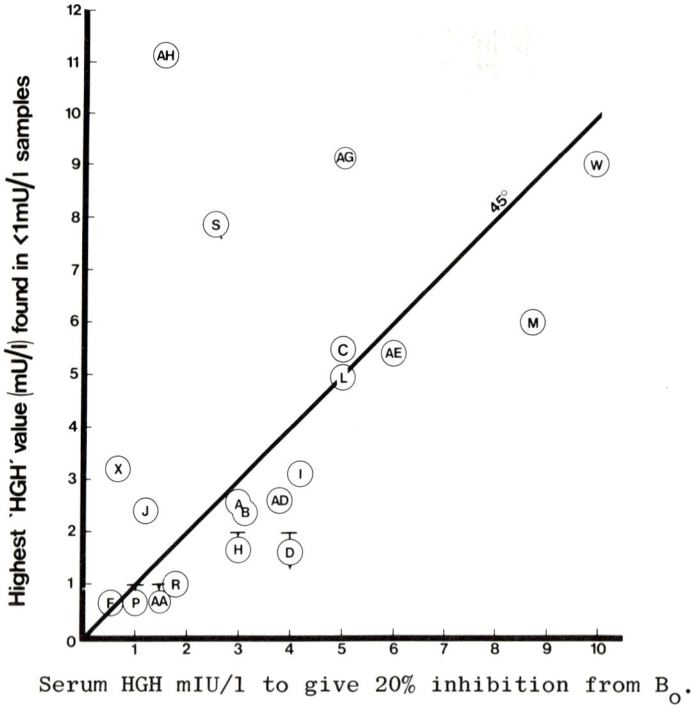

Fig. 2. Relationship between level of spurious HGH found and concentration range of standard curves. Laboratories AG and AH were anomalous in using preprecipitated antibody.

Thus, many assayists had an unrealistic view of the lower limit of their working range - laboratory W, for example, would have been safer if they had reported numerical estimations above 10 mIU/l and values below this as <10 mIU/l. They would, of course, have missed the lower 5% of acromegalics. These spurious responses provide an example of a fatal combination: (i) an assay with inadequate sensitivity; (ii) some, albeit proportionately quite small, source of non-specific response (e.g. effect of serum on the separation stage or a 'matrix' effect, i.e. one in which serum effectively inhibits the Ag Ab reaction); (iii) failure to recognise the effects as non-specific.

The only solution was for the errant participants to improve assay sensitivity and Fig. 3 shows how successful they were in so doing.

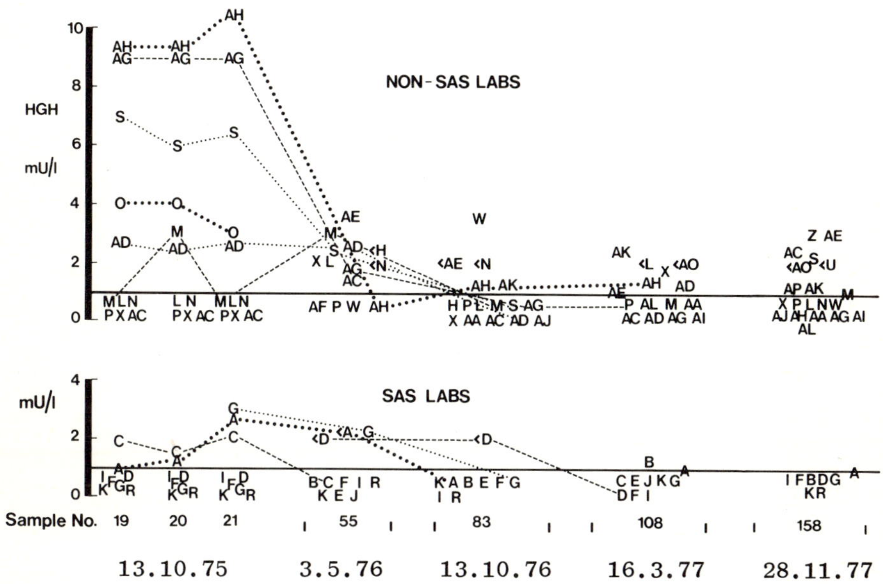

Fig. 3. Values found in zero (<1 mIU/l) samples at different times.

We were also able to relate performance on low pools to clinical interpretation and to show that inadequate sensitivity/specificity resulted in laboratories failing to recognise an acromegalic picture. Initially 50% of the non-SAS laboratories and 30% of SAS laboratories would have regarded the HGH levels in patients below the 5th centile for untreated acromegaly as 'normal', i.e. those with post glucose HGH in the range 3-10 mIU/l. 30% of non-SAS laboratories failed to recognise an acromegalic picture in the 5-20 centile range (10-20 mIU/l), while SAS performance was secure at these levels. By the end of the first year these systematic inadequacies had been removed and since then interpretative failures have been almost entirely due to recognisable errors in numerical results.

Accuracy: importance of providing working standards

While the baseline problem was being tackled, accuracy was also tested by distributing pools of essentially zero HGH content to which HGH standard had been added. During the first 6 months recoveries for the SAS laboratories were 109 ± 17(SD)% and for the 15 other laboratories 137 ± 45%. At this point the bias appeared to be accounted for by inadequacies in baseline performance since we did not subtract individual laboratories' (spurious) values for the unspiked material.

In 1977, by which time baseline performance was much improved (see Fig. 3), recovery was tested again and to our surprise considerable positive bias, averaging +16%, was found. The most likely explanation was that standards were being incorrectly made up and/or (more probably) were losing activity during storage. Ampoules of IRP contain sufficient material for 5,000 assays and frozen solutions are generally stored for long periods. We therefore asked participants to describe how they prepared their standards and to furnish evidence of the stability of their frozen solutions. A few laboratories were using incorrect procedures for preparing solutions. Positive bias, exceptionally as high as +10%, could arise from this. Only 15/34 laboratories produced evidence on stability - they were asked to give the potency of their stored standards against that of a newly opened ampoule (taken as 100%). The results were 70, 76, 87, 89, 90.9, 95-102% (8 laboratories), 107 and 112%. Only one laboratory provided confidence limits! Negative bias of standards gives rise to positive bias in unknowns and clearly we had identified the most probable source of our problem.

In June 1978 some 2000 ampoules of a freeze-dried 'Working Standard' were prepared from an ampoule of the IRP. These contained 160 μU of IRP and several ampoules were checked and found to have retained this activity as judged by very precise RIA in our own laboratory. These ampoules were then assayed by all participants after addition of 10 ml of their diluent. They were to expect a concentration of 10-20 mIU/l. 21 Laboratories returned results and their mean value was 17.77 ± 2.83 (SD) mIU/l, i.e. mean bias was +11.1% confirming the finding that participants' frozen standards were losing activity.

We therefore recommended that participants use the HGH Working Standard either as their routine laboratory standard or to check the activity of their solution of IRP at intervals. 3 Laboratories undertook to assay ampoules of Working Standard against new ampoules of IRP at intervals. By April 1979 19 laboratories were using the Working Standard and all but two of the remainder had asked for regular supplies. A 25 mIU/l recovery pool was distributed in January-February 1979 and mean recoveries were 98.52 ± 2.0 (SD)% for 3 distributions. The new standard was proving effective.

Precision: within-laboratory within-batch

We have not checked this rigorously but our evidence suggests that serious outliers run at about 3% between laboratories. These errors are due to technical, arithmetic and clerical mistakes. After outlier rejection within-laboratory within-batch CV was 6.2 - 25.7, median 11.3. Removing the two laboratories with the worst performance reduced this to 6.0 - 14.1. These estimates of precision are optimistic because they are blind to drift.

Within-laboratory between-batch variability

Routine testing and calculation of this has been a major feature of the Scheme. 7 Laboratories were clearly less precise on pools <5 mIU/l but several have improved on this with time. There was no apparent dose-dependence above this and for pools >5 mIU/l the median running 6 months cumulative CV fell from 23 to 15% over the first two and a half years.

Between-laboratory agreement

The CV for all laboratories on pools >3 mIU/l ran at 40-45% during the first year, 30-40% in the second and 25-35% in the third. The current value (February-March 1979) is 21%. It is interesting to note that between-laboratory agreement was worse on high pools (>50 mIU/l) despite the fact that within-laboratory precision was unimpaired. This probably reflects the acceptance of results too close to the lower asymptote (high hormone) and it indicates that accuracy rather than precision should dictate the upper limit of the working range.

Recommended Procedure

Several laboratories have obtained major improvements in performance as a result of adopting the Recommended Procedure. Two cautions are required: (a) Some laboratories who indicated that they were (now) using the Recommended Procedure were found to have made major changes to it. (One used different first and second antibodies and four times the specified dilution of sample!) (b) Some people will do anything badly!

CONCLUSIONS

Major improvements in accuracy, precision and between-laboratory agreement can be brought about by intensively interactive quality control schemes. A common standard is essential and should consist of ampoules used for one or only a small number of assays. Accuracy and agreement were not good enough to allow the overall means to serve as target values but a group of 11 laboratories were sufficiently accurate to provide a 'reference group mean' to so serve. Gross non-specificity was related to poor assay design and was quickly eliminated. Within-laboratory between-batch variability was much worse than that normally claimed for simple protein hormone RIA. The main differences between 'good' and 'poor' laboratories was that the former kept between-batch CV down to 1.5 x within-batch, while the latter had 3 times their within-batch figure.

A full report on this Scheme will appear shortly in Annals of Clinical Biochemistry and we are grateful to the Editors and publishers for permission to reproduce Fig. 2 and 3.

Radioimmunology 1979, Ch. A. Bizollon, editor.

DEVELOPMENT OF STATISTICAL AND ANALYTICAL TECHNIQUES FOR USE IN NATIONAL QUALITY CONTROL SCHEMES FOR STEROID HORMONES

D.W. WILSON, S.J. GASKELL, D.R. FAHMY, B.G. JOYCE, G.V. GROOM, K. GRIFFITHS, K.W. KEMP,[+] A.B.J. NIX[+] and R.J. ROWLANDS[+]

Tenovus Institute for Cancer Research, Welsh National School of Medicine, Cardiff, CF4 4XX, [+]Department of Mathematical Statistics and Operational Research, University College, Cardiff, CF1 1XL

INTRODUCTION

National quality control (NQC) schemes are designed, *inter alia*, to impartially evaluate the analytical performance of individual laboratories and to assess their degree of concordance with each other. This information, together with suggestions and constructive criticisms of the co-ordinator, provides the means by which laboratories can improve or re-assess their analytical technique. Quite apart from the responsibility that each laboratory has towards users of their service, these NQC schemes may ultimately be instrumental in the mandatory certification of laboratory competence without which laboratories would not be able to practise. Therefore it is important that each laboratory can recognize and reduce known sources of error in their analytical procedure. In this situation, the statistical analysis of NQC data would then be predominantly concerned with the elucidation of those analytical reagents or procedures which would be expected to produce 'acceptable' standards of quality for a particular assay. A corollary of this would be the introduction and use of 'matched' reagents which would intuitively confer greater uniformity on the analytical performance of participating laboratories.

Adopting the rationale that the improvement of intra-laboratory performance will enable the assessment of NQC schemes to become more meaningful, this group has developed statistical and analytical techniques for the improvement of accuracy, precision and monitoring of error for the determination of steroid hormones. These developments are now described and their relevance to NQC schemes discussed.

GAS CHROMATOGRAPHY-MASS SPECTROMETRY (GC-MS) METHODS FOR STEROID HORMONES

The preparation of plasma pools with values assigned from 'accurate' analytical techniques are of particular value in NQC schemes. The choice of the GC-MS technique is favoured by many researchers for assessing steroid hormone radioimmunoassays.[1-6] The principal reason is related to the high degree of specificity that can be achieved with good precision. In the development of these reference methods, several distinct stages of the technique are recognized which merit particular attention. These are the use of an internal standard to assess recovery losses, the extraction procedure for removing the steroid from the bulk of the plasma matrix, the subsequent purification stage (usually some form of chromatography), sample derivatization and then GC-MS analysis.

The incorporation of an *internal standard* to offset procedural losses is of crucial importance in the assessment of the precision and accuracy of the GC-MS method. Isotopic variants of the compounds to be analysed are frequently the internal standards of choice by virtue of the similarity of their physico-chemical properties. Consequently the variants that have been considered for the measurement of cortisol, oestradiol-17β, testosterone and progesterone have included [9,11,12,12-$^{2}H_{4}$]-cortisol, [2,4-$^{2}H_{2}$]-oestradiol-17β or [16,16,17-$^{2}H_{3}$]-oestradiol-17β, [16,16,17-$^{2}H_{3}$]-testosterone and [18,18,18-$^{2}H_{3}$]-progesterone. In practice, the internal standard contained in 10 μl of ethanol is added to an aliquot of the plasma pool and then allowed to equilibrate overnight at 20°C before extraction.

Judicious choice of *extraction solvent* enables a reasonable degree of specificity and high recovery of the steroid to be achieved. For example, cortisol is extracted from plasma (0.5 ml) with purified dichloromethane (10 ml) whereas oestradiol-17β which requires a less polar solvent is extracted from plasma (1.0 ml) with purified diethyl ether (8 ml).

The *purification of steroid extracts* is of paramount importance if ambiguous GC-MS results are to be avoided. The use of microcolumns (4 cm x 0.5 cm in diameter) of lipophilic Sephadex gels is of particular value in achieving this objective. In the oestradiol-17β method, for example, sequential chromatography on Lipidex 5000 (reversed phase) and Sephadex LH-20 (straight phase) affords the necessary sample purity. In this example, the residue from the ether extract is applied to the Lipidex 5000 column contained in chloroform/water/methanol (2:1:9) and the 0-3 ml fraction collected. The solvent is removed under nitrogen and the residue applied to a column of Sephadex LH-20 contained in methylene chloride/ petroleum ether/methanol/water (100:80:15:1) and the 2-6.5 ml fraction collected for subsequent derivatization and GC-MS analysis.[7]

Selective derivatization procedures may also be of value in permitting improved specificity at the preliminary purification stage. Certain steroids such as testosterone may be converted *in situ* (that is, prior to extraction) to the corresponding 3-oxime which, following solvent extraction, may be selectively recovered by virtue of its basicity using an ion exchange derivative of Sephadex (Axelson and Sjövall, 1976; Gaskell and Finlay, unpublished data).

Derivatization of steroid hormones is generally essential for the improvement of subsequent gas chromatographic behaviour, such as the minimization of adsorption losses, and for the optimization of mass spectrometric properties that confer specificity and sensitivity on the analytical technique. In the oestradiol-17β method, used in these laboratories, an internal GC-MS standard, dihydroequilenin is added to the residue from the column eluate and the resultant residue dissolved in 10 μl of *bis*-(trimethylsilyl)trifluoroacetamide/trimethylchlorosilane (99:1). Analysis of the bis-trimethylsilyl ethers of oestradiol-17β, deuterated oestradiol-17β and dihydroequilenin allows the oestradiol-17β content of the plasma pool to be measured by a two-stage GC-MS procedure with single ion monitoring. For selected ion monitoring, *tert*-butyldimethylsilyl ethers provide a useful variant on the widely used trimethylsilyl ethers. Their value is attributable to their stability and the general property that the facile loss of $C_4H_9^{\cdot}$ under electron impact gives extremely intense $|M-57|^+$ ions which generally account for a high proportion of the total ion current. These and related derivatives are currently being evaluated for use in reference methods for testosterone. In the cortisol method, purification of the extract by column chromatography is not necessary. The residue from the dichloromethane solvent extraction is allowed to react with 30 μl of methoxyamine hydrochloride in pyridine (15 g/L) overnight at 20°C. The solvent is evaporated under reduced pressure, the residue dissolved in 10 μl of *bis*-(trimethylsilyl)trifluoroacetamide/trimethylbromosilane/pyridine (90:5:5 by volume) and allowed to react for 15 minutes before GC-MS analysis.

GC-MS analysis provides the means by which considerable specificity in the overall analytical technique can be achieved. Judicious choice of derivatives such as those described, the use of carefully selected stationary phases (1% OV-1 on Gas Chrom Q at 290°C for cortisol) and subsequent analysis using selected ion monitoring have been invaluable in assigning 'accurate' values for steroid hormones in plasma pools for use in NQC schemes.

The advantage of selected ion monitoring at high mass spectrometric resolution (m/Δm 8,500), developed and routinely used in these laboratories, is that ions with a known exact mass and therefore specific elemental composition are monitored, rather than ions of given nominal mass. In the cortisol method, two gas chromatographic-mass spectrometric analyses are performed on the derivatized extract. In the first analysis, m/z 605.3626 [$(M-31)^+$ for cortisol-3,20-*bis* (methyloxime)-11,17,21-*tris*(trimethylsilyl ether)] and m/z 619.3782 [$(M-43)^+$ for cortisol-3,20-*bis* (ethyloxime)-11,17,21-*tris*(trimethylsilyl ether)] were sequentially monitored. In the second analysis, ions of m/z 608.3814 [$(M-31)^+$ for [$^2H_3$]cortisol-3,20-*bis*(methyloxime)-11,17,21-*tris*(trimethylsilyl ether)] and m/z 619.3782 were sequentially monitored. The peak height ratios of m/z 605/608 for the plasma pool allowed the quantification of the cortisol content by reference to a calibration curve established for each analytical series.

Alternative means of achieving a high degree of specificity in mass spectrometric analysis have been made by metastable peak monitoring. Metastable ions are those of intermediate stability which are emitted from the mass spectrometric ion source intact but fragment before mass separation and detection. Using a double-focussing mass spectrometer, 'daughter' ions derived from these metastable ions may be detected free from 'normal' ions by adjusting the accelerating voltage. The crucial feature of the metastable analysis, from an analytical point of view, is that focussing conditions are dependent on the masses of both the precursor and daughter ions. These techniques are expected to find applicability in the 'accurate' measurement of steroid hormones in plasma. The identification of sources of random and systematic error in GC-MS techniques and their subsequent treatment is particularly important where 'certified reference plasmas' are to be used for assessing the 'accuracy' of radioimmunoassays. A complete treatise on this topic is beyond the scope of this report but errors associated with the calibration curve and subsequent dose interpolation are worthy of mention. The calibration curve is usually a plot of the relative peak height ratios (Y_i) of analyte to internal standard as a function of the analyte mass (X_i). A physico-chemical model has been derived for GC-MS (Wilson and Gaskell, unpublished data) which is of the form

$$Y_i = \frac{k_1}{k_2} \frac{(X_i + \alpha b)}{(b + \beta X_i)} + \varepsilon_i$$

where k_1, k_2, α, β and b are assumed to be constant. This model reduces to

$$Y_i = P_1(X_i + P_2)/(P_3 + X_i) + \varepsilon_i$$

$$\text{where } P_1 = k_1/(k_2\beta),\ P_2 = \alpha b \text{ and } P_3 = b/\beta.$$

Regression analysis of the calibration data, using the method of least squares, provides estimates for some of the physico-chemical parameters together with the fiducial limits associated with the calibration curve which are important for subsequent dose interpolation. Alternatively an empirical approach can be used for the analysis of the calibration curve and a power function of the form $Y_i = aX_i^b$ has been found to be particularly useful for routine analysis. The choice of the function must be related to the goodness-of-fit, the number of degrees of freedom, the distribution of the signs of the residuals and the usefulness of the physico-chemical parameters in the GC-MS procedure. Whichever method is used, an estimate of the analyte concentration together with its fiducial limits must be available to potential users of this material.

These GC-MS methods, together with their attendant statistical methods, provide the means by which 'accurate' values for certain steroid hormones can be assigned to plasma pools used in NQC schemes.

THE PRACTICE OF STATISTICAL INFERENCE IN PROCESSING RADIOIMMUNOASSAY DATA

Major sources of error in NQC schemes arise from inadequate analysis of radioimmunoassay data. Manual plotting and subsequent drawing of the standard curve often appear comparable with statistical methods in estimating plasma potencies. However when the calibration co-ordinates depart from an 'ideal' situation, difficulties arise from subjective assessments of the data which introduce bias into the results. Furthermore, statistical assessments of goodness-of-fit, a rationale for the rejection of outliers, and a reasonable assessment of precision are not possible with the manual method. The use of desk calculators or larger computers considerably reduces errors associated with inadequate data processing. Suggested methods for the treatment of radioimmunoassay data using computer programs have been reported elsewhere.[9] It must be emphasized that there is no single mathematical function that is 'best' for fitting the coordinates of standard curves for all radioimmunoassays, just as there is no universal procedure for the rejection of outliers. In these laboratories, the 4-parameter logistic model has found wide applicability for many different types of assays whereas outlier rejection of standard hormone counts is based on the deviation of the individual counts from the fitted curve. The rejection of samples is based on the coefficient of variation associated with either the individual or mean coefficients of variation of the hormone concentration. The maximum acceptable value for the coefficient of variation, within the working range of the standard curve, is usually 15%. The computer program should preferably provide other information such as the minimum detectable hormone concentration, the optimizing procedure for assay conditions and graphical options for examining the standard curve and its associated precision profile. It is important that participating laboratories are able to supply this type of information to the co-ordinator of the NQC scheme and that statistical calculations (for example, the intra- and inter-assay variation), are correctly calculated. It is this type of information which forms the background against which results from the NQC scheme are compared and inferences drawn.

EFFICIENT DESIGN OF QUALITY CONTROL PROCEDURES FOR MONITORING ASSAY PERFORMANCE

The use of inadequate internal quality control procedures for monitoring assay performance is responsible for a large proportion of the intra-laboratory error as judged from NQC data. This group has compared the three most commonly used quality control procedures used in clinical endocrinology. This section is concerned with the identification of the 'best' quality control procedure for use in hormone assays. The procedures investigated were Shewhart, modified Shewhart ('2 from N') and the Cumulative Sum (CUSUM) technique.

The assessment of each control procedure was based on the concept of average run length. Formally, the average run length, L, of a given scheme is the average number of assay batches run before action is taken. Consequently it is necessary that each control procedure satisfy the following criteria. The average run length should be *small* when the system is out-of-control (L_2) and *large* when it is in-control (L_1). Since many schemes satisfy these conditions, it is important to select those which are 'optimal' in a sense to be described.

An optimal scheme with parameters denoted by $\underset{\sim}{\alpha}^*$ satisfies the following equations with respect to other parameters $\underset{\sim}{\alpha}$ such that for specified values of L_2

$$L_2(\underset{\sim}{\alpha}) = L_2(\underset{\sim}{\alpha}^*)$$

$$\text{and} \quad L_1(\underset{\sim}{\alpha}^*) \geqslant L_1(\underset{\sim}{\alpha})$$

Thus for a specified out-of-control run length ($L_2(\underset{\sim}{\alpha})$), the scheme ($\underset{\sim}{\alpha}^*$) is selected which has the maximum in-control run length L_1.

Assume data for the Shewhart chart has a standardized Normal distribution when the assay is in-control and a Normal distribution with mean θ and unit variance when out-of-control. Let β denote the probability of any particular observation made on the control statistic being rejected, then for Shewhart schemes the average run length is given by the reciprocal of β.

For in-control situations

$$\beta = \beta_1 = L_1^{-1} = 1 - \Phi(k_1) + \Phi(-k_2)$$

and for out-of-control

$$\beta = \beta_2 = L_2^{-1} = 1 - \Phi(k_1 \pm \theta) + \Phi(-k_2 \pm \theta)$$

The ± sign is used to denote an increase and decrease in the mean value of a quality control pool. The optimization procedure reduces to the maximization of the in-control run length L_1 where

$$L_1 = \beta_1^{-1} = (1 - \Phi(k_1) + \Phi(-k_2))^{-1}$$

subject to the constraints

$$L_2 = (1-\Phi(k_1-\theta)+\Phi(-k_2-\theta))^{-1}$$
$$L_2 = (1-\Phi(k_1+\theta)+\Phi(-k_2+\theta))^{-1}$$

This is a constrained maximization problem with the obvious symmetrical solution $k_1 = k_2$, their common value being determined by the equation

$$L_2 = (1-\Phi(k_1-\theta)+\Phi(-k_1-\theta)^{-1}$$

and by a further substitution gives the maximum in-control run-length

$$L_1(\underset{\sim}{\alpha}^*) = (1-\Phi(k_1)+\Phi(-k_1))^{-1} = (2\Phi(-k_1))^{-1}$$

As can be seen, the optimizing process depends only on the availability of an expression for the average run length for a quality control procedure. In addition to Shewhart, values for $L_1(\underset{\sim}{\alpha}^*)$ have been calculated for the '2 from N' and the CUSUM procedures for controlling the mean.

TABLE 1

COMPARISON OF OPTIMAL CONTROL SCHEMES FOR THE MEAN

$L_2(\alpha^*)$	Control scheme	$L_1(\alpha^*)$ Acceptance Criterion θ 0.5	1.0	1.5	2.0
	S	6.7	15.5	52.1	222.8
5	SAW	6.7(3)	16.2(3)	67.1(3)	485.0(4)
	C	5.6	23.9	268.5	11,108
	S	15.2	44.8	184.9	-
10	SAW	15.4(3)	53.0(4)	376(5)	-
	C	18.9	342.7	75,097	-

Key:- S - Shewhart; SAW - Modified Shewhart; C - CUSUM; and parentheses contain optimal values of N.

For the control of the mean, the acceptance criterion, θ, which is the 'change' permitted for the target mean usually expressed in standard deviation units of the assay variation, is generally about 1.5. Table 1 illustrates that for an average out-of-control run length L_2 equal to 5, the CUSUM method is 4-5 times more efficient. When L_2 is 10, a situation which can readily occur in a clinical chemistry laboratory of high through-put, the value of the average in-control run length is orders of magnitude different.

For control of the error, the permitted 'change' in the coefficient of variation could be 50%. This corresponds to a change, for example, in the coefficient of intra-assay variation from 10% to 15%. The value of L_2 chosen in these laboratories is usually about 10. Thus for duplicate and triplicate determinations of a quality control plasma pool the CUSUM technique is 1.4 and 3.02 as efficient respectively as the 'optimal' Shewhart scheme as shown in Table 2.

In conclusion, this group advocates the use of the CUSUM procedure for controlling the internal quality control of steroid hormone assays.[10,11] These schemes have been embodied in a computer program (Rowlands, Nix, Kemp, Wilson & Griffiths, unpublished data) for use in the clinical endocrinology laboratory and its use is expected to produce more meaningful NQC results.

TABLE 2

COMPARISON OF OPTIMAL CONTROL SCHEMES FOR THE ERROR

$L_1(\underset{\sim}{\alpha}^*)$

Order of Replication	$L_2(\underset{\sim}{\alpha}^*)$	Control Scheme	Tolerance Level β 1.50	1.75	2.00
2	5	S	18.3	40.1	96.4
		C	-	45	128
		%RE	-	112	133
	10	S	73.5	250.3	997.1
		C	103	650	8,177
		%RE	140	260	820
3	5	S	37	138	625
		C	45	260	2848
		%RE	122	188	456
	10	S	178	1155	10,000
		C	538	-	-
		%RE	302	-	-

Key:- S - Shewhart, C - Cusum, %RE - Percentage Relative Efficiency

DEVELOPMENT OF ROBUST ANALYTICAL METHODS FOR IMMUNOMETRIC ASSAY OF STEROID HORMONES IN HUMAN PLASMA

These laboratories have developed a number of simple and robust immunometric assays for the measurement of steroid hormones in plasma, the reagents for which can be despatched to area laboratories in the form of matched-reagent packs. The assay techniques satisfy 'normal' criteria for sensitivity, precision, specificity and, if GC-MS methods are available, accuracy. Consideration has also been given to reducing the running costs and improving the overall efficiency of these analytical procedures. The term robustness is defined here as 'that quality conferred by the analytical procedure which reduces the effect of perturbations on the final result brought about by manipulative, physical and chemical processes associated with the assay system'. This is an important property if the matched-reagent packs are to be used by analysts in other laboratories who may have varying degrees of proficiency.

Two examples of matched-reagent packs currently being evaluated by laboratories in the United Kingdom are discussed.

The cortisol method is a solid phase assay performed directly on diluted unextracted plasma using conditions of low pH where the effect of endogenous binding proteins is negligible. The pack contains cortisol-3-(O-carboxymethyl)-oxime ^{125}I-histamine radioligand, a specific cellulose linked antiserum, 3 quality control plasmas labelled with the cortisol content estimated by GC-MS and 'standard' cortisol solutions in dexamethasone-suppressed plasma. Full details for the measurement of cortisol in human plasma using this match-reagent pack have been described elsewhere.[4] Preliminary results from reputable laboratories in the United Kingdom show a marked improvement in their inter-laboratory coefficient of variation.

The progesterone method, which has been developed for non-specialist laboratories, employs an enzymeimmunoassay procedure. This technique uses progesterone-11α-hemisuccinyl-horseradish peroxidase conjugate as the 'label' and an antiserum raised in New Zealand white rabbits, using 11α-hydroxyprogesterone-11-hemisuccinate coupled to bovine serum albumin as the immunogen. The antiserum was then coupled to microcrystalline cellulose ready for use in the solid-phase enzymeimmunoassay procedure. Details of the analytical protocol, which involves a petroleum ether extraction step, are available from the authors (B.G. Joyce & D.R. Fahmy, unpublished data). The constituents of this pack, which are routinely used to assess luteal function, have provided values for National external quality control plasma pools which are in agreement with consensus values from those laboratories using conventional radioimmunoassays. Further development of this solid-phase enzymeimmunoassay procedure now allows an assessment of 'total' progestin during the luteal phase of the cycle directly from diluted unextracted plasma. Since preliminary data indicates that the profiles for 'total progestin' and progesterone are similar (B.G. Joyce & D.R. Fahmy, unpublished data) this improved assay method may be suitable for the assessment of luteal function directly from plasma. The advantages of solid-phase enzymeimmunoassay, such as the elimination of any radioactivity hazzard and time-consuming counting procedures, reduced running costs, their adaptability to standard automated systems and the long shelf-life of the enzyme label, make enzymeimmunoassays likely candidates for the next generation of immunometric methods.

It is important that these and other matched reagent packs are evaluated with the same rigour as the more conventional radioimmunoassays. All reagent packs must contain comprehensive statistical information that is truly representative of the product and where possible statements that indicate accuracy of the method should be included.

NATIONAL QUALITY CONTROL SCHEMES FOR OESTRADIOL-17β AND PROGESTERONE

Data from the NQC schemes for oestradiol-17β and progesterone, organized from these laboratories, have been analysed from 1976 - 1979. The result of these studies, wherein the co-ordinator has exercised both an analytical and an educational role, has been an increase in the degree of uniformity of assay performance between participating laboratories. The availability of oestradiol-17β levels assigned to quality control plasma pools from GC-MS analysis has been an important factor in achieving this goal. GC-MS values for plasma progesterone have been more time consuming to develop but values are now becoming available.

The use of certified reference materials in external quality control programmes is considered to be a major advance in assessing laboratory performance. In the case of steroid hormones, their use obviates the need to rely solely on the consensus value of the participating laboratories.

The choice of reference material for this purpose is of crucial importance if the maximum benefits are to be gained. This material by definition is 'a substance or material one or more properties of which are sufficiently well established to be used for the calibration of an apparatus or for the verification of a measurement method. Consequently the plasma matrix of the reference material should be representative of those plasma samples which are to be routinely analysed. For example, a certified reference plasma with abnormal steroid concentration ratios may produce biased results by virtue of different degrees of cross-reaction in a particular immunometric assay. With these reservations borne in mind, the use of certified reference plasmas are expected to play a major rôle in the validation of assay procedures especially for steroid hormones.

CONCLUSION

In this report, attention has been focussed on some of the factors necessary for improving standards of quality in immunometric assays and their relevance to laboratories participating in NQC schemes as described. These have included the 'accuracy', precision and robustness of assay procedures as well as improved methods for internal quality control.

ACKNOWLEDGEMENTS

The authors acknowledge the generous financial assistance of the Tenovus Organization.

REFERENCES

1. Siekmann, L. (1974) J. Steroid Biochem. 5, 727.
2. Breuer, H. and Siekmann, L. (1975) J. Steroid Biochem. 6, 685.
3. Wilson, D.W., John, B.M., Groom, G.V., Pierrepoint, C.G. and Griffiths, K. (1977) J. Endocr. 74, 503.
4. Riad-Fahmy, D., Read, G.F., Gaskell, S.J., Dyas, J. and Hindawi, R. (1979) Clin. Chem., in press.
5. Zamecnik, J., Armstrong, D.T. and Green, K. (1978) Clin. Chem. 24, 627.
6. Gaskell, S.J. and Pike, A.W. (1978) Gas-chromatography-high-resolution mass spectrometry in the analysis of steroids in physiological fluids. In: Quantitative Mass Spectrometry in Life Sciences II, p.181. Eds. A.P. de Leenheer, R. Roncucci and C. Van Peteghem. Elsevier, Amsterdam.
7. Siekmann, L., Siekmann, A. and Breuer, H. (1978) Fresenius Z. Anal. Chem. 290, 122.

8. Axelson, M. and Sjövall, J. (1976) J. Chromatogr. 126, 705.

9. Wilson, D.W. and Tan, S.E. (1978) In: Tumour markers "Determination and Clinical Significance." Eds. K.G. Griffiths, C.G. Pierrepoint and A. Munro-Neville. Alpha Omega Alpha, Cardiff.

10. Kemp, K.W., Nix, A.B.J., Wilson, D.W. and Griffiths, K. (1978) J. Endocr. 76, 203.

11. Wilson, D.W., Griffiths, K., Kemp, K.W., Nix, A.B.J. and Rowlands, R.J. (1979) J. Endocr. 80, 365.

Radioimmunology 1979, Ch. A. Bizollon, editor.

AN INTERLABORATORY QUALITY CONTROL IN FRANCE : A TWO YEAR SURVEY

COHEN R., BIZOLLON C. A.
Service de Radiopharmacie et de Radioanalyse. Centre de Médecine Nucléaire
LYON - FRANCE

In february 1977, an interlaboratory quality control system was proposed for different hospital laboratories which were specialized in radio immunology. The aim of this paper is : 1) to summarize the results obtained during 1977-1978 and 1978-1979. 2) interpret these results and 3) examine the advantages and the limitations of the system developed.

PRINCIPLE AND PRACTICAL APPLICATION

The organization of our system has been previously detailed [1]. Thus we will only present the principles used which guided its development and the general scheme of its application :

1-This is done on a voluntary basis (PROBIOQUAL). No other conditions are needed for membership. At the present time, nearly 50% of the french laboratories (i.e. : 65) are included in this organization.

2- Most (i.e. : 90%) of these laboratories used commercially available kits, and the control covers 16 different parameters :

Insulin	Aldosterone
GH	Cortisol
ACTH	FSH
IgE	LH
TSH	Prolactine
T_3	Testosterone
T_4	Estradiol
Renin - Angiotensin	Progesterone

3- Each study lasts for one year, separated into 4 equal time periods. At the beginning of the study, we sent the members the different control sera. These are lyophilized, undosed, and we make sure that they are devoid of Australia antigen. Each serum contains one or several substances to measure, and they belong to the following different types :

. some are of identical composition but have different code numbers. They are used to control reproducibility

. some differ either by spiking them with a known amount of pure product or with a standard preparation, or by diluting concentrated serum with buffer or with plasma free of hormones. These are used to detect and quantify systematic errors.

. others are spiked with substances which can interfere with the product to be dosed and are used to measure the specificity of the binding reagent.

. finally, some do not contain the substances to be measured : either plasma taken from patients who do not secrete it or artificially produced.

4- During each of the 4 periods in the study, each laboratory must determine each substance in 3 control sera. Thus, during a one year investigation, each substance is measured 12 times (4x3).

5- We insisted that the work be done with utmost care for the controlsera to avoid uncertain results and the difficult problem of their statistical treatment. The loss of information could be eliminated by the permanent intralaboratory quality control scheme that we feel complementary and propose to our members.

THE BENEFIT FOR EACH PARTICIPATING LABORATORY

On the basis of the data obtained by all the laboratories, it is possible for each of the members :

1- to compare its data to those obtained by other laboratories using the same technique or to data obtained in the entire group with different methods.

2- to verify if the results of the above described comparison is identical :

. for the different concentrations checked during one period,

. for the different controls made during one study,

. for sera spiked or diluted.

Table 1 shows the results of such an investigation on the basis of the data obtained by some laboratories using the 12 controls measured during one year.

TABLE 1

BIAS EVOLUTION DURING THE SECOND INVESTIGATION OF QUALITY CONTROL FOR SOME OF THE LABORATORIES.

The results from each laboratory are expressed as a percentage of the mean in relation to the labs using the same technique.

lab \ Serums	1	2	3	4	5	6	7	8	9	10	11	12	Mean
A (GH : technique AB)	198	133	117	131	138	166	128	123	148	140	137	126	140
B (GH : technique AB)	99	87	117	119	95	120	97	114	90	118	92	93	103
C (INSULIN : technique BX)	148	139	154	134	110	124	148	119	113	118	108	134	129
D (INSULIN : technique FB)	110	83	48	/	103	103	78	67	42	89	77	112	83
E (FSH : technique FA)	106	97	96	25	17	30	101	98	104	97	102	101	73

It can be noted, for example, that laboratories A and C showed a positive bias whatever the assay period or serum was, while laboratory B had no bias. Finally, laboratory E had some trouble during the second period of the year (i.e. : controls 4, 5 and 6) and laboratory D showed a negative bias for only some sera.

The results concerning spiked sera are in table 2.

TABLE 2

THYROXIN : RECOVERY TEST (% of recovery ± 1 S. D.)

Techniques	N	Sérum 1	Sérum 2
DA, DX	9	96,6 ± 20,0	99,1 ± 16,0
FG	5	86,2 ± 12,0	87,5 ± 10,0
AA, AX	3	102,0	96,7
EB	2	86,4	84,3

It appears that techniques coded DA and AA are satisfactories, while FG and EB are not .

3- to appreciate :

. the intrassay reproducibility of its data by comparing the results of duplicates for each control which allows it to determine its intrassay precision profile.

. the interassay reproducibility of its results by using the data obtained with identical controls at different period of the study. As previously the interassay precision profile is determined.

As it can be noted, a large amount of information can be obtained with this system. On the basis of personnal data, and those of the other members, each laboratory is allowed to :

. rapidly evaluate the analytical quality (bias, reproducibility, specificity) of the commercial kits used.

. the evolution of the kits as a function of time (modification of binding reagent or standards, alteration of the tracer,...)

With this information in hand each laboratory could make positive criticisms on their own methodology.
In the long run this information could equally help to decide the validity of the different kits used.

REFERENCE

1. BIZOLLON C.A., COHEN R. and FROGET D. - Mise en place et premiers résultats d'un programme de Contrôle et de Qualité National Français en Radioimmunologie. *Radioimmunoassay and related procedures in Medicine* 1977, Volume II International Atomic Energy Agency, VIENNE 1978, pp 91-103.

Radioimmunology 1979, Ch. A. Bizollon, editor.

THE MUNICH-MODEL AS EXTERNAL QUALITY-CONTROL EDUCATION PROGRAMME

W.G. WOOD, M.BAUER and I.MARSCHNER
Laboratories for Clinical Chemistry and Endocrinology,
Medizinische Klinik Innenstadt, D-8000 Munich 2, FRG.

INTRODUCTION

Most external quality control schemes (EQCS) are able to show the participant his performance in terms of bias, but are unable to analyse methodological errors. The Munich Model of EQCS has its strong point in being able to pin-point the weak points of an assay, but is at the same time restricted to one or two hormones in any one survey. Since 1974, EQCS for TSH[1], Insulin[2], T_3+T_4[3], hGH, Cortisol and Gastrin have been carried out. The EQCS for TSH, T_3 and T_4 have been repeated after an interval of 2 years. This report uses the results of the cortisol and second TSH surveys as examples.

BASIC PRINCIPLES OF THE MUNICH-MODEL

Each participant receives 20 sera which include a hidden standard curve in hormone-free serum (where possible), 3 or 4 tubes containing the same sample for intra-assay control, possible cross-reacting substances and sera from relevant clinical situations. Table 1 shows the composition of the sera used in the cortisol EQCS.

SERUM No.	CONTENTS.	SERUM No.	CONTENTS.
1	Dexamethasone suppression test	11	690 $nmol.liter^{-1}$standard
2	0 $nmol.liter^{-1}$standard	12	Serum 1 + corticosterone 700 $nmol.liter^{-1}$
3	Pregnancy pool - 21-40 weeks	13	Charcoal-treated serum (stripped serum)
4	Intra-assay c.v. pool	14	Intra-assay c.v. pool
5	138 $nmol.liter^{-1}$standard	15	Serum 13 + Serum 19 1:1 mixture
6	1725 $nmol.liter^{-1}$standard	16	Unselected pool serum from 100 patients
7	448 $nmol.liter^{-1}$standard	17	Intra-assay c.v. pool
8	276 $nmol.liter^{-1}$standard	18	Serum 1 + 11-deoxycorticosterone 725 $nmol.l^{-1}$
9	46 $nmol.liter^{-1}$standard	19	ACTH stimulation test
10	Cushing's disease	20	Pool serum - upper normal range 0900 value.

TABLE 1. Content of the cortisol EQCS sera.

The 20 sera are sent in lyophilised form by post to the participants together with a detailed questionnaire requesting assay method (kit - where used), method of construction of standard curve, laboratory normal range, internal quality-control measures, the laboratory standard curve with concentrations and raw counts (or for enzyme immunoassays) and the concentrations and raw counts from the 20 sera. The purpose of the raw data is to allow a standardisation of all laboratory standard curves using a spline-approximation[4] as well as to allow the plotting of the hidden standard curve to compare results read off both curves.

DATA PROCESSING

The data from the returned questionnaires is checked, coded and transferred to punched-cards (30-35 per participant) for computer processing. The computer programmes, some 35-40 in number, are constructed on a modular basis to allow different surveys to be performed with the minimum number of changes to the programmes. The computer programmes are concerned with:

1. Construction of standardised laboratory curves (S.C.) and hidden standard curve (H.C.) from the raw data supplied, together with a regression analysis of results given by the participant (O.C.), S.C. and H.C.

2. Comparison of a participant's results with all participants and with those using the same kit using O.C., S.C. and H.C.

3. Computation of the intra-assay coefficient of variation (c.v.)

4. The drawing of histogrammes for all 20 sera read off S.C. and H.C. together with the participant's own results.

The histogrammes showed where each participant lay, as well as the performance of each kit for all samples. Fig. 1 shows the histogramme for sample 18 in the cortisol EQCS. The serum was from dexamethasone suppressed patients spiked with 11-deoxycorticosterone (725 $nmol.liter^{-1}$). Only kits 2 and 6 showed little or no crossreactivity and gave results where expected (ca.55 $nmol.liter^{-1}$).

A second example of the usefulness of this type of EQCS is demonstrated in Figs. 2a and 2b. The results are from the second TSH EQCS. The trouble with many commercial TSH-kits is their

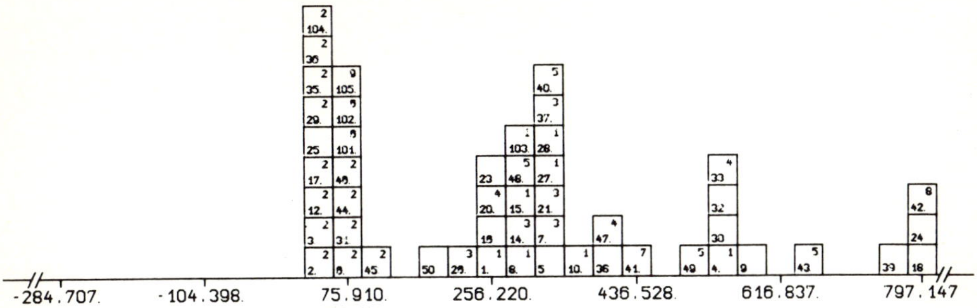

Fig. 1. Performance in the cortisol EQCS sample 18 (see Tab. 1). x-axis shows mean $\pm$ 3s range in nmol.liter^{-1}.

inability to measure correctly in the low concentration range, i.e. under 3 mU.liter^{-1}. This can be due to non-human serum in which the TSH standards are dissolved, non-optimised incubation systems, e.g. no pre-incubation, or standards not calibrated against the MRC 68/38 reference preparation for hTSH. Fig. 2a shows the results as given by each participant from his own standard curve for a serum containing ca. 3 mU.liter TSH. Kits 5, 11 and 12 give results closest to those expected, whereas other kits such as no. 14 gave values which were far too high. Fig. 2b shows the same serum but with values read off the hidden standard curve. Here the "good" kits again give values close to those expected. The kits with standards in buffer solution or non-optimised standards perform better. The kits in which no pre-incubation step was used showed little or no improvement in performance.

Each participant receives a computer print-out (6 pages) and an explanatory letter describing the set-up of the EQCS, together with tables summarising the most important data and showing where the participant's assay needs improvement. Each participant is invited to level criticism at the EQCS and is also invited to discuss any points which are unclear with the organisers.

CONCLUSIONS

The advantage of this type of EQCS is its ability to pin-point methodological weak points and also acts as an "automatic policeman without truncheon" for the commercial kit-producers. The disadvantage of the method is that it only assesses the "day-of-assay" performance and the frequency with which each component can be tested is at least only once in 2 years. The Munich-Model must therefore be viewed as an additional EQCS to be used in conjunction with regular 2 or 3 sample EQCS as run for example by the Supraregional Assay Service in the UK[5] and a good laboratory-internal quality-control programme.

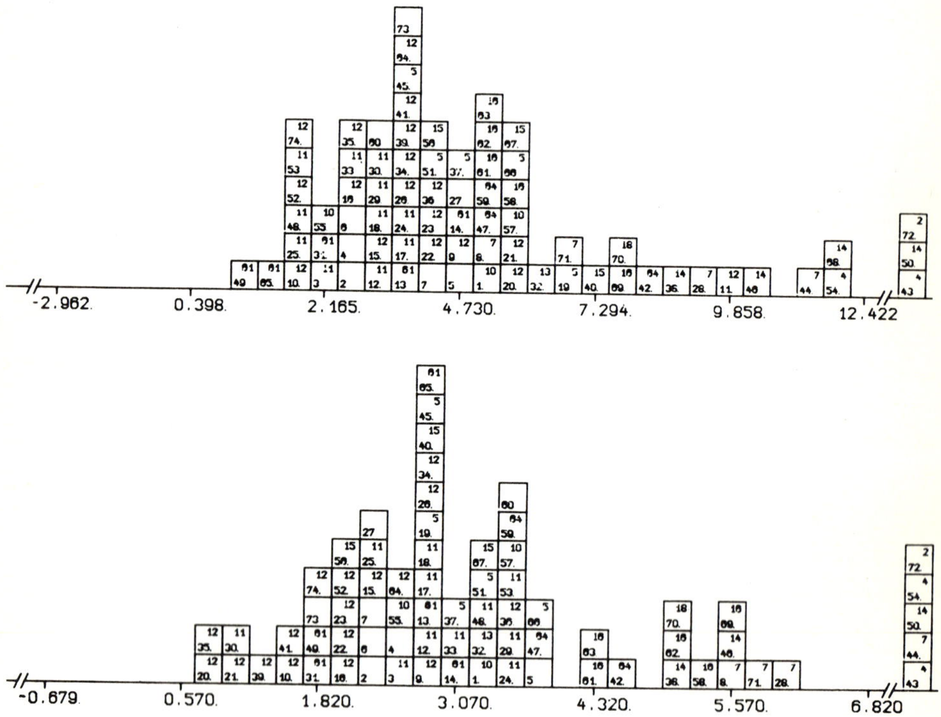

Figs. 2a (above) and 2b (below). Results from TSH-EQCS. x-axis shows mean $\pm$ 3s range in mU.liter^{-1}.

REFERENCES

1. Marschner, I. et al.(1976) J.Clin.Chem.Clin.Biochem. 14,345-351.
2. Marschner, I. et al.(1974) Horm.Met.Res. 6, 293-296.
3. Horn, K. et al. (1976) J.Clin.Chem.Clin.Biochem. 14, 353-360.
4. Marschner, I. et al. (1974) In: Radioimmunoassay and Related Techniques in Medicine, IAEA Vienna, pp 111-122.
5. Hunter, W.M. and McKenzie, I. (1979) This volume pp

AUTHOR INDEX

SUBJECT INDEX